Informatik aktuell

Reihe herausgegeben von

Gesellschaft für Informatik e.V. (GI), Bonn, Deutschland

Ziel der Reihe ist die möglichst schnelle und weite Verbreitung neuer Forschungs- und Entwicklungsergebnisse, zusammenfassender Übersichtsberichte über den Stand eines Gebietes und von Materialien und Texten zur Weiterbildung. In erster Linie werden Tagungsberichte von Fachtagungen der Gesellschaft für Informatik veröffentlicht, die regelmäßig, oft in Zusammenarbeit mit anderen wissenschaftlichen Gesellschaften, von den Fachausschüssen der Gesellschaft für Informatik veranstaltet werden. Die Auswahl der Vorträge erfolgt im allgemeinen durch international zusammengesetzte Programmkomitees.

Christoph Palm · Katharina Breininger ·
Thomas M. Deserno · Heinz Handels ·
Andreas Maier · Klaus Maier-Hein ·
Thomas Tolxdorff
(Hrsg.)

Bildverarbeitung für die Medizin 2025

Proceedings, German Conference on Medical Image Computing, Regensburg March 09–11, 2025

Springer Vieweg

Hrsg.
Christoph Palm
Fakultät für Informatik und Mathematik
Ostbayerische Technische Hochschule Regensburg
Regensburg, Deutschland

Thomas M. Deserno
Peter L. Reichertz Institut für Medizinische Informatik
Technische Universität Braunschweig und Medizinische Hochschule Hannover
Braunschweig, Deutschland

Andreas Maier
Lehrstuhl für Mustererkennung
Friedrich-Alexander-Universität Erlangen-Nürnberg
Erlangen, Deutschland

Thomas Tolxdorff
Institut für Medizinische Informatik
Charité - Universitätsmedizin Berlin
Berlin, Deutschland

Katharina Breininger
Center for Artificial Intelligence and Data Science (CAIDAS)
Universität Würzburg
Würzburg, Deutschland

Heinz Handels
Institut für Medizinische Informatik
Universität zu Lübeck
Lübeck, Deutschland

Klaus Maier-Hein
Medical Image Computing E230
Deutsches Krebsforschungszentrum (DKFZ)
Heidelberg, Deutschland

ISSN 1431-472X ISSN 2628-8958 (electronic)
Informatik aktuell
ISBN 978-3-658-47421-8 ISBN 978-3-658-47422-5 (eBook)
https://doi.org/10.1007/978-3-658-47422-5

Die Deutsche Nationalbibliothek verzeichnet diese Publikation in der Deutschen Nationalbibliografie; detaillierte bibliografische Daten sind im Internet über https://portal.dnb.de abrufbar.

Dieses Werk wurde durch die Universität Augsburg und das Bayerische Staatsministerium für Wirtschaft, Landesentwicklung und Energie (Förderkennzeichen: DIK-2310-0004// DIK0556/02) gefördert.

Planung/Lektorat: Petra Steinmueller
Springer Vieweg ist ein Imprint der eingetragenen Gesellschaft Springer Fachmedien Wiesbaden GmbH und ist ein Teil von Springer Nature.
Die Anschrift der Gesellschaft ist: Abraham-Lincoln-Str. 46, 65189 Wiesbaden, Germany

Bildverarbeitung für die Medizin 2025

Veranstalter

OTH	Ostbayerische Technische Hochschule Regensburg

Unterstützende Fachgesellschaften

CURAC	Computer- und Roboterassistierte Chirurgie
DGBMT	Fachgruppe Medizinische Informatik der Deutschen Gesellschaft für Biomedizinische Technik im Verband Deutscher Elektrotechniker
GI	Gesellschaft für Informatik – Fachbereich Informatik in den Lebenswissenschaften
GMDS	Gesellschaft für Medizinische Informatik, Biometrie und Epidemiologie
IEEE	Joint Chapter Engineering in Medicine and Biology, German Section

Kooperationspartner

BAIOSPHERE	The Bavarian AI Network

Tagungsvorsitz

Prof. Dr. Christoph Palm
Regensburg Medical Image Computing (ReMIC), OTH Regensburg

Tagungssekretariat

Sümeyye Yildiran
ReMIC, OTH Regensburg

Anschrift:	Seybothstraße 2, D-93053 Regensburg
Telefon:	+49 941 943 7172
Email:	`orga-2025@bvm-conf.org`
Web:	`https://bvm-conf.org`

Lokale BVM-Organisation

Sümeyye Yildiran, Leonard Klausmann, Alexander Leis, David Rauber, Christoph Palm, u. a.

Lokale BVM-Unterstützung

	Verein der Freunde der OTH Regensburg e.V.
RCAI	Regensburg Center for Artificial Intelligence
RCBE	Regensburg Center of Biomedical Engineering
RCHST	Regensburg Center of Health Sciences and Technology

Verteilte BVM-Organisation

Begutachtung	Heinz Handels und Jan-Hinrich Wrage – Institut für Medizinische Informatik, Universität zu Lübeck
Mailingliste	Klaus Maier-Hein – Medical Image Computing, Deutsches Krebsforschungszentrum (DKFZ) Heidelberg
Special Issue	Andreas Maier – Lehrstuhl für Mustererkennung, Friedrich-Alexander Universität Erlangen-Nürnberg
Tagungsband	Thomas M. Deserno und Paulo Haas – Peter L. Reichertz Institut für Medizinische Informatik, TU Braunschweig
Web & News	Christoph Palm und Sümeyye Yildiran – Regensburg Medical Image Computing (ReMIC), OTH Regensburg

BVM-Komitee

Prof. Dr. Katharina Breininger, Center for Artificial Intelligence and Data Science (CAIDAS), Universität Würzburg

Prof. Dr. Thomas M. Deserno, Peter L. Reichertz Institut für Medizinische Informatik der TU Braunschweig und der Medizinischen Hochschule Hannover

Prof. Dr. Heinz Handels, Institut für Medizinische Informatik, Universität zu Lübeck

Prof. Dr. Andreas Maier, Lehrstuhl für Mustererkennung, Friedrich-Alexander-Universität Erlangen-Nürnberg

Prof. Dr. Klaus Maier-Hein, Medical Image Computing, Deutsches Krebsforschungszentrum Heidelberg

Prof. Dr. Christoph Palm, Regensburg Medical Image Computing (ReMIC), OTH Regensburg

Prof. Dr. Thomas Tolxdorff, Institut für Medizinische Informatik, Charité–Universitätsmedizin Berlin

Programmkomitee

Marc Aubreville, Hochschule Flensburg
Katharina Breininger, Universität Würzburg
Thomas Deserno, TU Braunschweig
Jan Ehrhardt, Universität zu Lübeck
Sandy Engelhardt, Universitätsklinik Heidelberg
Nils Forkert, University of Calgary, Canada
Jürgen Frikel, OTH Regensburg
Michael Götz, Universitätsklinikum Ulm

Horst Hahn, Fraunhofer MEVIS, Bremen
Heinz Handels, Universität zu Lübeck
Tobias Heimann, Siemens Healthineers Erlangen
Mattias Heinrich, Universität zu Lübeck
Anja Hennemuth, Charité-Universitätsmedizin Berlin
Alexander Horsch, The Arctic University of Norway, Tromsø, Norwegen
Brijnesh Jain, OTH Regensburg
Dagmar Kainmüller, MDC Berlin
Bernhard Kainz, FAU Erlangen-Nürnberg
Ron Kikinis, Harvard Medical School, Boston, USA
Andreas Kist, FAU Erlangen-Nürnberg
Dagmar Krefting, Universität Göttingen
Andreas Maier, FAU Erlangen-Nürnberg
Klaus Maier-Hein, DKFZ Heidelberg
Lena Maier-Hein, DKFZ Heidelberg
Andre Mastmeyer, Hochschule Aalen
Dorit Merhof, Universität Regensburg
Jan Modersitzki, Fraunhofer MEVIS, Lübeck
Nassir Navab, TU München
Christoph Palm, OTH Regensburg
Bernhard Preim, Universität Magdeburg
Annika Reinke, DKFZ Heidelberg
Karl Rohr, Universität Heidelberg
Daniel Rückert, TU München
Sylvia Saalfeld, Universitätsklinikum Schleswig-Holstein
Dennis Säring, FH Wedel
Julia Schnabel, Helmholtz München & TU München
Ingrid Scholl, FH Aachen
Stefanie Speidel, HZDR/NCT Dresden
Nicolai Spicher, Universität Göttingen
Thomas Tolxdorff, Charité-Universitätsmedizin Berlin
Klaus Tönnies, Universität Magdeburg
Hristina Uzunova, DFKI Lübeck
Gudrun Wagenknecht, Forschungszentrum Jülich
René Werner, UKE Hamburg
Thomas Wittenberg, Fraunhofer IIS, Erlangen
Ivo Wolf, Hochschule Mannheim

Sponsoren und Unterstützer der BVM 2025

Wir freuen uns sehr über die langjährige kontinuierliche Unterstützung mancher Firmen sowie auch über das neue Engagement anderer. Die BVM wäre ohne diese finanzielle Unterstützung in ihrer erfolgreichen Konzeption nicht durchführbar.

Platin-Sponsoren

- **ID GmbH & Co KGaA**, Platz vor dem Neuen Tor 2, 10115 Berlin

Gold-Sponsoren

- **Erbe Elektromedizin GmbH**, Waldhörnlestraße 17, 72072 Tübingen

Silber-Sponsoren

- **BioPark Regensburg GmbH**, Am BioPark 13 (BioPark III), 93053 Regensburg
- **solectrix GmbH**, Dieter-Streng-Straße 4, 90766 Fürth
- **NEXUS/CHILI GmbH**, Friedrich-Ebert-Str. 2, 69221 Dossenheim

Bronze-Sponsoren

- **MVA.ai: 3rd bit from the left GmbH**, Staudingergasse 17-19/22, A-1200 Wien
- **SZENARIS GmbH**, Otto-Lilienthal-Str. 1, 28199 Bremen

Sponsoren

- **AKTORmed GmbH**, Neugablonzer Straße 13, 93073 Neutraubling
- **Satisfai Health Inc.**, 1050 Homer Street, Suite 390, Vancouver, BC, V6B 2W9, Canada

Preisträgerinnen und Preisträger der BVM 2024 in Erlangen

BVM Award CHILI

Camilla Gonzalez
(Technische Universität Darmstadt)
Lifelong Learning in the Clinical Open World – Doktorarbeit
Christoph Bender (DKFZ Heidelberg)
Hardware-Related Biases in Machine Learning Algorithms for Photoacoustic Image Analysis – Masterarbeit

Beste wissenschaftliche Arbeiten

1. **Paul Kaftan**
   (Universität Ulm)
   Heinrich MP, Hansen L, Rasche V, Kestler HA, Bigalke A
   Volumetric Medical Images with Sparse Keypoints for Efficient Geometric Segmentation of Lung Fissures with a Graph CNN
2. **Patrick T. Haft**
   (Technical University Munich)
   Huang W, Gastao C, Rueckert D, Zimmer VA, Hammernik K
   Neural Implicit k-Space with Trainable Periodic Activation Functions for Cardiac MR Imaging
3. **Merlin Nau**
   (FAU Erlangen-Nürnberg)
   Vija AH, Reymann MP, Gohn W, Maier AK
   Improving Hybrid Quantum Annealing Tomographic Image Reconstruction with Regularization Strategies

Pitt-Meinzer-Vortragspreis

Luisa Gallée
(Universität Ulm)
Beer M, Götz M
Interpretable Medical Image Classification Using Prototype Learning and Privileged Information

Bestes Poster

Fenja Falta
(Universität zu Lübeck)
Heinrich MP, Himstedt M
Addressing the Bias of the Dice Coefficient: Semantic Segmentation of Peripheral Airways in Lung CT

Vorwort

Die German Conference on Medical Image Computing (Bildverarbeitung für die Medizin, BVM) wird seit fast 30 Jahren an wechselnden Orten Deutschlands veranstaltet. Sie findet nach einer virtuellen Ausrichtung im Jahr 2021 nun erstmal tatsächlich an der OTH Regensburg statt. Inhaltlich fokussiert sich die BVM dabei auf die computergestützte Analyse medizinischer Bilddaten. Die Anwendungsgebiete sind vielfältig, z.B. im Bereich der Bildgebung, der Diagnostik, der Operationsplanung, der computerunterstützten Intervention und der Visualisierung.

In dieser Zeit hat es bemerkenswerte methodische Weiterentwicklungen und Umbrüche gegeben – insbesondere im Bereich des Maschinellen Lernens und der Künstlichen Intelligenz – an denen die BVM-Community intensiv mitgearbeitet hat. In der Folge dominieren inzwischen Arbeiten in diesem Zusammenhang die BVM. Auch diese Entwicklungen haben dazu beigetragen, dass die Medizinische Bildverarbeitung an der Schnittstelle zwischen Informatik und Medizin als eine Schlüsseltechnologie zur Digitalisierung des Gesundheitswesens etabliert ist.

Zentraler Aspekt der BVM ist neben der Darstellung aktueller Forschungsergebnisse schwerpunktmäßig aus der vielfältigen, deutschlandübergreifenden BVM-Community insbesondere die Förderung des wissenschaftlichen Nachwuchses. Die Tagung dient vor allem Promovierenden aber auch Studierenden mit hervorragenden Abschlussarbeiten als Plattform, um ihre Ergebnisse zu präsentieren, dabei in den fachlichen Diskurs mit der Community zu treten und Netzwerke mit anderen Forschenden zu knüpfen. Trotz der vielen Tagungen und Kongresse, die auch für die Medizinische Bildverarbeitung relevant sind, hat die BVM deshalb nichts von ihrer Bedeutung und Anziehungskraft eingebüßt.

Inhaltlich kann auch bei der BVM 2025 wieder ein attraktives und hochklassiges Programm geboten werden. Es wurden aus 94 Einreichungen über ein anonymisiertes Review-Verfahren mit jeweils drei Reviews 29 Vorträge, 37 Posterbeiträge und zwei Softwaredemonstrationen angenommen. Die besten Arbeiten werden auch in diesem Jahr mit Preisen ausgezeichnet.

Die Webseite der Konferenz findet sich unter:

`https://www.bvm-conf.org`

Das Programm wird durch Tutorials und drei eingeladene Vorträge ergänzt, für die wir uns herzlich bedanken. Als Referentin und Referenten für die Keynote-Vorträge begrüßen wir herzlich:

- Ivana Išgum
  qurAI group, University of Amsterdam, Netherlands
- David Hawkes
  UCL Centre for Medical Image Computing, University College London, Great Britain
- Dirk Wilhelm
  MITI Research Group, Technical University of Munich, Germany

An dieser Stelle möchten wir allen, die bei den umfangreichen Vorbereitungen zum Gelingen der Konferenz beigetragen haben, unseren herzlichen Dank für ihr Engagement aussprechen: der und den Vortragenden der Keynotes, den Verfasserinnen und Verfassern der wissenschaftlichen Beiträge, den Lehrenden der Tutorien, den Industrievertretenden, dem Programmkomitee, den Fachgesellschaften, den Mitgliedern des BVM-Organisationsteams und allen Mitarbeitenden des Labors Regensburg Medical Image Computing (ReMIC) der OTH Regensburg.

Wir wünschen allen Teilnehmenden der Konferenz BVM 2025 spannende neue Kontakte und inspirierende Eindrücke aus der Welt der medizinischen Bildverarbeitung.

Januar 2025

Christoph Palm (Regensburg)
Katharina Breininger (Würzburg)
Thomas M. Deserno (Braunschweig)
Heinz Handels (Lübeck)
Andreas Maier (Erlangen)
Klaus Maier-Hein (Heidelberg)
Thomas Tolxdorff (Berlin)

Die Originalversion des Buchs wurde revidiert. Ein Erratum ist verfügbar unter https://doi.org/10.1007/978-3-658-47422-5_80

Inhaltsverzeichnis

Die fortlaufende Nummer am linken Seitenrand entspricht den Beitragsnummern, wie sie im endgültigen Programm des Workshops zu finden sind. Dabei steht V für Vortrag, P für Poster, K für Keynote und S für Softwaredemonstration.

Keynote

Session 1: Image Registration

Session 2: Video Analysis

Session 3: Shape Modelling

Session 4: Generative Models

Session 5: Improving Reliability

Session 6: Ultrasound & OCT

Session 7: Digital Pathology

Session 8: Segmentation

Postersession 1

Postersession 2

Keynote: AI for Analysis of Coronary Artery Disease

Ivana Išgum

Quantitative Healthcare Analysis (qurAI) GROUP at University of Amsterdam
i.isgum@amsterdamumc.nl

Coronary artery disease is a leading cause of morbidity and mortality worldwide. Coronary CT is a non-invasive tool enabling analysis of the coronary arteries and providing important diagnostic information. However, current clinical analysis typically remains limited to visual evaluation of the coronary artery tree as the extraction of the detailed quantitative information requires high level of expertise and it is a time-consuming process. Besides the information about the coronary arteries, these images also contain information about the whole heart and body composition that may be valuable for the prediction of cardiovascular risk. Manual extraction of this information requires segmentation of the target structures, which is highly time-consuming rendering the analysis infeasible. Hence, such analysis is not routinely performed.

Numerous studies have shown that deep learning-based image analysis can facilitate automatic extraction of this relevant information thereby shortening the analysis times and improving reproducibility. This presentation will show our recent developments on the automatic analysis of coronary CT scans towards detection of cardiovascular disease and extraction of cardiovascular risk. The analysis includes extraction of the coronary arteries that provides the basis for the downstream assessment of the vessel morphology. This is followed by the segmentation of the artery lumen and segmentation of the atherosclerotic plaque components. The amount of plaque and stenosis of the lumen indicate the risk and provide the basis for clinical decision-making. Subsequent merging the findings from different vessels in the coronary tree allows standardized risk reporting. Moreover, deep leaning methods for the analysis of the whole heart, i.e. cardiac structures and large arteries, as well as methods for assessment of body composition will be outlined.

The presentation will also showcase how the analysis can be extended to CT scans made for other purposes that visualize the heart and offer the possibility to quantify markers indicating the presence or risk of cardiovascular disease. Next to the opportunities these methods offer, the presentation will discuss current challenges towards trustworthy utilization and present the work on addressing these.

C. Palm et al. (Hrsg.), *Bildverarbeitung für die Medizin 2025*, Informatik aktuell,
https://doi.org/10.1007/978-3-658-47422-5_1

Keynote: Fifty Years of Medical Image Computing and my Small Part

David Hawkes

University College London (UCL)
d.hawkes@ucl.ac.uk

Reluctantly abandoning my career in rock-and-roll and inspired by the elegant mathematics of reconstruction in computed tomography I started working in medical imaging as a clinical scientist. Working in the clinical environment I appreciated how much in medicine was unknown. I became convinced that a physics and engineering approach could contribute to improving healthcare and that this must be done in close collaboration with clinical colleagues in order to be relevant. I also became convinced that real impact in healthcare engineering would only come about by working closely with industry. Only this would enable wide dissemination. Clinical translation of new technologies involves engaging with complex regulatory pathways, validation and clinical trials. Late in the day I also learnt that the patient has a voice that needs to be heard in order to better direct scarce resource to solve the problems that really matter.

This talk will describe how I was fortunate to be inspired by giants in the field. I will run through my early journey from nuclear medicine and X-ray computed tomography to medical image computing, with initial emphasis on imaging as a tool for measurement. I realized that the resources required for development of imaging hardware would be difficult to come by in the academic research environment. On the other hand computing costs were dramatically reducing and compute power was rapidly increasing. I believed that academia was the place both to develop the underpinning mathematics and algorithms, as well as the computer implementations and experimentation needed to have impact. This led to the formation of the Computational Imaging Sciences Group (CISG) at Guy's Hospital (later KCL) and subsequently the Centre for Medical Image Computing (CMIC) at UCL. With the rapid development of MR and wide availability of other modalities probing different aspects of structure and function, we were motivated to find ways of combining information. This led to the need to tackle image registration. With integration of real-time imaging and video this led naturally to work on image guided interventions. This led to the foundation of the Welcome EPSRC Centre for Interventional and Surgical Sciences (WEISS). Close collaboration with pathologists resulting from our work with surgeons opened my eyes to the world of cellular microscopy. This led to our efforts in trying to relate the macroscopic (millimeter) scale of medical imaging to the microscopic world of histology, where cancer and other diseases are ultimately diagnosed and staged.

I retired just as machine learning and artificial intelligence were taking off and this promised a revolution as profound as that which I had witnessed in the early days of medical imaging. I will describe how I learnt from the many frustrations and failures that are inevitable in a research career in a rapidly evolving field, but also the excitement and inspiration as to what to do next. I will try to draw parallels with the promises and

C. Palm et al. (Hrsg.), *Bildverarbeitung für die Medizin 2025*, Informatik aktuell,
https://doi.org/10.1007/978-3-658-47422-5_2

excitement, but also the disappointments that might lie ahead in the field of machine intelligence and AI, to inspire the next generation in computation applied to medicine.

Finally everything I have described is collaborative, involving many disciplines, and I gratefully acknowledge the many students, post-docs, visiting scientists and faculty that have made this all possible, along with the long term support of our funders. This area is truly multidisciplinary and medicine by its nature crosses all international boundaries. It has been an exciting and rewarding journey.

Keynote: Autonomous Surgery from a Surgeon's Perspective

Dirk Wilhelm

Technical University of Munich (TUM)
dirk.wilhelm@tum.de

In addition to continuously rising costs, the healthcare system is currently characterised by an increasing shortage of staff. It is currently estimated that by the year 2023 there will be a shortage of 500,000 nurses and 6,000 doctors in Germany alone. Consequences of this are delays in medical treatment, lack of operation in individual departments resulting in medical undersupply and overworked staff. In addition to the recruitment of specialists from abroad and process optimisation, the use of robotic systems is a possible approach to solving this system. For these to relieve the workload, they must have autonomous functions to be able to take over work. While this is already feasible today for logistical tasks and patient transport, for example, the limits of this approach are still unclear. A survey of AI experts currently assumes that surgical skills could be taken over by artificial intelligence by 2050-2055 already [1] - and the success story of surgical robotics and companies such as Intuitive Surg. Inc. shows that robots have already replaced humans on the patient side. But are effective robotic systems and powerful AI algorithms sufficient to reproduce surgical procedures autonomously? Do we already have the necessary components of autonomous surgery?

When revising the current literature, one might assume that this indeed is the fact and that we are about to replace humans also for very delicate tasks. One can find for example reports on autonomous suturing and knot tying systems, robotic appendectomy and retraction and many more. But is this what we understand as an intervention already and can we easily jump from these success stories to full surgeries?

From a surgeons perspective and although sub-processes of an operation can already be automated, a surgical procedure however poses a much greater challenge. This not only is due to the complexity of the process, but also to the fact that operations can only be described or predicted in abstract terms, but have aspects of a highly complex system at a granular level. We assume that these can only be resolved through comprehensive standardisation of surgeries and a comprehensive approach that includes the individual patient, the underlying disease, but numerous other factors alike. The presentation will not only attempt to provide a status quo to this topic, but also approaches to how the problem can be tackled in the long term.

References

1. Grace K, Salvatier J, Dafoe A et al. When will AI exceed human performance? Evidence from AI experts. J Artif Intell Res. 2018;62:729–54.

C. Palm et al. (Hrsg.), *Bildverarbeitung für die Medizin 2025*, Informatik aktuell,
https://doi.org/10.1007/978-3-658-47422-5_3

Image Registration for a Dynamic Breathing Model

Pia F. Schulz[1], Andra Oltmann[2], Johannes Bostelmann[1], Ole Gildemeister[1], Franz Wegner[2,3], Jan Lellmann[1,4], Philipp Rostalski[2,5], Jan Modersitzki[1,4]

[1]Institute of Mathematics and Image Computing, University of Lübeck, Germany
[2]Fraunhofer IMTE, Fraunhofer Research Institution for Individualized and Cell-Based Medical Engineering, Germany
[3]Institute for Interventional Radiology, UKSH, Germany
[4]Fraunhofer Institute for Digital Medicine MEVIS, Germany
[5]Institute for Electrical Engineering in Medicine, Universiy of Lübeck, Germany
pia.schulz@uni-luebeck.de

Abstract. Respiratory surface electromyography measures the electrical muscle activity during breathing non-invasively. Electrophysiological modeling of the respiratory cycle is a valuable tool for analysis of the signals. A promising approach for dynamic simulations is based on knowing the deformation of the torso at a finite number of time steps between expiration and inspiration. In order to provide a foundation for such models, we present a new image registration method that determines the torso transformation during the respiratory cycle. For this purpose, we extend a ResNet-LDDMM based 3D/3D registration approach. We modify the network structure and add 2D data taken during respiration into the registration to include information about the breathing motion. Our experiments show that these modifications improve the registration quality, thereby providing a step towards a more realistic model of electrical transfer behavior over the respiratory cycle. The code is publicly available at `https://github.com/schulz-p/Image-Registration-for-a-Dynamic-Breathing-Model`.

1 Introduction

Respiration is caused by muscle contraction, which generates airflow into the lungs. Respiratory surface electromyography (sEMG) measures the electrical muscle activity generated during these contractions non-invasively and thus promises to quantify respiratory effort, e.g. in order to improve mechanical ventilation [1]. In various areas of sEMG research, modeling has proven to be a valuable tool for testing novel signal processing algorithms and better understanding the underlying physiology. Built upon magnetic resonance imaging (MRI), most of these models calculate the electrical transfer behavior for static, isometric muscle contractions [2]. However, breathing is a dynamic process, with complex shape variations and a large range of movement. As recently shown by [3] on forearm movements, sampling the motion by a limited number of discrete finite element models can be a valid method for dynamic simulations.

Motivated by the need of dynamic sEMG models, we consider the task of deriving a finite number of deformations of the torso between the end-expiratory and end-inspiratory phase. As the acquisition of volumetric MRI data over the respiratory cycle is an error-prone task, we use image registration to generate the deformations of the

C. Palm et al. (Hrsg.), *Bildverarbeitung für die Medizin 2025*, Informatik aktuell,
https://doi.org/10.1007/978-3-658-47422-5_4

torso at intermediate time points of the breathing cycle. We base our method on 3D MRI data acquired at static end-expiratory and end-inspiratory phase as well as 2D cine-MRI scans recorded during the respiration cycle to obtain information about the thorax movement. In particular, we perform a 3D/3D registration while incorporating additional 2D data corresponding to intermediate time points.

For this purpose, we build upon the successful LDDMM (large deformation diffeomorphic metric mapping) approach, as summarized e.g. in [4, 5]. Transformations resulting from this procedure provide a time-continuous deformation path between the coordinate systems of the initial and final images, which allows to obtain a smooth interpolation at intermediate time points. Specifically, we rely on a ResNet-LDDMM approach similar to the one proposed in [6], where the authors showed that incorporating Deep Residual Neural networks [7] into the LDDMM framework can provide a significant performance boost. However, their approach is based on point cloud data, which is not readily available in our case. Moreover, their model does not incorporate data at intermediate time points.

In this work, we extend the ResNet-LDDMM registration approach [6] in the following aspects to meet the requirements of the application at hand:

1. Instead of point cloud registration, we perform an intensity-based registration to calculate a transformation of the torso from the end-expiratory to the end-inspiratory phase. The transformation is modeled by a Neural Implicit Representation.
2. We incorporate intermediate 2D data to include information about the torso movement across the breathing cycle.
3. We modify the network architecture of the ResNet-LDDMM procedure [6]: Instead of 3 linear layers with one ReLU activation function per residual block, we utilize sinusoidal activation functions and include them twice in each residual block to represent deformations with higher frequencies.

Our new registration approach allows to determine a finite number of deformations of the torso between the end-expiratory and end-inspiratory phase. These intermediate transformations provide the basis for the calculation of electrical transfer behavior with a dynamic breathing model in future work.

2 Material and methods

2.1 Dataset

In order to enable calculating a dynamical breathing model as mentioned in the introduction, the deformation of specific thorax parts at a finite number of time steps between end-expiration and end-inspiration is required. The parts relevant for this are the diaphragm, the lung, the heart, the liver, the rib cage and the thorax itself. The given data consists of 3D T1-weighted MRI sequences of the torso recorded in the end-expiratory and end-inspiratory phase and a set of eleven 2D T2-weighted TRUFI MRI sequences (with TE = 1.67 ms and TR = 236.43 ms) of the frontal and sagittal plane taken during breathing. Additionally, a semi-automatic data segmentation of the mentioned thorax parts is generated with Materialise Mimics 24.0 (Materialise NV, Leuven, Belgium) in the 3D images.

2.2 Method

We can formulate the emerging registration problem as follows: Given are two 3D images $I_m, I_f : \Omega \subset \mathbb{R}^3 \to \mathbb{R}$, which we call the moving and fixed image, respectively, as well as a set of 2D images $I_{(n,j)} : \Sigma_{(n,j)} \subset \mathbb{R}^2 \to \mathbb{R}$, $n = 1, ..., N, j = 1, ..., M_n$, where each $\Sigma_{(n,j)}$ is embedded into Ω. Here, N is the number of time intervals between end-expiration and end-inspiration, and M_n denotes the number of images associated with time step n. The goal is to find transformations $\phi_n : \mathbb{R}^3 \to \mathbb{R}^3$ such that

$$I_m \circ \phi_N \approx I_f, \quad P_{(n,j)}(I_m \circ \phi_n) \approx I_{(n,j)} \quad \text{and} \quad \phi_0 = id \tag{1}$$

for $n = 1, .., N$ and $j = 1, ..., M_n$, where the operator $P_{(n,j)} : \mathbb{R}^3 \to \mathbb{R}^2$ extracts for each time step a slice of the warped 3D volume corresponding to the 2D image $I_{(n,j)}$. The LDDMM method calculates diffeomorphic time-dependent transformations $\phi : [0, 1] \times \mathbb{R}^3 \to \mathbb{R}^3$ based on the flow equation

$$\partial_t \phi(t, x) = v(t, \phi(t, x)), \quad \phi(0, x) = x \quad \text{for all } x \in \mathbb{R}^3, t \in [0, 1] \tag{2}$$

with a corresponding velocity field $v : [0, 1] \times \mathbb{R}^3 \to \mathbb{R}^3$. Forward Euler discretization with N time steps and step size $1/N$ yields

$$\phi_n(x) = \phi_{n-1}(x) + 1/N \cdot v_n(\phi_{n-1}(x)) \text{ for } n = 1, ..., N, \quad \phi_0(x) = x \tag{3}$$

where we use the notations $\phi_n(x) := \phi(t_n, x)$ and $v_n(x) := v(t_n, x)$.

This discretization scheme is captured in the network architecture of a ResNet-LDDMM approach (Fig. 1). The residual blocks (ResBlocks) correspond to v_n, representing the velocity field at the discrete time step n. Each block consists of three fully connected layers of width q with sinusoidal activation function after the first and second layer (Fig. 1, bottom). Note that in contrast to the ResNet-LDDMM approach of [6], we incorporate sinusoidal activation functions instead of ReLU and use the activation function twice rather than once to also capture deformations with higher frequencies.

To guarantee that the transformations ϕ_n described by the Neural Implicit Representation in Fig. 1 fulfill (1), we train the network such that it minimizes the energy

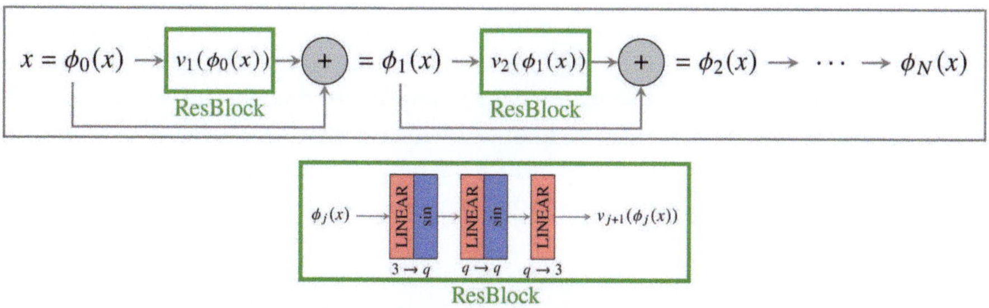

Fig. 1. Top: ResNet-LDDMM architecture, used for representing the registration transformation. Bottom: One residual block, the main component of the ResNet-LDDMM framework.

$$J[\phi_1, ..., \phi_N] = D^{3D}(I_m \circ \phi_N, I_f) + \alpha_1 \sum_{n=1}^{N} \sum_{j=1}^{M_n} D^{2D}(P_{(n,j)}(I_m \circ \phi_n), I_{(n,j)})$$
$$+ \alpha_2 S[\phi_1, ..., \phi_N] + \alpha_3 Q[\phi_N] \quad (4)$$

with similarity measures D^{3D} and D^{2D}, a regularizer S and a penalty Q. As similarity term of the 3D data, the mean squared error (MSE) is used. To account for the different intensity modalities between 3D and 2D MRI data, we choose normalized cross-correlation (NCC) as 2D distance measure. For regularization, the gradient of the velocity fields is penalized by

$$S[\phi_1, ..., \phi_N] = \sum_{n=1}^{N} \int_{\Omega} ||\nabla v_n(x)||_2^2 dx \quad (5)$$

where $v_1, ..., v_N$ are the underlying velocity fields of $\phi_1, ..., \phi_N$ in the sense of (3).

Note that the movement of the rib cage differs significantly from the rest of the considered thorax parts. While the diaphragm, lung, heart and liver move mainly downwards, the rib cage expands and moves upwards. To ensure a physically meaningful deformation of the rib cage, a rigidity term Q as proposed by [8] is evaluated on the rib cage and added to the loss.

2.3 Experiments and evaluation

We implemented the registration with GPU acceleration in PyTorch. As weighting parameters in (4), we empirically determined $\alpha_1 = 0.003$, $\alpha_2 = 0.1$ and $\alpha_3 = 0.01$. By setting $N = 5$, we allow for reconstruction of the breathing movement at four intermediate time steps. The dimensionality of the latent spaces inside the ResBlocks was set to $q = 100$. We used Adam as a stochastic gradient descent scheme for optimization, setting the learning rate to 0.001 and evaluating the model after 10^4 epochs. In each epoch, we randomly sampled 1% of the voxels in the 3D images and 1% of the 2D pixels in 5% of all 2D images.

In the evaluation, we focus on two aspects: Firstly, if the quality of the registration is satisfactory, and secondly, if the registration benefits from the incorporation of intermediate 2D data. To measure the quality of the 3D/3D registration, we consider the MSE between the fixed and the fully transformed moving image as well as the Dice scores of the given segmentations. We repeated the same experiments using the original residual blocks proposed by [6] with a learning rate to $3 \cdot 10^{-5}$ and compare the results. Whether the deformation calculated with our method is physically meaningful is examined by human inspection of the deformed segments at all discrete time steps. To test whether incorporating the 2D data is advantageous for the registration, we compare the 2D NCC before registration, after registration without 2D data and after registration with 2D data.

3 Results

First we quantify the performance of the sole 3D/3D registration. The MSE between fixed and moving image is improved from 0.012 before registration to 0.002 after registration. Using the residual blocks as in [6], only a higher MSE of 0.005 is achieved.

Segment	Dice before registration	Dice after registration [6]	Dice after registration (ours)
Diaphragm	0.174	0.414	0.552
Lung	0.838	0.934	0.963
Heart	0.85	0.864	0.912
Liver	0.678	0.887	0.905
Rib cage	0.246	0.381	0.524
Thorax	0.965	0.982	0.986

Tab. 1. Dice scores of segments before and after registration with the ResNet-LDDMM approach. The residual blocks used in our method outperform the original residual blocks of [6] in all segments.

Tab. 1 summarizes the Dice scores of the segments important for calculating the dynamic breathing model. Our procedure outperforms the results achieved with the residual blocks of [6] in all cases. The Dice scores of the lung, heart, liver and thorax, calculated with our method, are all greater than 0.9 after registration, indicating a good alignment of these parts. In contrast, though much improved by the registration, the Dice scores of the diaphragm and rib cage fall considerably behind. However, as these are rather thin structures, already a small misalignment impacts the Dice significantly.

To calculate a realistic breathing model, the deformation is not only required at the final time, but at intermediate time steps as well. The visual inspection of Fig. 2, showing the transformed segments at each discrete time step, indicates that the estimated intermediate transformations are physically plausible, meaning e.g. that rigid structures such as the ribs do not bend.

Next, we investigate the effect of integrating the intermediate 2D data into the registration framework. Using the 2D data is necessary for incorporating information about the torso movement during the breathing process. The mean 2D NCC between

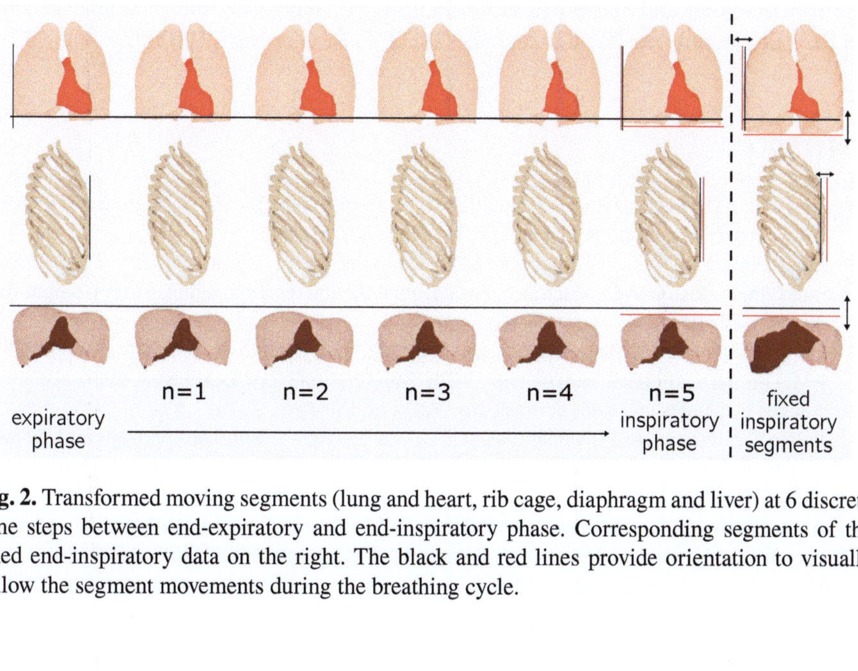

Fig. 2. Transformed moving segments (lung and heart, rib cage, diaphragm and liver) at 6 discrete time steps between end-expiratory and end-inspiratory phase. Corresponding segments of the fixed end-inspiratory data on the right. The black and red lines provide orientation to visually follow the segment movements during the breathing cycle.

the 2D images and the corresponding slice of the moving image before registration is 0.325. After the registration based only on the 3D data, an NCC of 0.351 is obtained. By including the 2D data into the registration, we achieve an NCC of 0.379 without noticing any changes in the 3D MSE. Thus, the use of the 2D information slightly improves the alignment with the 2D data during the breathing process without any restrictions on the quality of 3D/3D registration.

Altogether, we showed that our method calculates a physically plausible deformation between the images in the end-expiratory and end-inspiratory phase. By adaptation of the residual blocks in the ResNet-LDDMM approach [6] and the incorporation of additional 2D data, we improved the registration.

4 Discussion

We presented a 3D/3D registration method to model the motion of the torso during breathing. In our framework, we extended the ResNet-LDDMM approach [6] by modifying the residual blocks and incorporating additional intermediate 2D data. Our method allows not only calculation of a physically meaningful deformation of the torso, but also to evaluate the transformed torso at intermediate time steps between end-expiration and end-inspiration. With this our work provides a step towards a more realistic model of the electrical transfer behavior for respiratory sEMG electrodes leads, which is the basis for the analysis and simulation of sEMG signals and will be presented in future work.

Acknowledgement. We would like to thank Prof. Alex Frydrychowicz for his valuable support and expertise in MRI data acquisition. Andra Oltmann and Philipp Rostalski were supported by European Union - European Regional Development Fund, the Federal Government and Land Schleswig-Holstein, Project: "Diagnose- und Therapieverfahren für die Individualisierte Medizintechnik (IMTE)", Project No. 12420002.

References

1. Jonkman AH, Warnaar RSP, Baccinelli Wa. Analysis and applications of respiratory surface EMG: report of a round table meeting. Crit Care. 2024;28(1).
2. Pereira Botelho D, Curran K, Lowery MM et al. Anatomically accurate model of EMG during index finger flexion and abduction derived from diffusion tensor imaging. PLoS Comput Biol. 2019;15(8):e1007267.
3. Ma S, Clarke AK, Maksymenko K et al. Conditional generative models for simulation of EMG during naturalistic movements. IEEE Trans Neural Netw Learn Syst. 2024.
4. Younes L. Shapes and diffeomorphisms. Vol. 171. Springer, 2010.
5. Polzin T, Niethammer M, Vialard FX et al. 13 - A discretize–optimize approach for LDDMM registration. Riemannian Geometric Statistics in Medical Image Analysis. Academic Press, 2020:479–532.
6. Amor BB, Arguillère S, Shao L. ResNet-LDDMM: advancing the LDDMM framework using deep residual networks. IEEE Trans Pattern Anal Mach Intell. 2022;45(3):3707–20.
7. He K, Zhang X, Ren S et al. Identity mappings in deep residual networks. Proc ECCV. 2016:630–45.

8. Modersitzki J. Image registration with local rigidity constraints. Proc BVM. 2007:444–8.

Abstract: ConvexAdam

Self-configuring Framework for Dual-Optimisation-based 3D Multitask Medical Image Registration

Christoph Großbröhmer[1], Hanna Siebert[1], Lasse Hansen[2], Mattias P. Heinrich[1]

[1]Institute of Medical Informatics, University of Lübeck
[2]EchoScout GmbH, Lübeck
mattias.heinrich@uni-luebeck.de

Effective medical image registration aims to align anatomical structures accurately and apply smooth, plausible transformations across diverse imaging tasks. Deep learning-based registration approaches require extensive training data and task-specific configurations, which limits their adaptability and usability across multiple modalities and anatomical regions. We present ConvexAdam [1], a dual-optimization framework that combines convex optimization for global alignment with Adam-based instance optimization for fine-tuning. By leveraging pretrained semantic or hand-crafted features, ConvexAdam achieves fast, precise registration with minimal reliance on extensive training, making it applicable to a wide range of clinical tasks. Recently, it has been shown that state-of-the-art general-purpose features can be directly leveraged to enhance performance [2], establishing ConvexAdam as a feature-agnostic meta-registration framework. A key component of the framework is an automatic hyperparameter selection scheme, which evaluates and ranks numerous parameter settings on validation data considering complementary metrics. This enables an optimal configuration for each specific registration task. Experiments on the Learn2Reg challenge datasets [3], covering modalities such as MRI, CT, and ultrasound, demonstrate that ConvexAdam achieves high rankings in registration accuracy, computational efficiency and generalization often outperforming conventional deep learning techniques. By offering high-precision deformable registration with minimal computational demands, ConvexAdam provides a scalable solution for time-sensitive clinical applications where rapid and versatile alignment across anatomical sites and imaging modalities is essential[1].

References

1. Siebert H, Großbröhmer C, Hansen L et al. ConvexAdam: self-configuring dual-optimisation-based 3D multitask medical image registration. IEEE Trans Med Imaging. 2024.
2. Dey N, Billot B, Wong H et al. Learning general-purpose biomedical volume representations using randomized synthesis. Preprint, Under review for ICLR 2025. 2024.
3. Hering A, Hansen L, Mok TC et al. Learn2Reg: comprehensive multi-task medical image registration challenge, dataset and evaluation in the era of deep learning. IEEE Trans Med Imaging. 2022.

[1]https://github.com/multimodallearning/convexAdam

C. Palm et al. (Hrsg.), *Bildverarbeitung für die Medizin 2025*, Informatik aktuell,
https://doi.org/10.1007/978-3-658-47422-5_5

Surrogate-based Respiratory Motion Estimation using Physics-enhanced Implicit Neural Representations

Jan Boysen[1], Hristina Uzunova[1], Jan Ehrhardt[1,2], Heinz Handels[1,2]

[1]German Research Center for Artificial Intelligence (DFKI), Lübeck
[2]Institute of Medical Informatics, University of Lübeck
jan.boysen@dfki.de

Abstract. Medical image registration plays a key role in radiation-based cancer treatment in the thorax. Naturally thorax image registration is highly patient-specific, requiring registration models to be trained patient individually. The available per-patient data is highly limited and often does not cover all potential scenarios occurring during treatment. In this work we create patient-individual implicit neural representations (INRs) that represent the displacement fields during a breathing cycle. We tackle the data shortage by including physical knowledge, while simultaneously improving generalization capabilities. Our results show that physical constraints can be well integrated into INRs. However, we find that extrapolation capabilities are highly dependent on the induced physical regularization.

1 Introduction

The success of cancer treatment in the human thorax through radiation therapy is highly dependent on the accuracy of the radiation beams coinciding with the tumor cells [1]. Thus, understanding the deformation of the lung and inner structures during a breathing cycle is of great clinical relevance for motion compensation techniques, like respiratory gating or tumor tracking [1, 2]. Direct observation of the relevant structures during treatment is technically complex and difficult to implement. Therefore, externally measured respiratory signals, so-called surrogates, are used together with patient-specific correspondence models to predict the internal motion. These correspondence models establish the relationship between external respiratory signals, such as spirometry, abdominal belts or camera observations, and the internal spatio-temporal motion measured using 4D image data, such as 4D-CT or 4D-MRI acquired ahead of the treatment [3].

Most correspondence models are two-stage approaches, where image registration is first used to estimate the internal respiratory motion from the given image data. In a second step, a correspondence model is created between the surrogate signals and the estimated motion fields [3]. However, in this paper we investigate the possibility of directly inferring patient-specific breathing models from the given images and surrogates within a single step. Deformable image registration is a common solution for capturing respiratory motion in radiotherapy [4]. Recently, implicit neural representations (INRs) showed a top-performing accuracy in intra-patient registration of inhalation-exhalation CTs [5]. Other studies use INRs for time-continuous motion estimation in spatio-temporal imaging data [6, 7]. In our work, we investigate the performance of INRs for surrogate-based respiratory motion prediction in interpolation and extrapolation scenarios. This is done

C. Palm et al. (Hrsg.), *Bildverarbeitung für die Medizin 2025*, Informatik aktuell,
https://doi.org/10.1007/978-3-658-47422-5_6

by considering the acquired surrogate signals as input to the INR next to the image coordinates in order to generate a motion estimate for the corresponding breathing state as output. To improve the physical correctness of the learned motion fields, a regularization with physical intuition about the tissue deformation characteristics is applied. This is closely related to physics-informed neural networks (PINNs) [8].

2 Materials and methods

In this work, we aim to perform patient-based image registration of 4D lung CTs in order to model the movement of the lung during the breathing phases of a patient. The proposed approach combines the strengths of two methods: INRs and PINNs, resulting in what we call a physics-enhanced implicit neural representation.

2.1 Surrogate-based motion estimation

For model training, we assume a given 4D image data set $(\boldsymbol{I}_j)_{j=1,\ldots,n_{ph}}$ consisting of n_{ph} image volumes $\boldsymbol{I}_j : \Omega \to \mathbb{R}$ ($\Omega \subset \mathbb{R}^3$) acquired at breathing phase j, and a set of corresponding surrogate measurements $\mathbb{S} = (\boldsymbol{s}_j)_{j=1,\ldots,n_{ph}}$, $s_j \in \mathbb{R}^{n_{\text{sur}}}$. In our application $\boldsymbol{s}_j$ consists of the air volume (measured by spirometry during the image acquisition) and an indicator for inhale (= 1) or exhale (= 0), i.e. $n_{\text{sur}} = 2$.

The goal of our model training is to learn the internal motion with respect to a reference breathing phase (here: maximum inhale $\boldsymbol{I}_1$) and represented by nonlinear transformations

$$\varphi : \Omega \times \mathbb{R}^{n_{\text{sur}}} \to \Omega \qquad \varphi(\mathbf{x}, \boldsymbol{s}) = \mathbf{x} + u(\mathbf{x}, \boldsymbol{s})$$

for spatial coordinates $\mathbf{x} \in \Omega$ and surrogates $\boldsymbol{s} \in \mathbb{S}$. The trained model should then be able to predict the motion for previously unknown signals $\boldsymbol{s} \notin \mathbb{S}$.

In our case, this deformation prediction is established as a patient-based image registration, where different volumes of a 4D series are warped to the reference breathing phase using a surrogate-conditioned per-patient INR network to learn the deformations with the general objective

$$L = L_{\text{image}} + \alpha L_{\text{reg}} \tag{1}$$

The image loss $L_{\text{image}} = \text{NCC}\left[\boldsymbol{I}_1, \boldsymbol{I}_j \circ \varphi(\mathbf{x}, \boldsymbol{s}_j)\right]$ represents the difference between the warped moving image $\boldsymbol{I}_j$ with $j = 2, \ldots, n_{ph}$ and fixed image $\boldsymbol{I}_1$, where $\text{NCC}[\cdot, \cdot]$ is the normalized cross correlation. The regularization loss L_{reg} ensures the plausibility of the displacement field weighted by a certain parameter α. Here, the regularizer is chosen based on a physically-enhanced approach.

2.2 Physics-enhanced implicit neural representation

The main idea of INRs [9] is to map spatial coordinates $\mathbf{x}$ to a signal by using the mapping function $f_{\text{INR}}(\cdot)$

$$\text{signal}(\mathbf{x}) = f_{\text{INR}}(\mathbf{x}) \tag{2}$$

The mapping function f_{INR} can be typically obtained by solving an optimization problem using a dense neural network (DNN), that takes spatial coordinates (and possibly additional conditional information) as input and returns the corresponding signal value.

To address the tendency of DNNs towards low-frequency signals, the commonly used rectified-linear unit activation is replaced by a sinusoidal activation resulting in so-called sinusoidal representation networks (SIRENs) [9]. Inspired by the intensity-based implicit deformable image registration (IDIR) [5] framework, we utilize INRs in order to establish patient-based image registration conditioned on surrogates. We predict a non-linear displacement field $u(\cdot)$ (to the fixed $\boldsymbol{I}_1$) from the input image coordinates $\mathbf{x}$ of a moving image and the given surrogate values $\boldsymbol{s}$ using SIREN as follows

$$f_{\text{SIREN}}(\mathbf{x}, \boldsymbol{s}) = u(\mathbf{x}, \boldsymbol{s}) \tag{3}$$

by minimizing the registration loss in Eq. 1. Through the consideration of the additional surrogate conditioning $\boldsymbol{s}$, we are able to expand the typically one-to-one INR architecture to a patient-based registration approach.

To improve the generalization capabilities of the network we include the physics-based loss from López et al. [7], that enforces neo-hookean hyper-elastic tissue behavior in the INR. This is closely related to PINNs [8], where the physically feasible behavior is directly induced during the training and, thus, learning is not only data-driven but also knowledge-based [10]. Our approach does not directly use PDE residuals, however, a physically inspired regularization term is used during optimization

$$L_{\text{reg}}(\varphi, \lambda) = \text{trace}(\boldsymbol{C}) - 3 - \log(|\boldsymbol{J}|^2) + \lambda(|\boldsymbol{J}| - 1)^2 \tag{4}$$

where with φ being the displacement field and λ the specific weighting parameter of the function. $|\boldsymbol{J}|$ is the determinant of the jacobian $\boldsymbol{J} = d\varphi/d\mathbf{x}$. $\boldsymbol{C}$ is defined as $\boldsymbol{C} = \boldsymbol{J}^T\boldsymbol{J}$. We apply the same physical constrains to our model by using the L_{reg} in Eq. 1.

2.3 Implementation details

The registration INR consists of three hidden layers with 256 neurons in each. The input layer with five neurons takes in a voxel coordinate, lung volume and a binary value for the breathing phase. For the whole training a batch size of 10,000 is chosen, corresponding to 10,000 randomly sampled coordinates from the input image. The lung volumes are blurred with uniform noise to prevent overfitting towards the volumes in the training set. The parameters λ and α are set to 1 and $1e^{-4}$, respectively. The maximum number of epochs during training is 2,500 with integrated early stopping. Before the main training of the network, a pre-training procedure inspired by López et al. [7] is conducted. Here, the network parameters are initialized such that the identity transformation is outputted. This is done by training the network for the registration between the same copied volume using the training loss from Eq. 1. The intuition behind this is that the network is not just supposed to learn a random identity transformation, but one that matches the introduced physical constraints and the optimization surface of the loss function. The pre-training ends, once the identity transformation is well approximated.

3 Experiments and results

3.1 Data

We use an adapted version of the 4D CT image dataset introduced by Wilms et al. [11] containing 12 patients. All patients have lung cancer with a visible tumor in the CT images. However, this study does not differentiate between the tumor and residual lung tissue. For each patient the dataset contains either 10 or 14 CT images of the lung at different breathing states during inhalation and exhalation. The lung volume at maximum exhalation is defined as zero. The lung volumes in the remaining images are inferred from this zero-definition. All images have a spatial resolution of 512x512x270 voxels with a non-isotropic spacing. Wilms et al. [11] defined landmarks for evaluation at four breathing states per patient.

3.2 Experiments

We are performing experiments on a NVIDIA GeForce GTX 1080 Ti on a per-patient basis and define three experiments per patient, that differ by the images in the test set. In all experiments the reference breathing phase is the "End-Inhale" (EI) state. The test set of the first experiment "End-Exhale" (EE) contains the end-exhalation state and additionally the one (in case of 10 images) or two (in case of 14 images) states with the next smallest lung volumes. In the other two experiments we leave out an intermediate state during inhalation in the experiment "Mid-Inhale" (MI) or an intermediate state of the exhalation phase in the experiment "Mid-Exhale" (ME) during training. The left-out images then form the test set. Our performance baseline is a multivariate regression approach proposed by Wilms et al. [11]. It is a classical two-stage approach with a nonlinear intra-patient registration for motion estimation [12] followed by an ordinary least squares (OLS) regression for correspondence modeling with the surrogate signal. In contrast to our line of work, Wilms et al. [11] use a diffeomorphic approach based

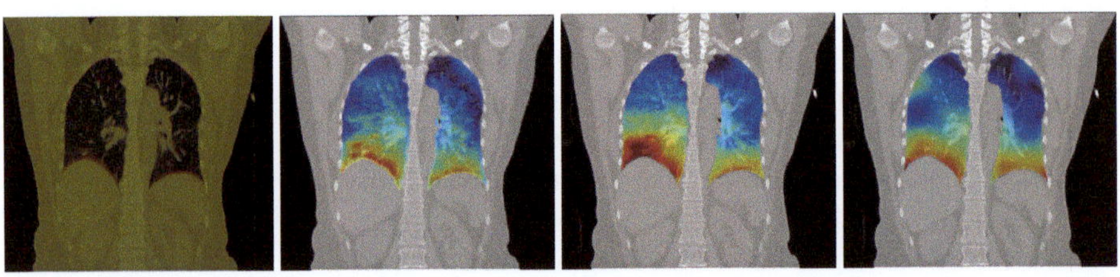

(a) Overlay of EI (green) and ME (red). **(b)** Registration-based motion estimate. **(c)** Motion predicted by OLS regression [11]. **(d)** Motion predicted by physics-enhanced INR.

Fig. 1. CT scans of two breathing states (EI and ME) for patient 31 (a) and color-coded magnitudes of the motion estimates generated by image-based intra-patient registration (b), surrogate-based regression using OLS [11] (c), and our surrogate-based motion estimate by a physics-enhanced INR (d). Note that only intra-patient registration uses ME image information and can therefore be considered a pseudo ground truth.

Tab. 1. Landmark-based euclidean error in mm between the fixed and moving images in the respective experiments. "N": Distance between fixed and non-warped moving image; "W": Distance between fixed and warped moving image using Wilms et al.'s approach [11]; "O": Distance between fixed and warped moving image using our approach.

Patient ID	EI → MI			EI → ME			EI → EE		
	N	W	O	N	W	O	N	W	O
Patient 01	3.98	1.68	1.96	2.08	1.48	1.54	4.25	1.29	2.54
Patient 02	5.08	1.65	2.10	2.51	1.32	1.97	6.29	1.56	2.85
Patient 03	4.43	1.83	1.92	2.41	1.83	1.99	5.45	1.74	2.81
Patient 04	4.95	2.24	2.08	2.52	1.77	2.14	6.19	1.76	3.34
Patient 23	3.76	2.42	2.04	2.42	1.78	2.20	6.79	2.34	4.26
Patient 31	4.56	2.15	1.84	1.98	1.87	1.72	6.44	1.46	4.61
Patient 35	3.80	1.78	1.74	1.92	1.97	1.82	4.31	1.61	2.87
Patient 36	6.68	2.59	2.11	3.84	2.08	2.16	10.76	2.66	5.83
Patient 41	4.11	2.02	1.77	2.76	1.70	1.77	6.40	1.74	3.64
Patient 44	4.03	1.68	1.90	2.07	1.43	1.90	6.06	1.60	4.41
Patient 48	5.87	1.90	6.21	2.56	1.61	4.48	7.98	1.70	6.56
Patient 53	6.71	2.24	2.50	2.94	1.77	2.00	2.94	2.65	3.07
Mean	4.74	2.03	2.00	2.50	1.73	1.93	5.99	1.86	3.66
Std	1.06	0.33	0.21	0.55	0.23	0.20	1.98	0.47	1.01

on static velocity fields. Tab. 1 presents the results of the three experiments for patient-specific surrogate-based motion estimation. The baseline results are shown in the "W" columns in Tab. 1. The "N" columns in Tab. 1 show the average landmark displacement between the fixed and moving image without registration. Columns "O" present the euclidean landmark distances between the fixed and moving image using our physics-enhanced INR. Tab. 1 shows that our physics-enhanced INR performs comparable to the baseline (see columns "EI→MI" and "EI→ME"). In the EE experiment our method exhibits a substantial performance gap compared to the baseline. Patient 48 in our dataset (highlighted in gray in Tab. 1) is neglected in the mean and standard deviation shown at the end of the table, because this patient represents an outlier within the dataset due to medical abnormalities in its lungs. Fig. 1a shows an overlay of the inhale and exhale CT images. The green area marks the inhale state (EI) and the red area the mid-exhale state (ME). Fig. 1c shows the magnitude of the displacement field from the work of Wilms et al. [11]. The magnitude of displacement increases from blue to red. Similarly, does Fig. 1d show the displacement field of our physics-enhanced INR.

4 Discussion

The MI and ME experiments both evaluate the interpolation capabilities of our physics-enhanced INR. The results show, that our approach performs competitive for in-domain data. The EE experiment evaluates the models extrapolation capabilities, as the moving image is out-domain of the INR. The results suggest, that our physics-induced loss works well in-domain, but struggles to utilize the physics information out-domain. We reason, that the principal cause for this is the absence of an optimization criterion along the temporal, respectively volumetric, dimension. Our used optimization criterion only regularizes displacement fields at specific breathing states, but not in the volumetric vicinity or even between different breathing states. However, our results show that physical knowledge can be integrated into INRs and optimize the INR's behaviour accordingly. The displacement field magnitude plots in Fig. 1 indicate, that both the baseline and the physics-enhanced INR infer the largest displacement at the bottom of the lung. Considering the biggest difference between the two breathing states is located at the bottom of the lung (see red area in Fig. 1a), we find both models inferring the correct displacement field. Further, we find the displacement field magnitudes of the INR to be smoother than the ones by Wilms et al. [11].

Addressing the out-domain performance of physics-enhanced INRs is one consideration for future work. This will require the investigation of temporal-dependent physics equations. Further, we plan to integrate a diffeomorphic parametrization of the motion fields to allow for easier inversion. Ultimately, this would allow us to use INRs for image generation by warping the fixed image with the inverse displacement field to any volume and breathing phase of the patient.

References

1. Keall PJ, Mageras GS, Balter JM et al. The management of respiratory motion in radiation oncology report of AAPM Task Group 76. Med Phys. 2006;33(10):3874–900.
2. Shirato H, Shimizu S, Kitamura K et al. Organ motion in image-guided radiotherapy: lessons from real-time tumor-tracking radiotherapy. Int J Clin Oncol. 2007;12(1):8–16.
3. McClelland JR, Hawkes DJ, Schaeffter T et al. Respiratory motion models: a review. Med Image Anal. 2013;17(1):19–42.
4. Ehrhardt J, Lorenz C, eds. 4D modeling and estimation of respiratory motion for radiation therapy. (Biological and Medical Physics, Biomedical Engineering). Springer, 2013.
5. Wolterink JM, Zwienenberg JC, Brune C. Implicit neural representations for deformable image registration. PMLR. 2022;172:1349–59.
6. Garzia S, Rygiel P, Dummer S et al. Neural fields for continuous periodic motion estimation in 4D cardiovascular imaging. arXiv: 2407.20728. 2024.
7. Arratia López P, Mella H, Uribe S et al. WarpPINN: cine-MR image registration with physics-informed neural networks. Med Image Anal. 2023;89:102925.
8. Raissi M, Perdikaris P, Karniadakis GE. Physics informed deep learning (part I): data-driven solutions of nonlinear partial differential equations. arXiv: 1711.10561. 2017.
9. Sitzmann V, Martel J, Bergman A et al. Implicit neural representations with periodic activation functions. Proc NeurIPS. 2020;33:7462–73.
10. Lawal ZK, Yassin H, Lai DTC et al. Physics-informed neural network (PINN) evolution and beyond: a systematic literature review and bibliometric analysis. Big Data Cogn Comput. 2022;6(4):140.
11. Wilms M, Werner R, Ehrhardt J et al. Multivariate regression approaches for surrogate-based diffeomorphic estimation of respiratory motion in radiation therapy. Phys Med Biol. 2014;59(5):1147.
12. Werner R, Schmidt-Richberg A, Handels H et al. Estimation of lung motion fields in 4D CT data by variational non-linear intensity-based registration: a comparison and evaluation study. Phys Med Biol. 2014;59(15):4247.

Comparison of Framewise Video Classification in Laryngoscopies

Ole Felber[1], Louis Bellmann[1,2], Philipp Breitfeld[1,2], Martin Petzoldt[2], Felix Rindt[2], René Werner[‡1,3,4], Maximilian Nielsen[‡1,3,4]

[1]Institute for Applied Medical Informatics, Univ. Medical Center Hamburg-Eppendorf (UKE)
[2]Center for Anesthesiology and Intensive Care Medicine, UKE
[3]Institute of Computational Neuroscience, UKE
[4]Center for Biomedical Artificial Intelligence (bAIome), UKE
m.nielsen@uke.de

Abstract. In this study, the performance of single-task and multi-task models, incorporating both static and temporal classification approaches, for various tasks in medical video laryngoscopy (VL) is assessed through a deep learning (DL) image encoder and LSTM networks. The data foundation is an in-house dataset of 464 individual recordings. In contrast to previous works, we consider the impact of multi-task learning and temporal dependencies in the data through video snippets. Results show that multi-task models outperform single-task models for tasks with sparse labels, indicating the benefits of shared learning across tasks. Moreover LSTM-based models significantly improve temporal consistency and performance for tasks with inherent temporal dependencies such the process state of VL.

1 Introduction

Airway management is a crucial part of emergency medicine and anesthesia, ensuring open airways and effective ventilation. As part of the intubation process, laryngoscopy is a key step that provides the clinician with a view of relevant anatomical structures prior to inserting the endotracheal tube. Video laryngoscopy (VL) has emerged as a valuable alternative to direct laryngoscopy, offering enhanced visualization that improves outcomes in difficult airway scenarios and reduces the risk of failed intubations [1]. Beyond patient-level benefits, VL generates video data of interventions that can be analyzed through deep learning video processing techniques, which may be used as an diagnostic assistance tool during intervention, for auto-reporting or retrospective quality assessments [2, 3].

The main challenges in VL analysis involve detecting critical anatomical structures such as the glottis and epiglottis, identifying medical devices, recognizing lesions, and assessing the *informativeness* (i.e. how usable it is for the operator to perform the intubation) of the view. Despite the wide range of tasks that originate from VL, much of the past research has focused on singular aspects, not considering the diversity of problem statements necessary for, analysis of the procedure [2, 3].

However, looking at the bigger picture, automatic analysis of VL is only a means to an end, e.g. systematic reporting of the procedure. Therefore it is necessary to address

[‡]These authors contributed equally the least to this work.

C. Palm et al. (Hrsg.), *Bildverarbeitung für die Medizin 2025*, Informatik aktuell,
https://doi.org/10.1007/978-3-658-47422-5_7

these diverse tasks adequately in the same framework. Furthermore, VL data consists of consecutive video frames, and while previous approaches have focused on single-frame predictions, temporal consistency across frames is a desired property for reliable analysis. In addition, certain information in VL, such as the procedural state (e.g., establishing a view, tube insertion, or tube placement) and special maneuvers performed by the clinician, are inherently time-dependent and cannot be effectively captured by static, frame-by-frame examination [2, 3].

This work aims to address two research questions:

- How does the incorporation of temporal information affect framewise prediction and temporal consistency of VL videos?
- How does fusing multiple tasks within a single encoder model impact overall performance?

To answer these questions, we first establish a baseline using a single-frame encoder for each task in the VL dataset. We then compare this approach to a multi-task encoder that jointly addresses seven tasks. In the next step, we integrate temporal context through 43 second long VL snippets which are then processed by a Long Short-Term Memory (LSTM) network on top of the encoder's latent space, enabling the model to process sequential information [4]. The scope of our study includes 24 different labels, that include mutually exclusive categories (multi-class) and binary labels (multi-label) of which several have not yet been investigated [2, 3].

To our knowledge, this is the first study on automatic VL analysis to consider multiple different unrelated tasks from whole VL videos and analyzing the effects of temporal context information. Based on the two open questions, our contributions are as follows:

- *Temporal information enhances performance:* We demonstrate that incorporating temporal information improves the predictive accuracy across all annotation categories.
- *Multi-task learning improves performance:* We show that leveraging a multi-task approach improves the performance of individual tasks, suggesting that shared information across tasks aids in the learning process.
- *Temporal processing improves temporal consistency:* By incorporating LSTM-based temporal processing, we show that VL predictions achieve greater temporal consistency.

2 Methods

This study conducts four experiments by combining two distinct experimental setups for VL classification in multiple tasks. Firstly, we compare multiple single-task approaches with a direct multi-task approach. Secondly, we evaluate static single-frame classification against temporal contextualised single-frame classification. The implementation is done in python using the pytorch deep learning framework.

2.1 Video laryngoscopy data

The VL recordings used in this study were collected as part of the work by Kohse et al. [5]. The study focused on patients with anticipated difficult airways. A total of 464 VL recordings were captured, of which 101 were annotated frame-by-frame by two medical experts.

We categorized the annotations into seven clinically motivated tasks, each designed to capture key aspects of the VL (percentages in brackets indicate relative frequencies calculated as: frames with positive label / total amount of frames):

- *Confounders*: Visual impairments that limit the assessability of anatomical structures, devices, etc. in a given frame. Confounders is a non-temporal and binary labeled task and has been formerly investigated. *Labels*: Saliva (27%)
- *Device*: Medical devices present in the frame. Non-temporal, multi-label, investigated. *Labels*: Tube (32%), cuff (18%)
- *Landmark*: Visibility of anatomical landmarks with high importance for intubation. Non-temporal, multi-label, investigated. *Labels*: Glottis opening (46%), epiglottis (54%)
- *Maneuver*: Special intubation maneuver performed by operator. Temporal, binary, investigated. *Labels*: Direct lifting (30%)
- *Placement*: Approximate position of the endotracheal tube in the patient's airway. temporal, multi-label, not investigated. *Labels*: Tip behind arytenoids (5%), tip behind cords (5%), cuff behind cords (2%)
- *Process*:Current phase of the intubation process. Temporal, multi-class, not investigated. *Labels*: Preparation (5%), establishing view (16%), accepted view (19%), inserting bougie (13%), placed bougie (9%), inserting tube (12%), placed tube (8%), extracting abort (2%), extracting intubated (2%), intubated (11%), scope disconnected (3%)
- *View*: Current view of the camera. Non-temporal, multi-class, investigated. *Labels*: Signal error (5%), outside (28%), pharynx (24%), larynx (43%)

To reduce computational cost, we downsample all videos to 224 by 224 pixels in the spatial dimension and reduce the temporal resolution to 3 frames per second. Furthermore the videos were split into snippets of 128 frames or 43 seconds. Fig. 1 provides a general impression of our dataset and highlights three single frames which are representative for a single-task and label. Since this is a multi-task problem, all shown frames are labeled for all other tasks.

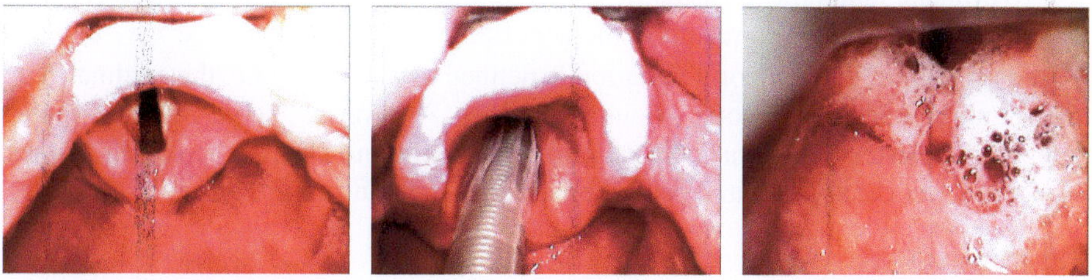

(a) Landmark: Glottis opening. **(b)** Device: Tube. **(c)** Confounder: Salvia.

Fig. 1. Representative frames showcasing key visual elements in the video laryngoscopy dataset, that showcase different tasks and labels.

2.2 Experimental setup

For all four experiments, we utilize the XCiT (Cross-Covariance Image Transformer) deep learning image encoder network [6] to generate frame-level embeddings from the video data. The experimental setup is structured to evaluate two key factors. The experimental approaches are as follows:

1. *Single-frame classification*: Frame-level embeddings generated by the XCiT encoder are directly fed into a linear layer (classification head) to predict the relevant labels without considering temporal dependencies.
2. *Temporal classification*: An additional LSTM network is integrated on top of the frame embeddings to capture temporal dependencies before classification [4].

For the multi-task vs. single-task comparison, the models are configured as:

1. *Multi-task classification*: A single classification head outputs predictions for all tasks (labels) simultaneously with representation from one single encoder model.
2. *Single-task classification*: Each task has its own dedicated encoder (and LSTM, if temporal context is used) model and classification head, resulting in 7 independent models.

In each experiment, the encoder (and LSTM, when applicable) and classification head are trained simultaneously with either categorical cross entropy for multi-class problems or binary cross entropy for multi-label problems.

All experiments are evaluated through a nested patient-level 5-fold cross-validation approach with an inner and outer loop:

- *Outer loop*: The dataset is split into 80% training (fitting) and 20% testing sets.
- *Inner loop*: The training set from the outer loop is further divided into 50% training and 50% validation subsets.

This process results in a total of 10 runs per experiment, with two predictions per sample. We further perform early stopping on the validation-set based on the balanced accuracy. As an additional metric we evaluate temporal consistency, which evaluates how stable the predictions are across sequential frames. The reported metrics are aggregated as a mean of case level metrics.

To evaluate temporal consistency, we first define the set of all time steps $i \in T$ with predictions $\hat{y}_i$ diverging in regard to the next frame as $\hat{y}_{i+1}$ as $Y_t := \{i \in T | \hat{y}_i \neq \hat{y}_{i+1}\}$. Based on this set, the temporal variation is defined as $t_{\text{var}} = \frac{|Y_t|}{n}$, i.e. the cardinality of the set normalized by the total amount of frames. A lower t_{var} score indicates higher temporal consistency, with a score of zero representing no changes across all frames. Hence, perfect consistency and perfect predictions are mutually exclusive.

3 Results

Fig. 2 provides an overview of the balanced accuracies across the different tasks for all four experiment configurations. For 4 out of the 7 tasks, balanced accuracies exceed 85%. Moreover, the tasks Placement and Process also achieve reasonably high performance, particularly considering the number of classes of the Task process and the low prevalence of Placement labels in the dataset. However, the task Confounder shows the weakest performance, with even the best configuration only achieving a 7% improvement over chance level.

When comparing single-task and multi-task models, both single-frame and LSTM-based configurations show similar performance for both approaches with differences generally below 2%. However, in the specific cases of the tasks Maneuver and Placement, multi-task models outperform their single-task counterparts. These two tasks have the fewest labeled frames, suggesting that the multi-task setup facilitates beneficial cross-learning across tasks with sparse labels resulting in better generalization.

This trend persists even with LSTM-based models, with one notable exception: The task Maneuver in the single-task setting shows a substantial performance drop (0.16) when using an LSTM. This is in contrast to temporal tasks, i.e. Process and Placement, which require temporal context. Here, LSTM-based models consistently outperform single-task models. Interestingly, this also applies to the non-temporal task Confounder, possibly through added context and temporal consistency (Fig. 3).

Furthermore, the inclusion of LSTMs notably improves temporal consistency. Across all tasks, LSTM-based models exhibit more stable predictions, with reduced frame-to-frame variability. The comparison between the two LSTM approaches show a slight advantage of single-task models over multi-task ones.

4 Discussion

In this study, we investigated the effects of temporal and multi-task learning for VL analysis on a set of complete VL videos annotated for a multitude, tasks partially not

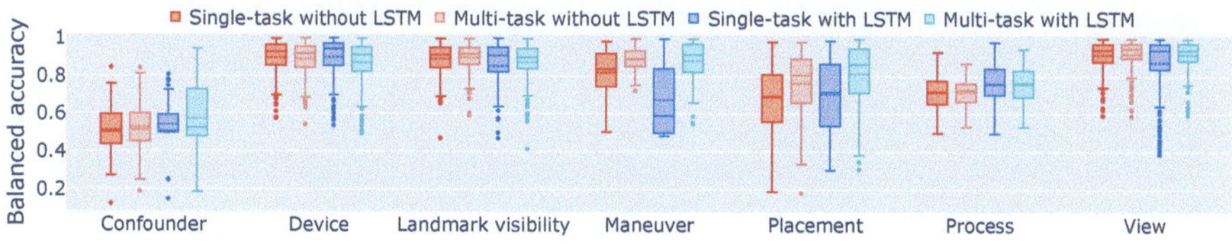

Fig. 2. Overview of task-wise performance for all 4 experiments.

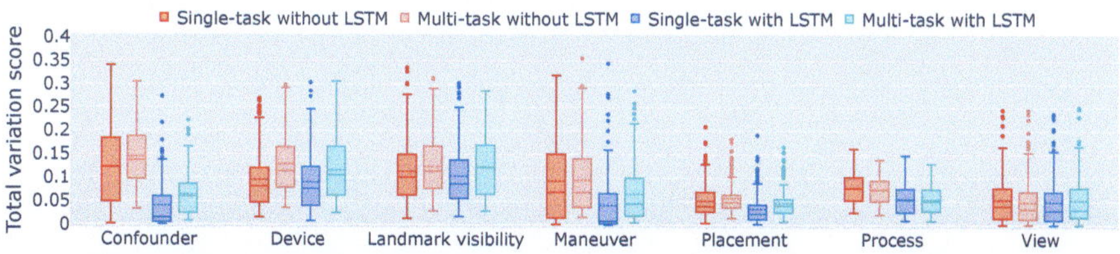

Fig. 3. Overview of task wise temporal consistency for all 4 experiments, lower values representing more consistent predictions.

yet investigated by others [2, 3]. The tasks span from time independent ones such as anatomical structures to highly time dependent ones such as the placement of the endotracheal tube. For the tasks already investigated our performance lines up with previous publications.

Circling back to the two key questions that guided our experiments: First, our study demonstrates that multi-task models outperform single-task models for tasks with sparse labels, such as Maneuver and Placement, suggesting that shared learning improves performance in these cases. Second, LSTM-based models consistently enhance both temporal consistency and task performance, particularly for tasks requiring temporal context, such as the Process label. Additionally, employing a combined multi-task model proves to be more efficient in terms of both training and inference. However, this comes at the expense of reduced flexibility, as adding new tasks or labels requires full retraining of the model.

References

1. Hansel J, Rogers AM, Lewis SR et al. Videolaryngoscopy versus direct laryngoscopy for adults undergoing tracheal intubation. Cochrane Database Syst Rev. 2022;(4).
2. Yao P, Usman M, Chen YH et al. Applications of artificial intelligence to office laryngoscopy: a scoping review. Laryngoscope. 2022;132(10):1993–2016.
3. Sampieri C, Baldini C, Azam MA et al. Artificial intelligence for upper aerodigestive tract endoscopy and laryngoscopy: a guide for physicians and state-of-the-art review. Otolaryngol Head Neck Surg. 2023;169(4):811–29.
4. Hochreiter S, Schmidhuber J. Long short-term memory. Neural Comput. 1997;9(8):1735–80.
5. Kohse E, Siebert H, Sasu P et al. A model to predict difficult airway alerts after videolaryngoscopy in adults with anticipated difficult airways–the VIDIAC score. Anaesthesia. 2022;77(10):1089–96.
6. Ali A, Touvron H, Caron M et al. Xcit: cross-covariance image transformers. Adv Neural Inf Process Syst. 2021;34:20014–27.

Real-time Fiberscopic Image Improvement for Automated Lesion Detection in the Urinary Bladder

Thomas Eixelberger[1,2], Karl Weingärtner[3], Philipp Maisch[4], Christian Bolenz[4], Thomas Wittenberg[1,2]

[1]Chair for Visual Computing, Friedrich-Alexander-Universität Erlangen-Nürnberg
[2]Fraunhofer-Institut für Integrierte Schaltungen IIS, Erlangen
[3]Abteilung für Urologie, Sozialstiftung Bamberg
[4]Abteilung für Urologie, Universitätsklinikum Ulm
thomas.eixelberger@fau.de

Abstract. Fiber endoscopes are flexible devices that use glass fibers for optical transmission of images out hollows such as the urinary bladder, trans-nasal cavities, or the lung. Even though bendable tip-chip endoscopes have been available for the past decades, fiberscopes are still in broad use, as they provide good images for a good price. However, images obtained from fiberscopes are particularly degraded by the honeycomb pattern related to the core and cladding of each fiber. To remove such honeycomb patterns for the human visual inspection of natural orifices as well as to condition such images to be used for machine and deep learning tasks, real-time compensation algorithms are needed. Using a large set of >15,000 fiberscopic images from the urinary bladder, two related approaches are investigated, namely (1) how to eliminate honeycomb patterns in real-time and hence improve the image quality, (2) to use such improved image data to train a deep-learning task to detect tumorous lesions in the urinary bladder. The investigated non-parametric filtering approach removes the honeycomb artifacts in the frequency domain using a DoG filter and thresholding. This filtering approach was evaluated on the fiberscopic images with and without visible honeycomb pattern using the BRISQUE image quality algorithm [1]. Secondly, the thus improved images were used as enhanced training dataset for a pre-trained deep neural networks (RT-DETR) for automated lesion detection in the urinary bladder. Based on the BRISQUE score, for approx. 10,000 cystoscopic images the fiber structures could be eliminated and the image quality could be improved. The BRISQUE score improved on average from 31.19 to 18.32. The F1-score for lesion detection using 572 cystoscopic improved from 0.623 to 0.802 using the honeycomb structured images for training, and to F1 = 0.830 with the images with the removed honeycomb structures. The investigated approach is on one hand capable to improve the fiberscopic honeycomb pattern in real-time, while on the other hand the honeycomb removal leads to improved rates for automated lesion detection in the urinary bladder.

1 Introduction

Fiber endoscopes are a special type of flexible endoscopes in which glass fiber bundles are used to transmit light into and images out of tight and bending hollows such as the urinary bladder [2, 3], trans-nasal cavities [4], or the lung [5] through natural

C. Palm et al. (Hrsg.), *Bildverarbeitung für die Medizin 2025*, Informatik aktuell,
https://doi.org/10.1007/978-3-658-47422-5_8

orifices such as the urethra, nose, or mouth. Although flexible tip-chip endoscopes have been available for the past decades, fiberscopes are still widely used in various medical fields such as gastroenterology, urology, or pulmonology. Nevertheless, the acquired fiberscopic images are usually degraded/affected by a so-called "honeycomb pattern" (Fig. 1). For the visual inspection of internal hollow organs such as the urinary bladder, larynx, or lung, these honeycomb patterns are partially eliminated by manual defocusing, whereas such defocused images cannot really be used for automated image analysis such as lesion detection. To digitally eliminate such honeycomb patterns and hence improve the related image quality, a real-time approach is necessary, both to support the visual examination of internal hollow organs as well as for automated assessment of the acquired fiberscopic image data. To this end, Winter et al. [6, 7] have investigated the compensation of the fiber-structures and came up with different filter approaches for digital removal of the honeycomb structures. Research by Smith et al. [8] identified specific distortion patterns and proposed corrective algorithms enhancing image clarity in real-time applications. Liu et al. [9] propose a two-step iterative shrinkage thresholding algorithm to remove honeycomb patterns in fiber-bundle endo-microscopy, hence improving image restoration and visualization. Recently, deep neural networks have also been suggested for fiberscopic bundle reconstruction [10]. Due to the insufficient learning data available for cancer detection in the urinary bladder [11], it would be beneficial to expand the pool of training data by adding fiberscopic images. However, these images are of reduced image quality and cannot be used directly without prior enhancement. Thus, the goal of this contribution is twofold, namely (1) to eliminate honeycomb patterns from fiberscopic images in real-time and hence improve the image quality, and (2) to use such improved image data for retraining of a deep-learning task to detect tumorous lesions in the urinary bladder.

2 Materials and methods

From the Urology department of the Sozialstiftung Bamberg, we received 15,158 cystoscopic images of the urinary bladder obtained with a fiber cystoscope. In total, images were captured from 2,289 patients and 3,151 investigations. The spatial resolution of the images is $w \times h = 768 \times 576$ pixels. Fig. 1 shows three cystoscopic images with a strong visible honeycomb fiber structure to less visible or no visible (left to right).

2.1 Removal of the honeycomb structures

The filtering approach addresses the removal of the degrading honeycomb structures from the fiberscopic images, which can be regarded as high-frequency components in the image data. High-frequency elements can typically be associated with rapid changes in intensity, which are often sharp edges, which are due to the core-cladding structures in the fiber-bundles and appear as the honeycomb pattern. As no known reference is available of how the hexagonal fiber bundle structure is oriented w.r.t. to the cartesian image sensor [7], a non-parametric filtering approach must be applied [6].

For the removal the RGB images are converted to the frequency domain using the discrete Fourier transform (DFT). In the next step, the magnitude image I_{mag} of the

DFT image is filtered with the difference of Gaussians (DoG) filter, where the difference between the two Gaussian-blurred images are obtained with kernels G_1 (σ_{x_1} = w/50 and σ_{y_1} = h/50) and G_2 (σ_{x_2} = w/5 and σ_{y_2} = h/5) with h and w denoting width and height of the image. The resulting image $I_{\text{filtered}}(x, y)$ is binarized using Otsu's approach and inverted to filter out the higher frequencies. To eliminate the last higher frequencies we set the corresponding pixels in the binary mask to zero using four circle patterns with a diameter of h/2. The centers of the circle are located at $(\pm f_{\text{highest}_x}/2, \pm f_{\text{highest}_y}/2)$. The filtered image is converted back to the spatial domain using the inverse DFT.

For evaluation the honeycomb removal, we employ the BRISQUE ('Blind / Referenceless Image Spatial Quality Evaluator)' approach. This is a robust tool for quantifying image quality without the need for a reference image, making it particularly valuable in various fields. BRISQUE is widely used in digital photography, online video streaming, as well as medical imaging. The approach operates by predicting human perception of image quality based on natural scene statistics, allowing it to provide insights into how images are likely to be perceived by human viewers. One advantages of BRISQUE is its efficiency, enabling its application in real-time scenarios where immediate feedback on image quality is necessary.

2.2 Deep neural networks for lesions detection in the urinary bladder

The fiberscopic image data is used to fine-tune a deep neural network for lesion detection in the urinary bladder, specifically a *real-time detection transformer* (RT-DETR) [3, 12] with a depth of 18 layers. To this end we pre-trained the RT-DETR network with the COCO dataset and retrained it with 35,699 colonoscopic white light images. To refine the network for cystoscopic data we use 12,066 cystoscopic images from 19 videos including 112 unique lesions [11]. The initial state T_{before} of the RT-DETR18 is evaluated on two test datasets D_1 and D_2. D_1 consists of 453 images *with* lesions and 277 *without* any occurrences, both coming from a pool of 110 patients, and were obtained with rigid and flexible cystoscopes. D_2 includes 67 with lesions and 32 images with negative findings, and was obtained with rigid cystoscopes . D_1 was collected by the Ulm Urology department and D_2 was collected by Fraunhofer IIS. All datasets were labeled manually by two experienced annotators using bounding box delineations and were then validated by urologists to ensure accuracy. To assess improvements using

Fig. 1. Example images with strong (left and center) to less honeycomb fiber structure (right).

fiberscopic data, we fine-tune the network T_{before} with the top 3,000 fiberscopic images, selected by BRISQUE score, including 1,553 images showing lesions. These images are used solely for training, not evaluation. We train a network with the original data *without* honeycomb removal $T_{\text{honeycomb}}$ and a second network T_{smooth} *with* removed honeycomb structure. To evaluate these networks we calculate the Precision, Recall, and F1-score at an IoU (Intersection over union) of 30%.

3 Results

This section presents the key findings of the study, highlighting the outcomes and insights gained from the analysis of the fiberscopic image data.

3.1 Honeycomb removal

In 10,496 of the 15,158 fiberscopic images, the BRISQUE score (0 = best quality, 100 = worst quality) decreased after using the DFT-based image enhancement, indicating improved image quality. The mean score dropped from $\mu = 31.19$ to $\mu = 18.32$, with an average decrease of $\mu = -12.87$ ($\sigma = 12.14$). In the remaining 4,662 images, the quality either decreased or remained the same, with BRISQUE scores rising from 12.98 to 18.01, resulting in an average increase of $\mu = 5.03$ ($\sigma = 4.11$). Fig. 2 shows exemplary image tuples *before* (left) and *after* (right) filtering with the DFT fiber compensation filter. For the first three images the image quality has increased, with less fibers visible. At the bottom right image the image quality decreased, with the resulting image being less sharp. The DFT-based fiber removal filter runs on an i7 processor with a Nvidia 2070 Super at 35 frames per second.

3.2 Lesion detection in the urinary bladder

Tab. 1 shows the performance metrics of the evaluated neural networks T_{before}, $T_{\text{honeycomb}}$, and T_{smooth}. Example predictions of the neural networks can be seen in Fig. 3.

Fig. 2. Pairs of images before (left) and after filtering (right) with the proposed honeycomb-compensation approach.

Network	Precision	Recall	F1-Score
T_{before}	0.718	0.5502	0.6230
$T_{\text{honeycomb}}$	0.770	**0.838**	0.802
T_{smooth}	**0.880**	0.786	**0.830**

Tab. 1. Results of RT-DETR18 evaluated on dataset D_1 and D_2.

4 Discussion

The proposed honeycomb removal filter effectively eliminates artifacts in fiberscopic images with visible fiber structures (Fig. 2). However, the filter can sometimes degrade image quality in already good images, causing blurriness and halos (Fig. 2 bottom right). Therefore it is essential to measure image quality before and after the proposed filtering, as there exists no clear threshold for acceptable quality. The filtering strength can be adjusted by changing the radius r of the circles in the mask after the thresholding filter. Increasing the radius removes more frequencies, smoothing the image but risking detail loss and blurriness or halos. We incrementally increased the radius r starting at $r = 0$ and stopping when quality decreased, and found the optimal performance at $r = \text{image width}/20$. For non-real-time applications, testing various radius values to find the best one for each image is advisable. Previous experiments indicate that changing the kernel sizes of the DoG filter has a negligible effect.

As shown in Tab. 1, the detection network's performance significantly improved when using the set of 3,000 fiberscopic images for the training. This increase can be explained by the composition of the training data. While the initial cystoscopic training dataset only contained white light images from rigid endoscopy, the fiberscopic images included also a large number of PDD (photo dynamic detection) images. As the test

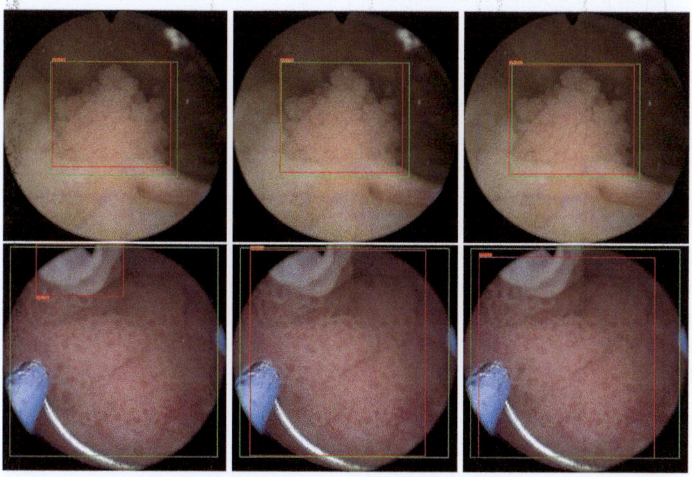

Fig. 3. Results of lesion detection: Left column depicts results from network T_{before}, center from network $T_{\text{honeycomb}}$, and right from network T_{smooth}. Images in the top row are fiberscopic images, images in the bottom row are from rigid cystoscopes. Green boxes indicate ground truth, while red boxes represent network predictions.

dataset D_2 also included such PDD images, the refined network enhances the detection rate through the learning process with fiberscopic PDD images. Furthermore, network T_{smooth}, using honeycomb removed images, outperformed network the $T_{honeycomb}$. Therefore, improving the image quality positively impacts the training of transformer-based networks.

Further work will evaluate our approach on a wider range of endoscopy images and investigate the usage for expanding the learning data pool for deep-learning based detection approaches.

Acknowledgement. This work has partially been supported by the Richard & Annemarie Wolf-Stiftung.

References

1. Mittal A, Moorthy AK, Bovik AC. No-reference image quality assessment in the spatial domain. IEEE Trans Image Proc. 2012;21(12):4695–708.
2. Kobayashi H, Kikuchi E, Mikami S et al. Long term follow-up in patients with initially diagnosed low grade Ta non-muscle invasive bladder tumors: tumor recurrence and worsening progression. BMC Urol. 2014;14(1).
3. Eixelberger T, Maisch P, Belle S et al. Comparison of YOLO and transformer based tumor detection in cystoscopy. Curr Dir Biomed Eng. 2024;10(4):228–31.
4. Rodriguez SA, Banerjee S, Desilets D et al. Ultrathin endoscopes. Gastrointest Endosc. 2010;71(6):893–8.
5. Prout BJ, Metreweli C. Pulmonary aspiration after fibre-endoscopy of the upper gastrointestinal tract. Bri Med J. 1972;4(5835):269–71.
6. Winter C, Rupp S, Elter M et al. Automatic adaptive enhancement for images obtained with fiberscopic endoscopes. IEEE Trans Biomed Eng. 2006;53(10):2035–46.
7. Winter C, Zerfaß T, Elter M et al. Physically motivated enhancement of color images for fiber endoscopy. Proc MICCAI. 2007:360–7.
8. Smith W, Vakil N, Maislin S. Correction of distortion in endoscope images. IEEE Trans Med Imaging. 1992;11(1):117–22.
9. Liu J, Zhou W, Xu B et al. Honeycomb pattern removal for fiber bundle endomicroscopy based on a two-step iterative shrinkage thresholding algorithm. AIP Adv. 2020;10(4).
10. Eadie M, Liao J, Ageeli W et al. Fiber bundle image reconstruction using convolutional neural networks and bundle rotation in endomicroscopy. Sensors. 2023;23(5):2469.
11. Eixelberger T, Maisch P, Kruck S et al. Deep learning by domain transfer for early tumor detection in the urinary bladder. Curr Dir Biomed Eng. 2023;9(1):53–6.
12. Zhao Y, Lv W, Xu S et al. DETRs beat YOLOs on real-time object detection. arXiv: 2304.08069. 2023.

Abstract: Universal and Flexible Framework for Unsupervised Statistical Shape Model Learning

Nafie El Amrani, Dongliang Cao, Florian Bernard

University of Bonn, Bonn, Germany
n.elamrani@uni-bonn.de

Statistical shape models (SSM) are an essential tool in medical image analysis and computational anatomy, facilitating a deeper understanding of anatomical variability across populations. Despite the evident utility of SSMs, their creation often comes with the drawback of depending on some form of human supervision, e.g. in the form of correspondence annotations. Although unsupervised learning-based 3D shape matching methods have made a major leap forward in recent years, the correspondence quality of existing methods does not meet the demanding requirements necessary for the construction of SSMs of complex anatomical structures. We address this shortcoming by proposing a novel deformation coherency loss to effectively enforce smooth and high-quality correspondences during neural network training, which we then fuse into a recent state-of-the-art shape matching method. Doing so allows us to unsupervisedly train a deep neural network that is able to predict high-quality correspondences that are suitable for SSM construction. We demonstrate that our framework outperforms existing methods in creating high-quality SSMs by conducting extensive experiments on five challenging medical datasets with varying anatomical complexities, including structures like the liver, pancreas, lung, spleen, and hippocampus. Our proposed method sets the new state of the art in unsupervised SSM learning, offering a universal solution that is both flexible and reliable. Our source code is publicly available at GitHub[1] [1].

References

1. Cao D, Eisenberger M, El Amrani N et al. Spectral meets spatial: harmonising 3D shape matching and interpolation. Proc IEEE CVF CVPR. 2024:3658–68.

[1] https://github.com/NafieAmrani/FUSS

C. Palm et al. (Hrsg.), *Bildverarbeitung für die Medizin 2025*, Informatik aktuell,
https://doi.org/10.1007/978-3-658-47422-5_9

Robust Statistical Shape Modelling with Implicit Neural Representations

Christoph Großbröhmer[1], Fenja Falta[1], Ron Keuth[1], Timo Kepp[2], Mattias P. Heinrich[1]

[1]Institute of Medical Informatics, University of Luebeck, Lübeck, Germany
[2]German Research Center for Artificial Intelligence, Lübeck, Germany
c.grossbroehmer@uni-luebeck.de

Abstract. We present a frameworkfor multi-label statistical shape modelling using implicit neural representations (INRs). By training a generalised INR alongside instance-specific latent codes to model individual shapes as continuous signed distance maps, the approach captures complex anatomical variations without relying on fixed landmarks. We further propose to employ the shape model for regularisation to obtain robust reconstructions of corrupted or incomplete data. Experiments on 2D chest X-ray segmentations demonstrate that this regularisation facilitates reconstructions under flawed data conditions, achieving high-fidelity segmentations. Conceptual examples highlight topological advantages of INR-based shape models over conventional point distribution models.

1 Introduction

Statistical shape models (SSM) [1] are an established method for the probabilistic description of anatomical structures. In addition to their use for direct quantitative population analysis, they also provide a comprehensible basis for the inclusion of statistical information as priors for various tasks in the field of medical informatics, such as semantic segmentation or shape completion. SSMs are typically modelled with point distribution models (PDM) [1] based on corresponding landmarks across a dataset. While the sparseness of points has advantages with regard to representation compactness, it is limited in terms of capturing topographical changes. Furthermore, the determination of corresponding landmarks is not trivial and is the subject of ongoing research using both classical and deep learning methods [2]. After PDM construction, principal component analysis (PCA) is often used to determine the direction and strength of variation modes.

The use of Implicit Neural Representations (INRs), which represent data as continuous functions that can be queried at arbitrary points, has gained popularity in recent years. While INRs were usually limited to individual instances, there are several approaches to generalise them across a population, e.g., by modulating instance-specific layers [3]. During training, a hypernetwork modulating these layers and patient-specific latent codes are jointly optimised alongside population-shared INR weights. Discrete shapes can be learned in an auto-decoder approach represented by spatially smooth signed distance functions (SDF) [4]. Applications include the reconstruction of vertebrae shapes from sparse inputs [5] and the construction of conditioned fetal brain atlas [6]. The latter could also show a correlation of patient-specific attributes with principal components of the optimised latent code. Raju et al. use a combination of

C. Palm et al. (Hrsg.), *Bildverarbeitung für die Medizin 2025*, Informatik aktuell,
https://doi.org/10.1007/978-3-658-47422-5_10

CNNs and an implicit SDF shape decoder trained on meshes to generate anatomically plausible segmentations [7]. Similar to our work, a statistical shape model of the target structure is defined by the optimised latent space and can be accessed with the means of PCA. However, current research in the field of implicit SSMs has been limited to single structures and under the assumption of complete and uncorrupted input data at test time.

Our main contributions are threefold: First, we investigate the conceptual advantages of non-linear INR-SSMs and, second, we construct multi-label implicit statistical shape models without any direct correspondence using segmentation maps. Finally, we introduce a novel probabilistic regularisation technique to address corrupted input data. Code and interactive examples are available at GitHub[1].

2 Materials and methods

Our method consists of three components: Constructing the shape model, fitting an unseen sample and shape regularisation employing a low-rank PCA (Fig. 1).

An SSM can be constructed by employing a principal component analysis (PCA) on a set of shape parametrisations with n parameters to obtain eigenvalues $\lambda_1, \ldots, \lambda_n \in \mathbb{R}$ and eigenvectors $\boldsymbol{v}_1, \ldots, \boldsymbol{v}_n \in \mathbb{R}^n$. Shapes can then be modelled based on the mean shape $\overline{\boldsymbol{s}}$ and a linear combination of $k \leq n$ eigenvectors $\boldsymbol{v}_1, \ldots, \boldsymbol{v}_k$ with the largest corresponding eigenvalues $\lambda_1, \ldots, \lambda_k$

$$\overline{\boldsymbol{s}} + \sum_{j=1}^{k} b_j \boldsymbol{v}_j \tag{1}$$

For a typical PDM approach, the shapes are parametrised by defining corresponding points across the shape's surface. Instead, we propose to learn the parametrisation through a generalised INR, which aims to reconstruct a multi-label segmentation $\boldsymbol{s}_i$

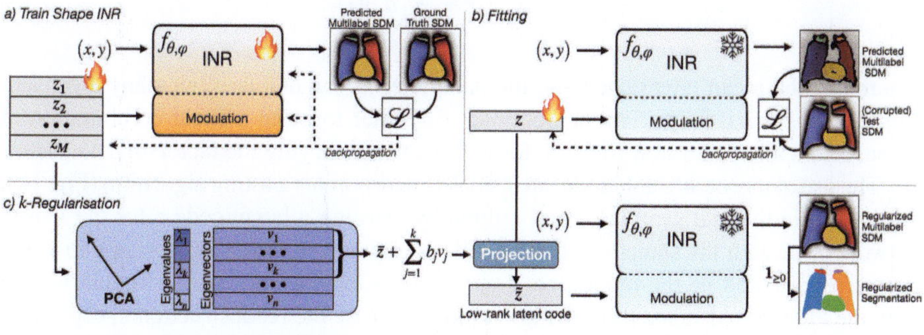

Fig. 1. Proposed self-regularising INR-SSM: a) A modulation-based generalised INR and patient-specific latent codes are jointly optimised. b) New samples are fitted using the frozen INR by optimising a new latent vector z. c) A PCA is performed on the trained latent codes to obtain a low-rank approximation $\tilde{z}$ of z, that is fed into the frozen INR to obtain a robust reconstruction.

[1] https://github.com/multimodallearning/INR-SSM

based on a n-dimensional latent code $z_i \in \mathbb{R}^n$. Since segmentations are binary and INRs represent continuous function, we do not directly predict the segmentations as output from the network, but the signed distance maps (SDMs) of these segmentations. The segmentations can be easily obtained from the SDMs with the Heaviside step function $\mathbf{1}_{\geq 0}$.

For the generalisable INR, we combine a multi-layer perceptron (MLP) g_θ, that maps coordinates $(x, y) \in \mathbb{R}^2$ to the corresponding SDM values, and a modulation hypernetwork h_φ, that adapts the parameters θ based on instance-specific latent codes $z_1, z_2, \cdots \in \mathbb{R}^n$, into a single network $f_{\theta,\varphi}$, such that $f_{\theta,\varphi}(x, y, z_i) = g_{h_\varphi(\theta,z_i)}(x, y)$. The shared parameters θ, φ are optimised alongside the latent codes, such that the network reconstructs the SDM of the associated segmentation s_i for each latent code z_i. For a reconstruction loss $\mathcal{L}$ the optimisation target is given by

$$\sum_i \mathcal{L}(\text{SDM}(s_i), f_{\theta,\varphi}(x, y, z_i)) \rightarrow \min \tag{2}$$

Following [6], the generalisation capability of $f_{\theta,\varphi}$ is realised by feeding the latent codes z_i into the hypernetwork h_φ, predicting scale and shift parameters for the linear layers of g_θ with a single linear layer each (Fig. 1a).

The reconstruction loss $\mathcal{L}$ in Eq. 2 is chosen such that the SDM reconstruction is penalised for differences between the resulting segmentation $\mathbf{1}_{\geq 0}(f_{\theta,\varphi}(x, y, z_i))$ and ground truth segmentations s_i. To obtain these resulting segmentations from the predicted SDM in a differentiable manner, the Heaviside step function $\mathbf{1}_{\geq 0}$ is approximated with a hyperbolic function.

After training of $f_{\theta,\varphi}$, a principal component analysis can be performed on the learned latent codes $z_1, z_2, \ldots$ of the training data to obtain n eigenvectors with corresponding eigenvalues, with n being the size of the latent codes (Fig. 1c). Equivalent to Equation 1, we model possible instances by inputting a linear combination of the eigenvalues into the trained network $f_{\theta,\varphi}$

$$f_{\theta,\varphi}(x, y, \bar{z} + \sum_{j=1}^{k} b_j \boldsymbol{v}_j) \tag{3}$$

where $\bar{z}$ is the mean latent code and the parameter $k \leq n$ defines how many eigenvectors are considered for variation. Applying $f_{\theta,\varphi}$ after forming a linear combination of eigenvectors allows for non-linear deformations when varying the factors b_j.

The use of a generalisable INR intrinsically incorporates a fitting algorithm (Fig. 1b): An unseen individual sample s can be fitted by learning a latent code z for the frozen network $f_{\theta,\varphi}$ with the same loss function. This way we gain the closest shape to s that can be represented by the model, i.e. $\mathbf{1}_{\geq 0}(f_{\theta,\varphi}(x, y, z))$. We propose k-Regularisation with the PCA-based shape model (Fig. 1c) to regularise the reconstruction z, especially for incomplete or corrupted inputs. For this, the residual $z - \bar{z}$ is projected onto the span of $k < n$ eigenvectors, resulting in a low-rank approximation $\tilde{z}$ of the latent code z. For $k = 0$, the approximation $\tilde{z}$ equals the mean latent code $\bar{z}$, and for $k = n$ we retain the original latent code $\tilde{z} = z$. We then gain a regularised fitted shape as $\mathbf{1}_{\geq 0}(f_{\theta,\varphi}(x, y, \tilde{z}))$.

We evaluate our method on the JSRT dataset, which comprises 247 X-ray scans with a total of 188 landmarks of the heart, lungs and claviculae [8, 9]. We preprocess the data by creating multilabel segmentation maps from landmarks in a frame of 256×256 pixels and select 160 and 87 samples for shape model training and evaluation respectively. To assess the robustness of reconstructions, we corrupt the data by removing segmentations in a randomly drawn 80×80 square (*Corrupted*) or for the entire right lung (*Incomplete*), as shown in the left column of Fig. 4. For the generalised INR, we use a 5-layer MLP with sinusoidal activation functions [10] and a hidden dimension of 128. To account for all 5 classes of the dataset, the first and last layers are modelled to process label-specific SDMs as individual channels. We employ a latent code of size $n = 14$ and chose to modulate the second, third, and fourth layer by employing MLPs accounting for scale and shift parameters, similar to [6], resulting in around 100k trainable parameters. Latent codes are initialised with $z \sim \mathcal{N}(0, 10^{-3})$. We use Adam to optimise both latent codes (with a warm-up period for 500 epochs) and $f_{\theta,\varphi}$ for a total of 2000 epochs with a learning rate of 10^{-3} for training and fitting new samples. The model achieves mean training Dice scores and 95th percentile of Hausdorff Distances (HD) of 97% and 0.80mm respectively.

3 Results

First, we demonstrate the advantages of our nonlinear and segmentation-based shape model compared to a linear PDM-based SSM by training the shape model on two different arbitrarily created datasets (Fig. 2): 1. Partial ring structures, that are a simple, but nonlinear deformation of each other, and 2. discs and rings that are topologically different and cannot be represented by the same set of keypoints. Compared to a PDM-based SSM as described in Sec. 2, the statistical latent code can already capture the main transformation by scaling only the first eigenvector in both scenarios.

We further evaluate the performance of the Statistical Shape Model and regularisation in three scenarios: Fitting (1) original, (2) corrupted and (3) incomplete out-of-training samples. For (2) and (3), we investigate both corruption-agnostic and -aware fitting. For the latter, we assume knowledge over the corrupted area and optimise the latent code with a loss computed for non-corrupted image parts, thus only using uncorrupted and available information.

On the JSRT dataset (Tab. 1, Fig. 3), our approach is able to reconstruct test segmentations to a mean Dice of 87.8% and HD of 3.6 mm, which is close to a correspondence-bound PDM-SSM model with $n = 14$ eigenvectors (Dice: 91.2%, HD: 2.70 mm).

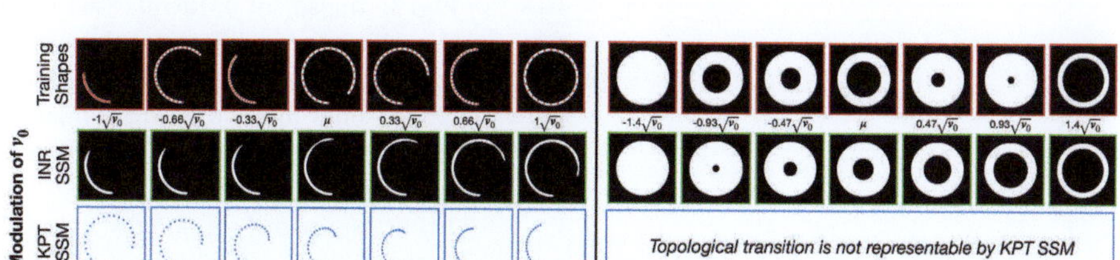

Fig. 2. Topological advantages of INR-SSMs shown for examples of partial ring structures (left) and disc-to-ring transition (right). Rows show excerpts of training data (red), and reconstructions based on scaled first eigenvector $\boldsymbol{v}_0$ for INR-SSM (green) and PDM-SSM (blue).

Tab. 1. Dice scores (DSC) and 95th percentile of Hausdorff-Distances (HD) in mm regarding all investigated scenarios. Results include reconstruction with the mean learned latent code ($k = 0$), un-regularised fitting ($k = n = 14$) and best-performing k-Regularisation per task.

	Original		Corrupted			Incomplete			
Corruption-aware	-	-	✓	×	×	✓	✓	×	×
k	0 ($\tilde{z} = \bar{z}$)	14 ($\tilde{z} = z$)	14	6	14	6	14	2	14
DSC ↑	65.6 ±12.0	87.8 ±5.6	86.5 ±6.7	77.5 ±7.5	70.6 ±8.3	84.4 ±5.7	88.1 ±5.6	67.4 ±10.5	58.7 ±6.1
HD ↓	9.5 ±3.1	3.6 ±1.6	4.1 ±1.9	7.5 ±2.4	∞	4.7 ±1.6	4.0 ±1.7	8.9 ±2.7	13.7 ±3.0

Shapes can be reasonably well recovered with corruption (86.8%) and incomplete inputs (82.7%) if the fitting loss is altered accordingly. The complex task of corruption-agnostic optimisation highly benefits from the proposed probabilistic k-Regularisation. The highest reconstruction metrics can be achieved by limiting the reconstruction to the first 6 and 2 eigenvectors respectively. When only evaluating the reconstruction of the missing lung, maximum accuracy is already achieved with only $k = 6$ eigenvectors (Fig. 3). These effects are also visible in the qualitative examples shown in Fig. 4, where the regularisation preserves the tapered shape of the lower lung region.

4 Discussion

Our method is able to fit new samples to the learned multi-label shape model without the need for corresponding keypoints, but reconstruction quality is highly sensitive to corrupted or missing information. We demonstrated that this can be mitigated with PCA-based k-Regularisation. While it has little effect on corruption-aware fitting, it provides an effective method of regularisation when this information is missing. The similarity in reconstruction accuracy between INR and PDM-SSM is particularly noteworthy, considering that the segmentations were directly obtained from the keypoints. Further improvements might be achieved by advanced INR generalisation techniques. Our conceptual experiments demonstrate the advantages of INR-based SSMs; however,

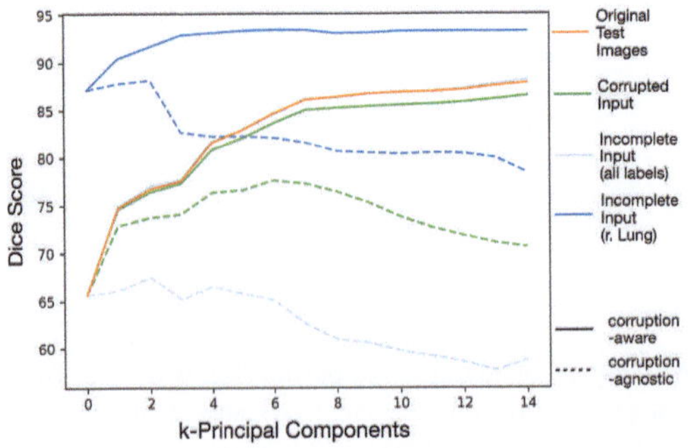

Fig. 3. Impact of k-Regularisation as Dice Scores for different values of k in all investigated scenarios. Solid and dashed lines indicate corruption-aware and corruption-agnostic fitting respectively. The results for $k = 0$ and $k = n = 14$ correspond to $\tilde{z} = \bar{z}$ and $\tilde{z} = z$ respectively.

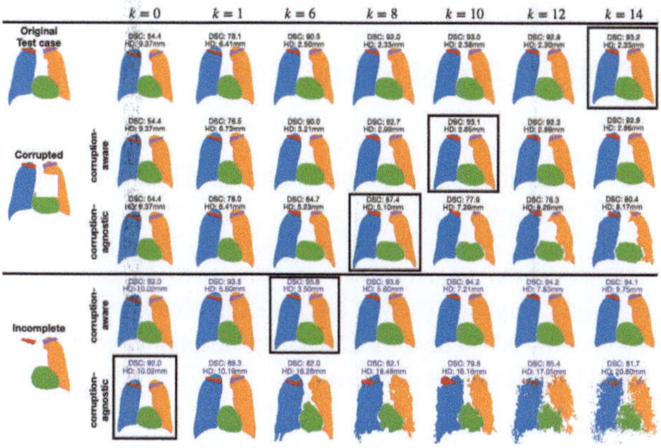

Fig. 4. Qualitative reconstruction results with mean (black) and right lung (blue) Dice scores (DSC) and 95th percentile of Hausdorff distances (HD) in mm for selected cases. Reconstructions with the highest Dice values are highlighted with black boxes.

future work should include broader application-based comparisons and datasets where their topological properties offer clear benefits.

Acknowledgement. This work has been partially funded by the Federal Ministry of Education and Research (BMBF, 13GW0578C).

References

1. Cootes TF, Taylor CJ, Cooper DH et al. Active shape models: their training and application. Comput Vis Image Underst. 1995;61(1):38–59.
2. Adams J, Elhabian S. Point2SSM: learning morphological variations of anatomies from point clouds. Proc ICLR. 2023.
3. Kim C, Lee D, Kim S et al. Generalizable implicit neural representations via instance pattern composers. Proc IEEE CVF CVPR. 2023:11808–17.
4. Park JJ, Florence P, Straub J et al. DeepSDF: learning continuous signed distance functions for shape representation. Proc IEEE CVF CVPR. 2019:165–74.
5. Amiranashvili T, Lüdke D, Li HB et al. Learning shape reconstruction from sparse measurements with neural implicit functions. Proc MIDL. 2022:22–34.
6. Dannecker M, Kyriakopoulou V, Cordero-Grande L et al. CINA: conditional implicit neural atlas for spatio-temporal representation of fetal brains. Proc MICCAI. 2024:181–91.
7. Raju A, Miao S, Jin D et al. Deep implicit statistical shape models for 3D medical image delineation. Proc AAAI. 2022;36(2):2135–43.
8. Shiraishi J, Katsuragawa S, Ikezoe J et al. Development of a digital image database for chest radiographs with and without a lung nodule. Am J Roentgenol. 2000;174(1):71–4.
9. Gaggion N, Mansilla L, Milone DH et al. Hybrid graph convolutional neural networks for landmark-based anatomical segmentation. Proc MICCAI. 2021:600–10.
10. Sitzmann V, Martel J, Bergman A et al. Implicit neural representations with periodic activation functions. Proc NeurIPS. 2020;33:7462–73.

iRBSM

A Deep Implicit 3D Breast Shape Model

Maximilian Weiherer[1,2], Antonia von Riedheim[3], Vanessa Brébant[3], Bernhard Egger[1], Christoph Palm[2]

[1]Visual Computing Erlangen, Friedrich-Alexander-Universtität Erlangen-Nürnberg
[2]Regensburg Medical Image Computing (ReMIC), OTH Regensburg
[3]Department for Plastic, Hand and Reconstructive Surgery, University Hospital Regensburg
maximilian.weiherer@fau.de

Abstract. We present the first deep implicit 3D shape model of the female breast, building upon and improving the recently proposed Regensburg Breast Shape Model (RBSM). Compared to its PCA-based predecessor, our model employs implicit neural representations; hence, it can be trained on raw 3D breast scans and eliminates the need for computationally demanding non-rigid registration, a task that is particularly difficult for feature-less breast shapes. The resulting model, dubbed iRBSM, captures detailed surface geometry including fine structures such as nipples and belly buttons, is highly expressive, and outperforms the RBSM on different surface reconstruction tasks. Finally, leveraging the iRBSM, we present a prototype application to 3D reconstruct breast shapes from just a single image. Model and code publicly available at https://rbsm.re-mic.de/implicit.

1 Introduction

Albeit emerging use cases, 3D generative shape models for the female breast, such as the one proposed in this work (Fig. 1), rarely exist. Most probably, this is due to the sensitivity of the data, making it challenging to acquire even small-sized datasets. Potential applications of 3D breast shape models include breast surgery planning and simulation, breast volume estimation from 3D scans, and post-operative outcome assessment and monitoring. Besides clinical applications, such models may also be of great interest to

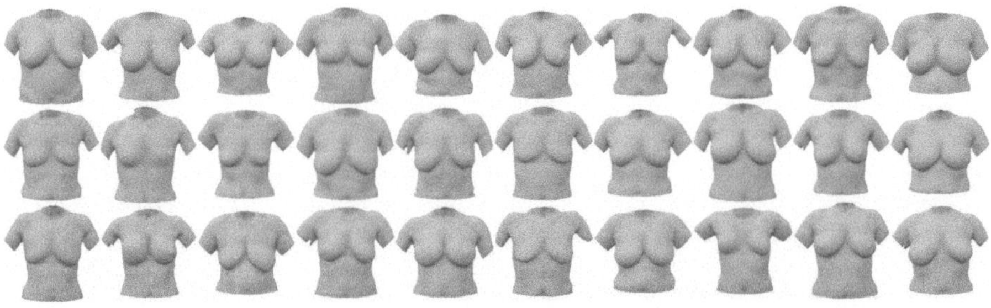

Fig. 1. Random samples from the proposed iRBSM. Our model is able to generate a large variety of plausible breast shapes, including fine details such as the nipples or belly buttons.

C. Palm et al. (Hrsg.), *Bildverarbeitung für die Medizin 2025*, Informatik aktuell,
https://doi.org/10.1007/978-3-658-47422-5_11

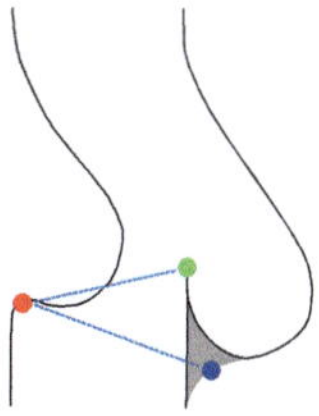

Fig. 2. The RBSM suffers from erroneous correspondences as a result of occlusions. As shown, for large and sagged breasts, occluded underbusts (grey region) yield incorrect correspondences when using template-based surface registration. Specifically, while the red and the green points are supposed to correspond semantically, due to the occlusion of the underbust in *surface-only* 3D breast scans, the red and the blue points will incorrectly match instead. This leads to distortions on the shape boundaries in the resulting shape model.

the fashion industry, enabling virtual try-on or custom bra design. To date, only a single publicly available shape model of the female breasts exists: the Regensburg Breast Shape Model (RBSM) [1]. The RBSM is a Principal Component Analysis (PCA)-based shape model and has been built from over a hundred 3D breast scans acquired in a standing position. While it represents an important step toward an expressive and large-scale breast model, it is not without limitations. First, it assumes semantically accurate point-to-point correspondence among registered 3D breast scans – an assumption that, in fact, can not be properly satisfied on *feature-less* breast shapes using standard surface registration techniques as used in [1]. The problem is amplified by severe occlusions in 3D breast scans (Fig. 2). Secondly, the RBSM lacks detail, often failing to capture fine structures such as nipples. This is a known problem in PCA-based models and results from the linearity of dimensional reduction. Finally, the proposed pipeline and mesh-based nature of the model itself lacks practicability, *always* requiring computationally expensive and error-prone non-rigid surface registration, including manual landmarking.

To address the aforementioned shortcomings, we introduce an *implicit* variant of the RBSM, dubbed iRBSM, which employs implicit neural representations. As opposed to the mesh-based representation of the RBSM, we model surfaces as the zero-level set of a signed distance function (SDF) which is parametrized by a latent-conditioned neural network. This representation has several key benefits over linear, PCA-based shape models. First, no fixed topology is required, enabling implicit models to naturally handle occlusions caused by sagged breasts without producing unwanted effects such as correspondence errors. Notably, this also renders surface registration (at all stages: during model building and at inference) unnecessary. Secondly, SDF-based generative models allow for a higher level of detail due to their non-linear nature. The result is an expressive model that can generate highly realistic and diverse breast shapes (Fig. 1).

In 2007, Seo et al. [2] were the first to build a classical, PCA-based 3D shape model from 28 breast scans to analyze breast volume and surface measurements. They assumed symmetric breasts. Recently, Mezier et al. [3] proposed a *rigged* breast model built from 55 artist-created blendshapes. Due to the synthetic nature of the data, their model generates rather unnatural-looking breast shapes.

2 Materials and methods

We will now describe the iRBSM in detail, starting with the training data that has been used to build our model, followed by the model formulation and implementation details.

2.1 3D breast scan database

Our model is trained on the same dataset already used for the RBSM but extended by 58 scans, totaling 168 consistently oriented scans. All scans have been taken in a standing position using the portable Vectra H2 system (Canfield Scientific, New Jersey, USA) which employs photogrammetry to reconstruct 3D surfaces from three photographs taken from frontal and lateral views. Data has been collected between 2020 and 2023 at the St. Josef Hospital Regensburg [1].

Our raw 3D breast scans are not closed, watertight surfaces – a necessary condition to be representable as SDF. To close the raw input scans, we use the following two-stage workflow. First, we offset the surface mesh in negative z-direction (*i.e.*, we copy the original mesh and translate it in negative z-direction) and connect corresponding border vertices. Next, we cut the mesh along (i) the frontal plane passing through the lateral breast pole [4] and (ii), the transversal plane passing through a point approximately 2 cm below the belly button. After each step, we again connect border vertices, eventually leading to a closed and watertight surface mesh.

2.2 Model formulation

We represent the iRBSM as a function $\phi : \mathbb{R}^3 \times \mathbb{R}^L \to \mathbb{R}$, mapping a 3-dimensional coordinate x and an L-dimensional latent code z to a signed distance, $\phi(x, z) = \Phi_\theta([x, z])$, where $\Phi_\theta : \mathbb{R}^{3+L} \to \mathbb{R}$ is a *latent-conditioned* SDF parametrized by a neural network with weights θ. Once ϕ is trained, the surface $\mathcal{S}_z \subset \mathbb{R}^3$ of a shape corresponding to the latent code z is given as the zero-level set of ϕ, that is, $\mathcal{S}_z = \{x \in \mathbb{R}^3 \mid \phi(x, z) = 0\}$. The surface $\mathcal{S}_z$ can be readily extracted as triangular mesh using marching cubes algorithm.

The auto-decoder framework [5] is used for training, in which we simultaneously optimize the network's parameters θ and latent codes z. Given a dataset of 3D breast scans each of which represented as an oriented point cloud, $X = \{x_1, x_2, \ldots, x_n\} \subset \mathbb{R}^3$ and associated per-point normals $N = \{n_1, n_2, \ldots, n_n\} \subset \mathbb{R}^3$, we employ the following loss proposed in [6] with slight modification

$$\mathcal{L}(\theta, z) = \sum_{i=1}^{n} |\phi(x_i, z)| + \|\nabla_{x_i}\phi(x_i, z) - n_i\|_2 + \\ \lambda_1 \mathbb{E}_{x \sim D}\left[\big| \|\nabla_x \phi(x, z)\|_2 - 1 \big| + \exp(-\alpha|\phi(x, z)|) \right] + \lambda_2 \|z\|_2 \quad (1)$$

where $D := [-1, 1]^3 \cup \{x_1 + \epsilon_1, x_2 + \epsilon_2, \ldots, x_n + \epsilon_n\}$ with $\epsilon_i \sim \mathcal{N}(0, \sigma^2)$ is a set of free-space points. Please note that we do *not* require ground truth SDF values for supervision; the whole model is trained solely on the raw 3D breast scans.

Given a 3D breast scan as *unoriented* point cloud, $X' = \{x'_1, x'_2, \ldots, x'_m\}$, at test-time, we obtain the corresponding latent code z^* by fixing the model's parameters θ and optimizing

$$z^* = \underset{z \in \mathbb{R}^L}{\arg\min} \left\{ \sum_{i=1}^{m} |\phi(x'_i, z)| + \lambda \|z\|_2 \right\} \quad (2)$$

Here, $\lambda \geq 0$ can be used to filter out noise. We refer to [5] for further details.

Tab. 1. Quantitative results for sparse surface reconstruction. Our model consistently outperforms the RBSM by a large margin. For comparison, we also report results on dense point clouds.

	Sparse (1,000 points)			Dense (≈ 20,000 points)		
	CD ↓	F-Score ↑	NC ↑	CD ↓	F-Score ↑	NC ↑
RBSM [1]	4.35 ± 1.27	43.3 ± 16.38	96.1 ± 1.89	4.27 ± 1.24	44.9 ± 16.73	96.1 ± 1.87
iRBSM (Ours)	1.66 ± 0.29	88.4 ± 6.54	98.6 ± 0.83	1.57 ± 0.28	90.7 ± 6.06	98.8 ± 0.75

2.3 Implementation details

We represent ϕ as an 8-layer fully-connected MLP with 512-dimensional hidden layers and skip connection to the middle layer. The final SDF value is regressed by applying the softplus activation function. Moreover, we use the geometric initialization scheme proposed in [6] and a latent dimension of 256. Latent codes are initialized from a zero-mean normal distribution with variance 10^{-4}. We trained for 10,000 epochs using a batch size of 16 and the Adam optimizer with a learning rate of 5×10^{-4} for model parameters and 10^{-3} for latent codes. Both learning rates are decayed by a factor of 0.5 every 2,000 epochs. We use 5,000 on-surface points and 5,000 free-space points sampled from D for each shape. We empirically set $\lambda_1 = 0.1, \lambda_2 = 0.01$, and $\alpha = 10$. All experiments are run on a single NVIDIA RTX A5000 with 24 GB of VRAM. Training the iRBSM took about 20 hours. At inference, we optimize Eq. (2) for 5,000 iterations using Adam. Additionally, we decay the learning rate by a factor of 0.5 every 1,000 iterations. We set $\lambda = 0.01$ in the noise-free case, and use $\lambda = 0.1$ for noisy inputs.

3 Results

Our evaluation is based on a test set of ten 3D breast scans held out during training. We start by evaluating our model's ability to reconstruct accurate surfaces from sparse point clouds. To do so, we randomly sample 1,000 surface points from each of our test scans to which we then fit our model (Sect. 2.2). We compare against the RBSM [1], which we fit to point clouds using landmark-based rigid alignment followed by model-based non-rigid surface registration.

We report Chamfer distance (CD), F-Score (with a threshold of 2.5 mm), and normal consistency (NC). To ensure fair comparison, we compute metrics only within the breast region, defined by cropping meshes using axis-aligned planes passing through the upper breast poles, along axillary lines, and approximately 5 cm below the lower breast poles.

Results can be found in Tab. 1 and Fig. 3. Our model quantitatively outperforms the RBSM by a large margin (over 2.5 times better in CD) while also leading to visually more pleasant results, overall being much closer to the ground truth (GT) than surface reconstructions obtained from the RBSM. Moreover, fitting the iRBSM took approximately 20 seconds on average and did *not* require any pre-processing; in contrast, fitting the RBSM required more than 23 seconds, *excluding* manual landmarking.

Next, we evaluate the iRBSM in a more realistic setting where only incomplete and noisy scans are available. To simulate holes in scans, we again randomly sample 1,000

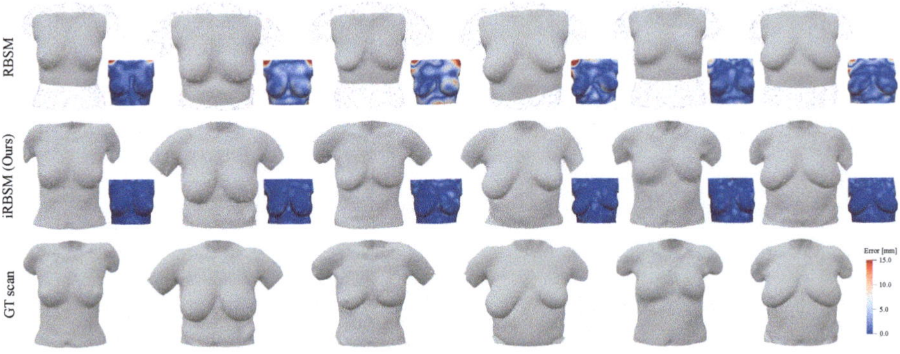

Fig. 3. Qualitative results for sparse surface reconstruction. We show surface reconstructions obtained from fitting the RBSM and our model to sparse point clouds. Our model leads to visually more pleasant reconstructions than its PCA-based counterpart.

surface points from each scan of our test set and then cut away a random patch by removing points within a sphere with a pre-defined crop radius, $r \geq 0$, centered on an arbitrary surface point. Noise is simulated by adding Gaussian noise with various standard deviations, $\sigma \geq 0$, to surface points. We compare against model-free approaches, Screened Poisson Surface Reconstruction (SPSR) [7], and a recent kernel-based reconstruction approach [8]. For SPSR, we did a modest parameter sweep, considering all possible combinations of the *octree depth* in $\{6, 7, 8, 9\}$ and *point weight* in $\{4, 100, 1000\}$. For [8], we varied the regularization weight $\lambda \in \{0, 10^{-13}, 10^{-12}, 10^{-11}, 10^{-10}\}$ and bandwidth $h \in \{0.5, 1, 2\}$.

Qualitative and quantitative results can be found in Fig. 4, demonstrating that the iRBSM is, among the methods tested, the best to handle large holes and even severe noise.

Fig. 4. Qualitative and quantitative results for incomplete (top) and noisy (bottom) inputs. In both scenarios, our model leads to visually more appealing yet plausible reconstructions. This is also reflected quantitatively (right) when compared to learning-free methods, SPSR [7] and Matérn [8]. Qualitative results are shown for $r = 100$ (top) and $\sigma = 10$ (bottom).

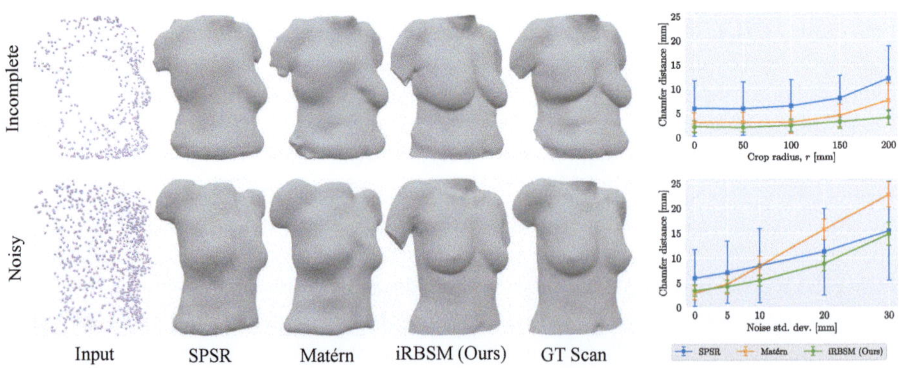

Fig. 5. Single image to 3D using the iRBSM. We employ our model to 3D reconstruct breast shapes from *single* images by first estimating depth using a state-of-the-art monocular depth estimation model [9] and then fitting the iRBSM to the unprojected depth map. This yields high-quality surface reconstructions with accurate normals in seconds and without special hardware.

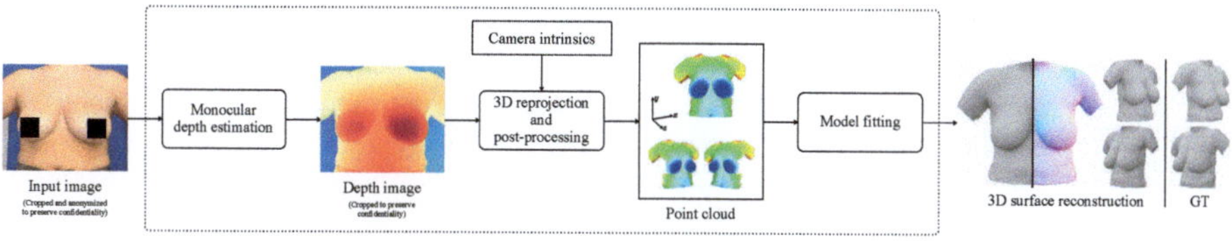

This demonstrates that the iRBSM is indeed a strong prior for 3D surface reconstruction of real-world point cloud data – a quite practical finding that we will exploit next.

We prototype an application to 3D reconstruct breast shapes from a *single* image (Fig. 5). Given an image from a calibrated camera, we employ a state-of-the-art monocular depth estimation model, Depth Anything V2 [9], reproject the depth map into 3D leveraging pre-computed camera intrinsics, and fit our model to the resulting point cloud. As shown, this workflow is capable of reconstructing high-quality surfaces.

4 Conclusion

The proposed iRBSM significantly advances expressive 3D breast models, being able to recover plausible breast shapes from sparse, incomplete, and noisy observations. The proposed application is a practical and robust method to acquire accurate 3D breast reconstructions from images without expensive hard- and software or special setups.

References

1. Weiherer M, Eigenberger A, Egger B et al. Learning the shape of female breasts: an open-access 3D statistical shape model of the female breast built from 110 breast scans. Vis Comput. 2023.
2. Seo H, Cordier F, Hong K. A breast modeler based on analysis of breast scans. Comp Anim Virtual Worlds. 2007.
3. Mazier A, Ribes S, Gilles B et al. A rigged model of the breast for preoperative surgical planning. J Biomech. 2021.
4. Hartmann R, Weiherer M, Schiltz D et al. A novel method of outcome assessment in breast reconstruction surgery: comparison of autologous and alloplastic techniques using three-dimensional surface imaging. Aesth Plast Surg. 2020.
5. Park JJ, Florence P, Straub J et al. DeepSDF: learning continuous signed distance functions for shape representation. Proc IEEE CVF CVPR. 2019.
6. Gropp A, Yariv L, Haim N et al. Implicit geometric regularization for learning shapes. ICML. 2020.
7. Kazhdan M, Hoppe H. Screened poisson surface reconstruction. ACM Trans Graph. 2013.
8. Weiherer M, Egger B. Matérn kernels for tunable implicit surface reconstruction. arXiv: 2409.15466. 2024.
9. Yang L, Kang B, Huang Z et al. Depth anything V2. Proc NeurIPS. 2024.

Diffusion Models for Conditional Brain Tumor MRI Generation with Tumor-induced Deformations

Mona Irsfeld[1,2], Heinz Handels[1,2], Hristina Uzunova[2]

[1]Institute of Medical Informatics, University of Luebeck
[2]German Research Center for Artificial Intelligence, Luebeck
mona.irsfeld@dfki.de

Abstract. Machine learning methods have achieved remarkable results in medical image processing but require large annotated training datasets, typically unavailable in the medical image domain. To overcome this issue, we propose a conditional diffusion model that generates brain MRIs with tumors directly with the corresponding ground truth annotations. An additional diffusion-based label modification approach is integrated in order to account for the tumor mass effect. Experimental results demonstrate that replacing up to 50% of real training data with generated samples does not significantly impact segmentation performance. Moreover, models trained exclusively on synthetic data still yield acceptable results, highlighting the potential of our approach to mitigate the problem of limited annotated data in medical imaging.

1 Introduction

Labeled data scarcity is a significant challenge in the field of medical image analysis. Since the acquisition, labeling and exchange of medical images are all highly time-consuming and costly tasks, alternative solutions often feature synthetic data generation.

By expanding the available training datasets and reducing the reliance on sensitive patient data for model training, this approach addresses both data scarcity and privacy concerns. However, generating realistic synthetic data is not a trivial task, especially when it comes to images containing pathologies. Specifically, in the case of brain tumors, their diffusive growth affects the surrounding healthy tissue causing complex interactions, including brain midline shift or infiltration of structures, which are generally referred to as the tumor mass effect [1].

Generating synthetic medical images has been widely explored using various models. Statistical shape and appearance models, for instance, have been effective in synthesizing images for training registration networks [2] but are limited in flexibility and generalization ability. Variational auto-encoders (VAEs) offer a more flexible deep-learning-based solution for data generation [3, 4] but tend to yield blurry images that lack the detail necessary for medical image applications. To cope with this issue, generative adversarial networks (GANs) were introduced, known for their ability to generate extremely realistic and high-quality images [5, 6]. Despite representing the state-of-art approach for a long time, GANs often face issues like mode-collapse, artifact hallucination, and low explainability and controllability of the latent space.

Despite various improvements achieved in these methods, in recent years, a new state-of-the-art generative approach emerged: denoising diffusion probabilistic models

C. Palm et al. (Hrsg.), *Bildverarbeitung für die Medizin 2025*, Informatik aktuell,
https://doi.org/10.1007/978-3-658-47422-5_12

(DDPMs) [7]. They have shown their ability to generate high-quality images with large variability on multiple instances [8, 9]. Up until now, some efficient DDPM-based approaches have demonstrated great success in generating MRI scans of healthy brains [10, 11]. Based on this success, this paper aims to utilize the expressivity, flexibility and control ability of DDPMs in order to synthesize realistic brain MRIs including tumors and the caused tumor-mass effect.

Here, we present a conditional DDPM named "Segmentation-based Image Generator with MAsking" (SIGMA), specifically designed to synthesize pathological axial slices of contrast-enhanced T1-weighted MRI brain scans. After training on images containing brain tumors, the model is able to generate images with glioblastomas and gliomas based on the anatomical conditioning of normal subjects. Furthermore, a diffusive tumor mask is integrated into the training process, allowing the network to learn the deformation of the peritumoral tissue, resembling the tumor mass effect. Compared to the Pix2PixHD GAN [12], our model yields more realistic images, quantitatively assessed by a lower FID score. Furthermore, the synthetic images can be applied in a downstream task for the training of a tumor segmentation network, showing that replacing up to half of the real training dataset does not impede the segmentation performance.

2 Materials and methods

The presented diffusion model aims to generate brain MRIs containing tumors conditioned on anatomical and pathological labels. Thus, the network is trained on tumor data with ground-truth tumor annotations and automatically generated anatomical segmentations. In the inference phase, however, the anatomical labels are extracted from healthy subject brains and the tumor labels are artificially placed, such that the trained DDPM can generate brain tumor MRIs in a fully controlled manner.

2.1 Wavelet DDPM

The proposed diffusion model is based on a DDPM variant denoted as "Wavelet Diffusion Model (WDM)" [11], which performs the diffusion process in the frequency domain of the images. Instead of directly passing the d-dimensional latents (matching the size of the training images) to the model, the inputs are first decomposed into 2^d (here: $d = 2$) frequency components using a discrete wavelet transform (DWT). In our approach, the diffusion process operates on the DWT-transformed image space, which is then passed to the U-Net backbone. This reduces computational costs in the early convolution layers by avoiding operations at full image resolution. The four resulting feature maps represent frequency components, which are then recomposed into a full-resolution image (192×192 pixels) via the inverse discrete wavelet transform (IDWT). The final reconstructed image corresponds to the predicted noise that is then removed from the noisy input image (Fig. 1).

2.2 Conditioning mechanism

SIGMA is trained to generate realistic pathological MRIs conditioned on anatomical and pathological labels. Since many pathological datasets do not include anatomical labels, those are automatically generated with Synthseg [13]. However, due to the tumor mass effect, multiple problems arise. Firstly, automatic anatomical segmentations around the tumor area are extremely imprecise due to the tissue displacement. Secondly, simply overlaying a tumor mask over healthy anatomical labels does not account for any tumor-induced deformations. Lastly, the tumor mass effect is extremely complex to explicitly model and depends on multiple parameters, mostly not known in the given datasets. Based on those considerations, we develop a mechanism to account for the tumor mass effect by considering the diffusive growth of tumors in the conditioning and learning the healthy tissue displacements. Specifically, we propose a masking approach that selectively suppresses the healthy tissue conditions near the pathology in a diffusive manner. This is achieved by applying a Euclidian distance transform to the tumor area, assigning each pixel a weight based on its relative distance to the closest tumor pixel (Fig. 2). The model incorporates these segmentation maps using Spatially Adaptive Normalization (SPADE) [14], which enables it to preserve more of the conditioning information than if the conditions were simply concatenated with the input.

2.3 Experimental setup

Fig. 1 shows the training procedure. A training image $\mathbf{x}_0$ from the BRATS dataset [15] is corrupted in the forward diffusion process by adding Gaussian noise $\epsilon \sim \mathcal{N}(0, \mathbf{I})$ controlled by a cosine noise schedule, utilizing $T = 1000$ diffusion steps and a randomly sampled timestep $t \sim U(0, T)$. The resulting noisy sample is decomposed into its wavelet coefficients, which are concatenated channel-wise and then passed to the U-Net-based backbone of the diffusion model, along with the label maps for pathological and healthy tissue. The output is reconstructed by IDWT, which produces the predicted noise to be removed from the original image. The DDPM is trained for 1000 epochs with a batch size of 32, mean squared error loss is used between the actual noise and the prediction.

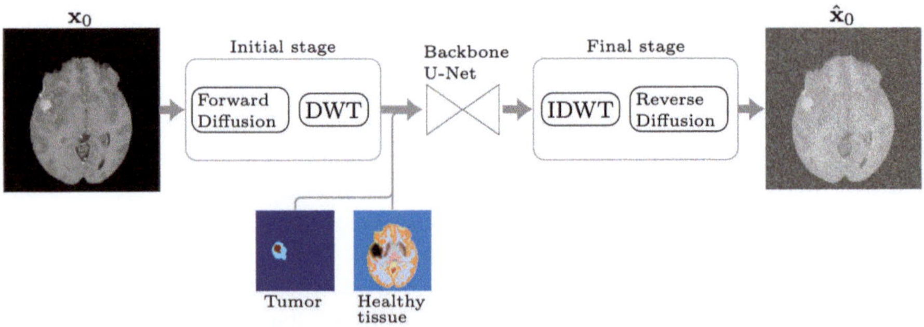

Fig. 1. Training procedure. Tumor data is corrupted with Gaussian noise and decomposed via DWT. The frequency components are fed into the U-Net backbone, which incorporates segmentation maps for both pathological and healthy structures (with diffusive masking around the tumor). The output is expanded with IDWT and reverse diffusion is applied to estimate the input noise.

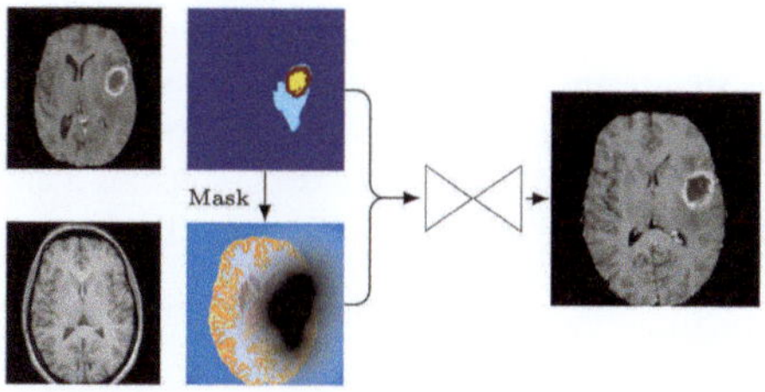

Fig. 2. Model inference. The tumor label from a pathological MR image is combined with segmentations of normal tissue from a healthy patient, with labels masked according to the tumor region. Combining these conditions results in a synthetic image that accurately reflects the locations of different tissue types.

In the inference phase, we combine the anatomical labels from healthy subjects from the IXI dataset[1], (obtained with Synthseg) with tumor labels from the BRATS dataset (Fig. 2). Random affine augmentation is additionally applied to the tumor labels, and a pre-registration ensures that the pathology remains within the brain area. The diffusive tumor mask conditioning is also applied to the anatomical labels. The trained DDPM then generates a synthetic image that accurately reflects the locations of both healthy and pathological structures as defined by the provided conditions and also accounts for the tumor mass effect surrounding the tumor.

3 Results

To assess whether the distribution of synthetic images aligns with that of real data, we compute the Fréchet Inception Distance (FID) between 20,000 MRI slices from the test section of the BRATS dataset and 4,300 of those generated by the trained DDPM.

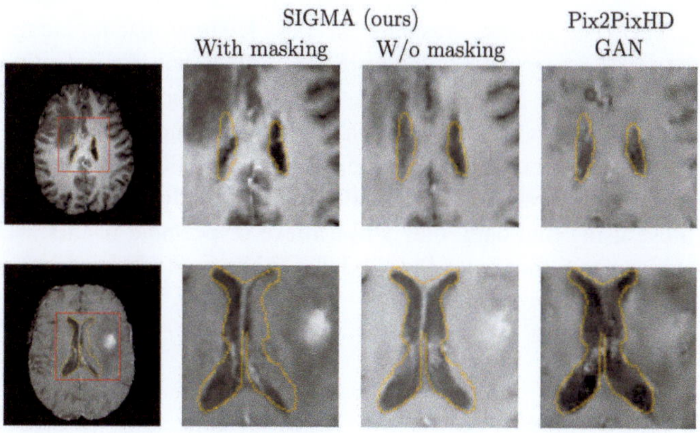

Fig. 3. Assessing tumor-induced deformations: Column 1: image generated by SIGMA with label masking; columns 2-4: images generated with label masking, without label masking, and by Pix2PixHD GAN [12], zoomed into the red-boxed region. While the ventricles' locations in the generated images remain close to their original positions (orange boundary), the masking approach introduces subtle shifts in the tumor region.

[1]https://brain-development.org/ixi-dataset/

Tab. 1. Mean dice scores (± std) for segmentation models trained on different dataset compositions. A paired Student's t-test was conducted to assess significant performance differences. The tests compare models trained (partially or completely) on data generated by SIGMA with those trained on real data (columns 2 and 4), as well as those trained on GAN-generated data (columns 3 and 5). Statistical significance is indicated by symbols: * (p<0.05), ** (p<0.01), *** (p<0.001).

	Real data	50% synthetic data		Synthetic data only	
		SIGMA	GAN [12]	SIGMA	GAN [12]
Tumor Core	0.733 (±0.28)	0.726 (±0.29)	0.713 (±0.29)*	0.712 (±0.29)***	0.662 (±0.31)***
Whole Tumor	0.749 (±0.19)	0.739 (±0.20)*	0.729 (±0.20)*	0.717 (±0.22)***	0.670 (±0.24)***
Active Tumor	0.733 (±0.25)	0.723 (±0.26)	0.713 (±0.27)	0.709 (±0.26)***	0.656 (±0.29)***
Mean Dice	0.715 (±0.22)	0.709 (±0.23)	0.697 (±0.23)**	0.688 (±0.24)***	0.633 (±0.26)***

SIGMA achieves a FID of *54.43*, considerably better than the FID of *289.95* obtained using a Pix2PixHD GAN [12] conditioned on the same labels as SIGMA.

Furthermore, the model is able to generate images that exhibit realistic tumor-induced deformations of healthy structures (Fig. 3), demonstrating the effectiveness of the masking approach. In contrast, the DDPM conditioned without label masking during training and inference as well as the Pix2PixHD GAN [12] fail to model the tumor mass effect adequately in the synthesized images.

To evaluate the potential of the generated images as training data for brain tumor segmentation, we train a U-Net to segment the tumor core, whole tumor, and active tumor regions. We compare segmentation models trained on differently composed datasets, each comprising 4,000 images: (1) real training data only, (2) 50% real and 50% synthetic samples, and (3) synthetic data only. Additionally, we conducted experiments using synthetic data generated by Pix2PixHD GAN [12] to benchmark against SIGMA's performance. The Dice scores, presented in Tab. 1, show that replacing up to 50% of training data with images generated by SIGMA does not significantly degrade the segmentation performance for most classes. The only significant decline is observed for the segmentation of the whole tumor, which includes surrounding edema. This is likely due to edematous areas being more visible in T2 or FLAIR sequences, rather than in T1-weighted images. Overall, although models trained solely on synthetic data perform worse than those using real data, they still achieve respectable results. Moreover, our approach significantly outperforms Pix2PixHD GAN across most settings.

4 Discussion

In this work, we introduced a conditional DDPM for generating transaxial MRI brain slices with tumors, guided by label maps for both pathological and normal anatomical structures. The approach effectively models realistic tumor-induced deformations of healthy brain tissue in the synthetic images and accurately reflects the location of structures as defined by the conditions. The generated data, along with the tumor conditions as corresponding labels, may therefore be used as additional or replacing training samples for tumor segmentation. Our experiments show that replacing up to 50% of real training data has no negative impact, and a model trained exclusively on synthetic data can still achieve acceptable performance. These results indicate the potential of our method to mitigate the problem of data scarcity for segmentation tasks. Future work should explore extending this approach to handle various MRI sequences or three-dimensional data, which may further enhance its utility in clinical contexts.

References

1. Lipková J, Menze B, Wiestler B et al. Modelling glioma progression, mass effect and intracranial pressure in patient anatomy. J R Soc Interface. 2022;19:20210922.
2. Uzunova H, Wilms M, Handels H et al. Training CNNs for image registration from few samples with model-based data augmentation. Proc MICCAI. 2017:223–31.
3. Volokitin A, Erdil E, Karani N et al. Modelling the distribution of 3D brain MRI using a 2D slice VAE. Proc MICCAI. 2020:657–66.
4. Uzunova H, Schultz S, Handels H et al. Unsupervised pathology detection in medical images using conditional variational autoencoders. Int J Comput Assist Radiol Surg. 2019;14:451–61.
5. Carver EN, Dai Z, Liang E et al. Improvement of multiparametric MR image segmentation by augmenting the data with generative adversarial networks for glioma patients. Front Comput Neurosci. 2021;14.
6. Uzunova H, Ehrhardt J, Handels H. Generation of annotated brain tumor MRIs with tumor-induced tissue deformations for training and assessment of neural networks. Proc MICCAI. 2020:501–11.
7. Sohl-Dickstein J, Weiss E, Maheswaranathan N et al. Deep unsupervised learning using nonequilibrium thermodynamics. Proc ICML. 2015;37:2256–65.
8. Ho J, Jain A, Abbeel P. Denoising diffusion probabilistic models. Proc NIPS. 2020.
9. Nichol AQ, Dhariwal P. Improved denoising diffusion probabilistic models. Proc ICML. 2021;139:8162–71.
10. Zhu L, Xue Z, Jin Z et al. Make-A-Volume: leveraging latent diffusion models for cross-modality 3D brain MRI synthesis. Proc MICCAI. 2023.
11. Friedrich P, Wolleb J, Bieder F et al. WDM: 3D wavelet diffusion models for high-resolution medical image synthesis. Proc MICCAI. 2024:11–21.
12. Wang TC, Liu MY, Zhu JY et al. High-resolution image synthesis and semantic manipulation with conditional GANs. Proc IEEE CVF CVPR. 2018.
13. Billot B, Greve DN, Puonti O et al. SynthSeg: segmentation of brain MRI scans of any contrast and resolution without retraining. Med Image Anal. 2023;86:102789.
14. Park T, Liu MY, Wang TC et al. Semantic image synthesis with spatially-adaptive normalization. Proc IEEE CVF CVPR. 2019:2332–41.
15. Menze BH, Jakab A, Bauer S et al. The multimodal brain tumor image segmentation benchmark (BRATS). IEEE Trans Med Imaging. 2015;34(10):1993–2024.

LLM-driven Baselines for Medical Image Segmentation
A Systematic Analysis

Jasmin Arjomandi, Luisa Neubig, Andreas M. Kist

Department Artificial Intelligence in Biomedical Engineering, Friedrich-Alexander-Universität Erlangen-Nürnberg (FAU), Germany
andreas.kist@fau.de

Abstract. Large Language Models (LLMs) are increasingly utilized in tasks such as code generation for medical image analysis. However, their specific influence on study outcomes remains under-explored. In this study, we provide a comprehensive evaluation of various open- and closed-source LLMs, comparing their performance across medical imaging datasets. Each LLM was tasked with generating code for a U-Net-based baseline for a semantic segmentation task, guided by a tailored prompt. We evaluated each LLM's generated model performance using the Dice coefficient and recorded all interactions with the LLM. Significant variations in baseline performance were observed among the LLMs, with differences of up to Δ 85.49% for the Bolus, 86.33% for the BAGLS, and 87.32% for the Brain Tumor test dataset. Additionally, we identified LLMs with minimal coding errors (best-performing LLMs: GPT o1 Preview and Claude 3.5 Sonnet with zero errors upon initial code execution; least-performing: Gemini 1.5 Pro and LlAMA 3.1 405B with 15 and 11 errors, respectively). In summary, careful selection of LLMs can significantly enhance medical image analysis code generation and establish reliable baselines for further algorithmic development.

1 Introduction

Large Language Models (LLMs) have made remarkable progress from natural language processing to code generation, and are now being explored in medical image analysis. One of the leading architectures in this field, U-Net, has proven to be a robust baseline for medical image segmentation. Despite this, there has been limited research on the direct impact of LLMs on code generation automation for medical image segmentation tasks. Understanding how different LLMs perform when tasked with generating baseline code for segmentation is critical for advancing algorithmic development in medical image analysis.

In this study, we investigate how multiple LLMs, both open and closed source, generate code for U-Net-based models for medical image segmentation. Each LLM was tasked to generate code for data loading, model architecture, training, validation, and testing, and a main script. As shown in Fig. 1, each U-Net-based architecture was trained and evaluated on three standard medical image segmentation datasets. The LLM-induced errors were tracked and fed back to the model to correct itself, until the code ran error-free (Fig. 1). The main evaluation criterion was the Dice coefficient, a standard measure of overlap between predicted and ground truth regions in segmentation tasks.

C. Palm et al. (Hrsg.), *Bildverarbeitung für die Medizin 2025*, Informatik aktuell,
https://doi.org/10.1007/978-3-658-47422-5_13

Additionally, we documented the interactions required to correct and finalize the code generated by each LLM.

This analysis helps identify which LLMs are better suited for medical image segmentation tasks, particularly when aiming to minimize human intervention in code generation and create strong, competitive baselines. By examining performance differences and error rates, we aimed to provide practical insights for researchers and developers on selecting the most suitable LLM for generating a reliable and functional baseline in medical image analysis.

2 Related works

Recent studies have explored LLMs in various medical applications. For example, Bai et al. introduced M3D, leveraging multimodal LLMs for 3D medical image analysis, demonstrating their capability to handle complex medical tasks [1]. Sun et al. proposed a training-free approach for segmentation using LLMs, highlighting their potential in semantic segmentation without the need for additional training data [2]. Wang and Ke expanded LLM capabilities with LLM-Seg, which bridges image segmentation and reasoning tasks, showcasing the increasing interest in LLMs for medical image processing [3].

However, most of these studies focus on using LLMs for analysis and reasoning, rather than for generating code for specific architectures like U-Net. Few studies have investigated the practical integration of LLMs for generating executable segmentation code that works across diverse medical datasets. By examining this underexplored area, our study provides a deeper understanding of how LLMs can be harnessed in medical image segmentation tasks with minimal user input beyond error correction.

3 Methods

We evaluated the LLM-generated code on three standard medical image segmentation datasets: the Benchmark for Automatic Glottis Segmentation (BAGLS, [4]), a Bolus Swallowing Dataset (without a pathological condition [5]), and an MRI Brain Tumor Dataset [6]. The BAGLS dataset consists of endoscopic video frames from laryngoscopy exams aiming for glottis segmentation. The Bolus Swallowing Dataset provides videofluoroscopic swallowing studies to assess swallowing disorders. The Brain Tumors dataset includes single-slice grayscale MR images with segmentation masks for different types

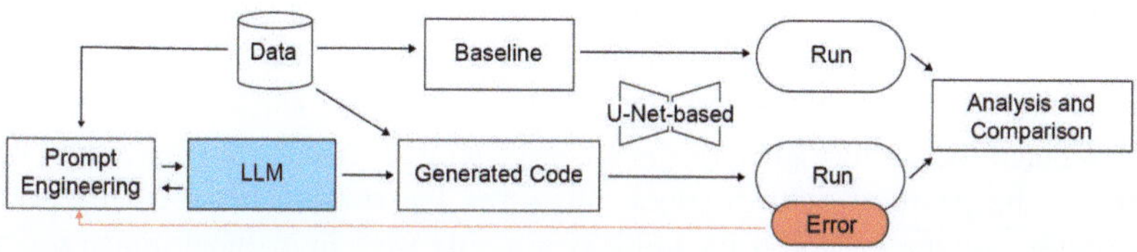

Fig. 1. Workflow of LLM-based semantic segmentation baseline generation for medical images.

of brain tumors, including Glioma, Meningioma, and Pituitary tumors, where in this study, we restricted ourselves to the Meningioma tumor images and their corresponding masks.

All datasets were preprocessed to fit the input requirements of the LLM-generated models. 5002 total images were selected for the BAGLS and Swallowing dataset and 999 for the Brain Meningioma tumor dataset, respectively. Images were resized and normalized to fit a range between 0 and 1 in the LLM-generated code. Each dataset was split into training (80%), validation (10%), and testing (10%) sets, with different methods defined by each LLM, either using `train_test_split` or `random_split`.

We selected eight state-of-the-art LLMs, including GPT-4, 4o and o1 Preview, Claude 3.5 Sonnet, Gemini 1.5 Pro, Github Copilot, Bing Microsoft Copilot (closed source), and LlAMA 3.1 405B (open source), to compare performance across different models. Each LLM was prompted with the same engineered query (prompt) to generate ready-to-run scripts (dataset.py, model.py, train.py, and main.py) needed to implement and train a U-Net-based semantic segmentation model.

The prompt engineering process was carefully designed to ensure clarity and avoid ambiguity, yet kept concise enough to avoid overwhelming the model or exceeding token limits, as longer prompts can sometimes confuse the model or lead to inefficient token utilization [7]. The prompt was refined iteratively through multiple experimental runs and by adding minimal required bullet-point instructions to generate all script parts, to ensure that each model would consistently generate similar results when the same prompt was reused, and reach a final prompt to use for all models. The LLMs were tasked with generating code (see above) and the interaction with each model was tracked. This includes the number of error messages, error types, LLM-suggested corrections, and any additional instructions provided to the LLMs when they encountered repeated error loops (see GitHub). The LLM-generated U-Net architectures used a series of convolutional layers for feature extraction, followed by upsampling strategies to recover spatial resolution, with skip connections between corresponding layers to help retain context information. For reference, we used a state-of-the-art U-Net-based variant, nnU-Net v2 [8]. Experiments were conducted on a machine equipped with NVIDIA GeForce RTX 3090 GPU running Python 3.10, pytorch 2.2.0 and CUDA 11.8. The number of interactions, errors, and modifications required to get each LLM-generated code running were recorded and compared.

For each LLM-generated model, the parameters such as batch size, learning rate, and loss function were directly derived from the output of the respective LLM. No additional fine-tuning or data augmentation was applied to any of the models to maintain the integrity of the comparison. The Adam optimizer was used across all models, and the Binary Cross-Entropy (BCE) or BCE with Logits Loss was used as the loss function, based on each LLM's suggestion. The nnU-Net was trained using CE+Dice loss as recommended by the authors' implementation. The number of training epochs was also decided by the LLM. More analyses are found in the Results section and on GitHub.

To evaluate the performance of the LLM-generated models, we used the Dice coefficient as the primary metric, which measures the overlap between the predicted segmentation and the ground truth and is commonly used in medical image segmentation tasks. We also tracked the training loss and validation loss for each epoch. The final

Dice scores were computed using one batch from the test set from each dataset, and visualizations of the segmentation outputs were generated for qualitative assessment. The LLM-generated code and our prompt engineering approaches, as well as further analyses on the gathered data, are available on the project's GitHub page[1].

4 Results

We first explored if the LLM-generated code can run "out of the box" or if errors occur. We found that only code generated by GPT-o1 Preview and Claude 3.5 Sonnet could successfully run without raising any errors (Fig. 2a). In contrast, Gemini 1.5 Pro and LlAMA 3.1 405B showed the highest number of errors, particularly RuntimeErrors, and ValueErrors, that we solved in a co-creation process with the LLM. Other models like Bing Microsoft Copilot and GPT4 faced a variety of issues, including NameErrors and AttributeErrors. In the cases of LlAMA and Gemini 1.5 Pro, minor additional information had to be provided to solve the respective errors to avoid producing the same errors. These results emphasize that some LLMs generated scripts require more extensive debugging, which could hinder efficiency in medical image analysis applications.

After ensuring that each LLM-generated code can be executed, we were interested in the training process of any U-Net model. While all LLMs use distinct training and architecture settings, we observe that the validation loss plots reveal key distinctions in model performance across epochs (Fig. 2b). GPT o1 Preview, GPT4, and Gemini 1.5 Pro achieved the lowest validation losses, converging quickly and showing effective learning with minimal overfitting. In contrast, Copilot and Bing Microsoft Copilot showed almost no convergence at very high loss values. LlAMA 3.1 405B displayed gradual convergence but remained less converged compared to other models. The nnU-Net baseline exhibits stable and low training loss across epochs, demonstrating its reliability as a baseline model for comparison.

Next, we investigated the performance of the individual models. As expected from the loss plots (Fig. 2b), we observe strong differences in performance on an unseen test

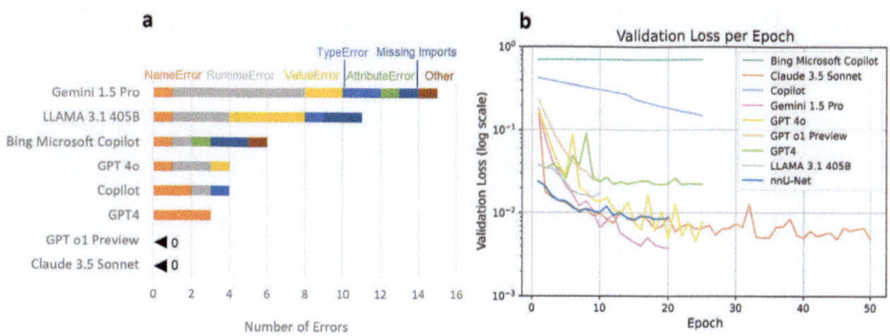

Fig. 2. From LLM-based code generation to successful training. a) comparing the number and type of errors and across LLMs. b) validation losses per epoch across LLM-generated models and nnU-Net (normalized loss shown), exemplarily for the BAGLS dataset.

[1]`https://github.com/ankilab/LLM_based_Segmentation.git`

set (Fig. 3). The GPT-based LLMs have shown high performance on all three datasets, especially GPT o1 Preview, which notably did not produce any errors during code generation. Interestingly, the Claude 3.5 Sonnet model also performed well, however, in general worse than the GPT-based models, but also showed no error during code generation. The LlAMA-based models could only perform reasonably well on the Bolus dataset. For us most surprisingly is the consistently poor performance of Bing and Github copilot. We do not only observe this effect quantitatively, but also qualitatively (Fig. 4).

We then compared the model architectures, hyperparameters used, the dataloaders, training, and main scripts across the models. Most models used four encoder/decoder stages, with GPT-4o having five and LlAMA 3.1 405B only three. DoubleConv blocks were common in GPT-4 and Claude. GPT-4o, Copilot, and Gemini 1.5 Pro incorporate BatchNorm2d after each convolution. Skip connections and ConvTranspose2d for upsampling were universally applied, following largely the original U-Net implementation. The bottleneck layer varies significantly across models, with GPT-4o, GPT-o1, Claude, and Gemini having larger bottlenecks (1024 channels), potentially allowing more complex representations. Meanwhile, LlAMA 3.1 405B has a relatively small

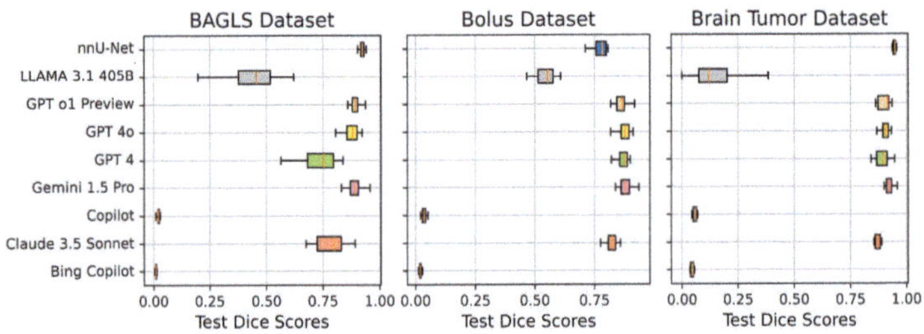

Fig. 3. Comparison of test Dice scores across different models, for each of the 3 datasets.

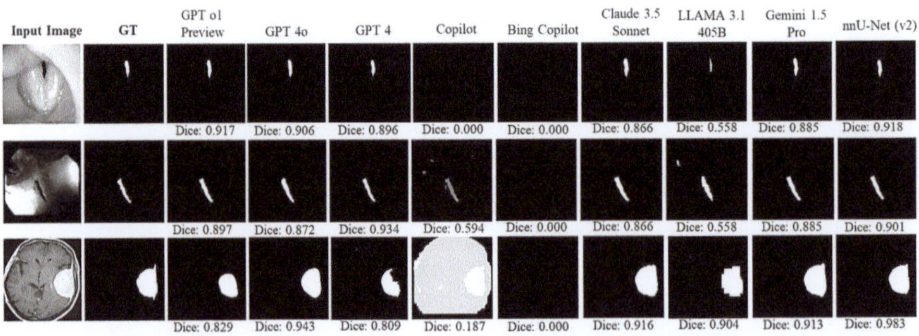

Fig. 4. Inference prediction masks comparison across models. Each horizontal set shows performance of each model on a sample image from each of the three datasets, namely BAGLS (top row), Bolus (middle row), Brain Tumor (bottom row).

bottleneck with 256 channels, likely affecting its capacity for encoding detailed spatial information.

All models except LlAMA 3.1 405B used smoothed Dice scores for evaluation. The loss was universally binary cross-entropy, in the case of GPT-4 computed on the logits. Post-processing strategies varied, with GPT-4o and Bing Copilot applying output interpolation before calculating Dice scores to ensure that the output matches the input and target image size. Batch sizes varied, with most using 16 samples, LlAMA 3.1 405B opting for 32, and GPT-4o and Gemini for 8. Data splitting methods also differed, likely affecting training efficiency. The number of trainable parameters differs considerably, with models like GPT-4o, GPT-o1, Claude, and Gemini featuring over 31 million parameters due to deeper layers and larger bottlenecks. In contrast, LlAMA 3.1 has the smallest parameter count (533,953), reflecting a more lightweight architecture.

5 Discussion and conclusion

The comparison of LLMs in medical image segmentation demonstrates that significant differences in model architectures, training strategies, and error handling affect performance. GPT o1 Preview and Claude 3.5 Sonnet performed well, requiring minimal modifications, while others like LlAMA 3.1 405B struggled with errors and inconsistent outputs.

From a ML specialist perspective, we would tune respective hyperparameters, especially batch size, learning rate, and number of epochs to allow better convergence. However, this study should reflect the out-of-the-box performance of LLM-generated code and models.

Future work could focus on further optimizing prompt engineering and incorporating more complex datasets. Moreover, integrating domain-specific fine-tuning for medical tasks with LLMs and exploring the combination of LLMs with transformer-based architectures could improve segmentation quality and consistency across different datasets.

References

1. Bai F, Du Y, Huang T et al. M3D: advancing 3D medical image analysis with multi-modal large language models. arXiv: 2404.00578. 2024.
2. Sun W, Du Y, Liu G et al. Training-free semantic segmentation via LLM-supervision. arXiv: 2404.00701. 2024.
3. Wang J, Ke L. LLM-seg: bridging image segmentation and large language model reasoning. Proc IEEE CVF CVPR. 2024:1765–74.
4. Gómez P, Kist AM, Schlegel P et al. BAGLS, a multihospital benchmark for automatic glottis segmentation. Sci Data. 2020;7(1):186.
5. Neubig L, Groh R, Kunduk M et al. Efficient patient orientation detection in videofluoroscopy swallowing studies. Proc BVM. 2022:129–34.
6. Akter A, Nosheen N, Ahmed S et al. Robust clinical applicable CNN and U-Net based algorithm for MRI classification and segmentation for brain tumor. Expert Syst Appl. 2024;238:122347.

7. Giray L. Prompt engineering with ChatGPT: a guide for academic writers. Ann Biomed Eng. 2023;51(12):2629–33.
8. Isensee F, Jaeger PF, Kohl SA et al. nnU-Net: a self-configuring method for deep learning-based biomedical image segmentation. Nat Methods. 2021;18(2):203–11.

Efficient Deep Learning-based Forward Solvers for Brain Tumor Growth Models

Zeineb Haouari[1,2], Jonas Weidner[1,2], Ivan Ezhov[1,2], Aswathi Varma[1,2], Daniel Rueckert[1,2], Bjoern Menze[3], Benedikt Wiestler[1,2]

[1]Technical University of Munich
[2]Munich Center for Machine Learning (MCML)
[3]University of Zurich
zeineb.haouari@tum.de

Abstract. Glioblastoma, a highly aggressive brain tumor, poses major challenges due to its poor prognosis and high morbidity rates. Partial differential equation-based models offer promising potential to enhance therapeutic outcomes by simulating patient-specific tumor behavior for improved radiotherapy planning. However, model calibration remains a bottleneck due to the high computational demands of optimization methods like Monte Carlo sampling and evolutionary algorithms. To address this, we recently introduced an approach leveraging a neural forward solver with gradient-based optimization to significantly reduce calibration time. This approach requires a highly accurate and fully differentiable forward model. We investigate multiple architectures, including (i) an enhanced TumorSurrogate, (ii) a modified nnU-Net, and (iii) a 3D Vision Transformer (ViT). The optimized TumorSurrogate achieved the best overall results, excelling in both tumor outline matching and voxel-level prediction of tumor cell concentration. It halved the MSE relative to the baseline model and achieved the highest Dice score across all tumor cell concentration thresholds. Our study demonstrates significant enhancement in forward solver performance and outlines important future research directions. Our source code is openly available at https://github.com/ZeinebZH/TumorNetSolvers

1 Introduction

Glioblastoma, the most prevalent malignant primary brain tumor, continues to have a dismal prognosis with a median overall survival of less than two years, despite extensive clinical trial efforts [1]. A significant challenge in improving treatment outcomes lies in the tumor's invasive nature, as it diffusely infiltrates surrounding brain tissue, rendering surgical resection of the entire tumor spread highly challenging. Consequently, postoperative radiotherapy (RT) has become a cornerstone of treatment, aimed at eliminating residual tumor cells while minimizing damage to healthy brain tissue. However, conventional imaging fails to detect these invading tumor cells, and RT planning relies on a uniform 15mm margin around the visible tumor to account for the diffuse spread, lacking patient-specific customization and limiting its effectiveness in addressing individual variations in tumor behavior [2].

Tumor modeling based on partial differential equations (PDEs) has emerged as a promising tool for providing personalized insights into tumor growth and invasion dy-

C. Palm et al. (Hrsg.), *Bildverarbeitung für die Medizin 2025*, Informatik aktuell,
https://doi.org/10.1007/978-3-658-47422-5_14

namics, driving the development of more targeted and effective treatment strategies. High-precision modeling techniques such as Markov Chain Monte Carlo have demonstrated potential in personalizing tumor simulations [3]. However, these methods involve numerous forward simulations, leading to extended runtimes, ranging from several hours to days, limiting their clinical applicability.

In contrast, deep learning (DL) methods present a faster alternative for solving this inverse problem by predicting tumor growth parameters without the need for iterative computations, thereby reducing runtimes to mere minutes [4, 5]. Despite their speed, DL models face significant challenges in generalizing to unseen cases, which restricts their broader applicability, particularly in critical clinical settings such as RT planning.

To overcome both these limitations, we recently proposed a novel idea that integrates the computational efficiency of DL models with the adaptability of gradient-based optimization [6]. Employing the DL-based forward solver TumorSurrogate [7], we conducted gradient-based optimization with respect to the input parameters of the tumor growth model. This iterative process minimizes the loss between the predicted and actual observed tumor distribution in the patient's MRI scans. In a cohort of nine glioma patients, our method significantly reduced the time required to solve the inverse problem from hours to minutes while achieving comparable modeling results.

Central to our novel gradient-based optimization approach is the DL-based forward solver. Here, we, therefore, systematically investigate distinct network architectures for their suitability as forward solvers. Our key contributions in this work are:

- Enhancing the solver's performance by exploring various network architectures.
- Systematically comparing these architectures regarding tumor outline matching and voxel-level tumor cell concentration prediction.

2 Materials and methods

2.1 Physical model

Within the reaction-diffusion formalism, brain tumor growth is modeled as a combination of two primary processes: proliferation and diffusion. This dynamic is governed by a partial differential equation (PDE) that describes changes in the normalized tumor cell density c over time

$$\frac{\partial c}{\partial t} = \nabla \cdot (D \nabla c) + \rho c(1 - c) \tag{1}$$

where $\nabla \cdot (D \nabla c)$ represents the spatial diffusion of tumor cells, and $c(1 - c)$ models logistic proliferation. The key parameters include the diffusion coefficient D, the proliferation rate ρ, and the tumor origin (x, y, z), collectively forming the parameter set $\theta = \{\rho, D, x, y, z\}$. Periodic boundary conditions are applied to ensure computational stability. Patient-specific anatomical information is integrated through segmentation masks of white matter (WM), gray matter (GM), and cerebrospinal fluid (CSF). Tumor diffusion is restricted to the WM and GM regions, with D assigned a fixed ratio between these tissues and set to zero in the CSF regions, following the framework outlined in [7].

2.2 Model architectures

The baseline model, TumorSurrogate [7], employs an encoder-decoder convolutional architecture with residual skip connections and bottleneck parameter integration. The encoder downsamples brain tissue data through convolutional blocks to generate a latent representation, which is then conditioned at the bottleneck by projecting and concatenating a biophysical parameter vector. The decoder subsequently maps this combined representation to a tumor simulation. Skip connections are employed symmetrically within both the encoder and decoder.

We adapted nnU-Net [8] for conditioned image regression by modifying it to handle continuous data. Key changes include adapting the preprocessing pipeline (Subsection 2.3), replacing the combined loss function (Dice + Cross-Entropy loss) with MSE loss, and adapting the dynamic U-Net architecture. Specifically, we removed the softmax activation layer to enable continuous value prediction and conditioned the network on the input biophysical parameter vector, in the exact same manner as the baseline. Unlike TumorSurrogate, this architecture features U-Net-style residual skip connections between the encoder and decoder, and is fully automatically configured based on dataset properties.

We adapted the image reconstruction ViT from Lin and Heckel [9] for 3D conditioned image-to-image regression by extending it to 3D and incorporating biophysical parameter conditioning. Volumetric, non-overlapping patches (16^3) were encoded as spatial tokens, and a biophysical parameter vector was incorporated as a distinct token within the shared embedding space. This combined representation enables the model to jointly leverage spatial structure and tumor-specific information for accurate brain tumor simulation. The model comprises 12 transformer blocks (6 attention heads, embedding dimension 384, MLP ratio 4).

2.3 Training setup and experiments

Models were trained and evaluated on a synthetically generated dataset (numerical solver [10], brain tissue atlas geometry [11]) comprising 10,000 training, 2,000 validation, and 2,000 test samples. Inputs consisted of tissue data paired with corresponding biophysical parameters, with tumor simulations serving as targets.

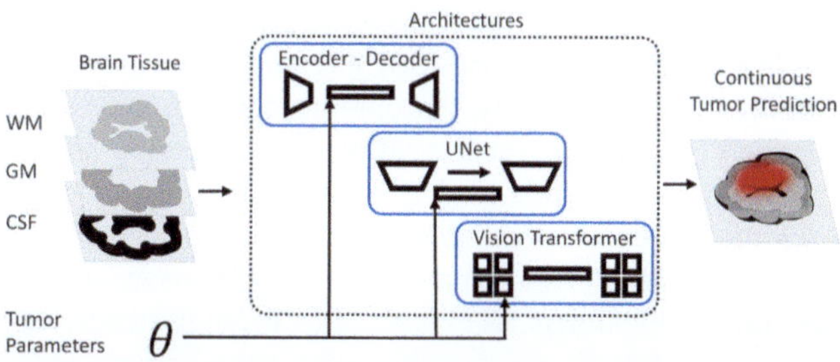

Fig. 1. Overview of our experimental pipeline. We input brain anatomy maps and tumor parameters θ into different networks (blue) and output the 3D tumor concentration (red).

Tab. 1. Training configurations for all models.

Pipeline	Preprocessing	Loss Function	Other Details
ViT	Both pipelines Data augmentation	MSE	-
nnU-Net	Both pipelines Data augmentation	MSE, Deep supervision	-
TS Baseline	Original preprocessing	Region-specific MSE [6]	-
TS Optimized	Both pipelines Data augmentation	MSE	Batch norm, Gradient clipping, Kaiming weight initialization

The original pipeline involved shifting the center of mass of the tumor to the image center, cropping to 120×120×120, and downsampling to 64×64×64 to reduce memory costs. We also adapted the nnU-Net preprocessing pipeline, retaining regression-suitable steps like normalization, resampling, and transposing while excluding segmentation-specific steps like foreground and class-based sampling.

The nnU-Net model follows the predefined configuration in [8], employing Stochastic Gradient Descent (SGD) with a momentum coefficient of 0.99 and Nesterov acceleration. A polynomial decay schedule manages the learning rate, starting from 1×10^{-2}. The TS Model is trained with the Adam optimizer, using a weight decay of 4×10^{-20} and parameters $\beta = (0.9, 0.999)$. A cosine annealing scheduler varies the learning rate between 10^{-6} and 10^{-4} as suggested in [7]. The ViT model is trained with the AdamW optimizer, with a learning rate range of 2×10^{-4} to 8×10^{-4} and a weight decay of 1×10^{-2}. Default β parameters $(0.9, 0.999)$ are used, and a one-cycle learning rate scheduler with a 10% ramp-up period is applied.

Data augmentation follows the nnU-Net framework, discarding intensity-based augmentations as they are unsuitable for tissue data, keeping rotations and mirroring. This results in four different pipelines (Tab. 1)

3 Results

3.1 Voxel-level prediction of tumor cell concentration

In Tab. 2, we compare voxel-level accuracy in predicting tumor cell concentration across different models (measured by MAE and MSE) as well as the global image similarity (SSIM) on the unseen test set. Notably, our optimized TumorSurrogate model consistently outperforms all other models across all metrics, achieving an MSE that is half that of the second-best model. While the ViT demonstrated superior performance over nnU-Net in voxel-level metrics, it exhibited the lowest overall global image similarity according to SSIM. Interestingly, the comparatively high errors in voxel-level prediction for nnU-Net were driven by outliers, as evidenced by the high standard error.

Tab. 2. Summary of model performances. We report mean and standard error.

Model	MSE $[10^{-3}]$ ($\downarrow$)	MAE $[10^{-3}]$ ($\downarrow$)	SSIM ($\uparrow$)
ViT	3.27 ± 0.06	15.57 ± 0.22	0.878 ± 0.001
nnU-Net	5.86 ± 0.26	17.75 ± 0.42	0.907 ± 0.001
TS Baseline	2.02 ± 0.04	12.27 ± 0.16	0.903 ± 0.002
TS optimized	0.98 ± 0.02	8.21 ± 0.09	0.912 ± 0.001

3.2 Tumor outline matching

To effectively apply the solver for planning radiotherapy in tumor patients, where only visible tumor margins are available for model fitting, it is crucial to assess how accurately the tumor outline is matched by the different models. In Fig. 2, we investigate the Dice overlap with the ground truth tumor cell distribution across various tumor cell concentration c thresholds. Again, our optimized TumorSurrogate model performs best overall. Notably, at low tumor cell concentration thresholds (up to $c \sim 0.3$), the ViT model performs almost on par with the optimized TumorSurrogate. However, its performance declines significantly at higher thresholds, translating to smaller tumor volumes, which may be attributed to the coarse tokenization employed (with patches sized 16×16×16).

4 Discussion

Our recently introduced gradient-based approach to solving the inverse problem [6] relies on a reliable, differentiable forward solver. This study explores three deep learning architectures: an encoder-decoder model (TumorSurrogate), a nnU-Net-based model, and a ViT-based model. Our optimized TumorSurrogate implementation outperformed the others in predicting voxel-level tumor cell concentration and matching tumor outlines. For clinical translation, matching the visible tumor outline (Dice score) is crucial.

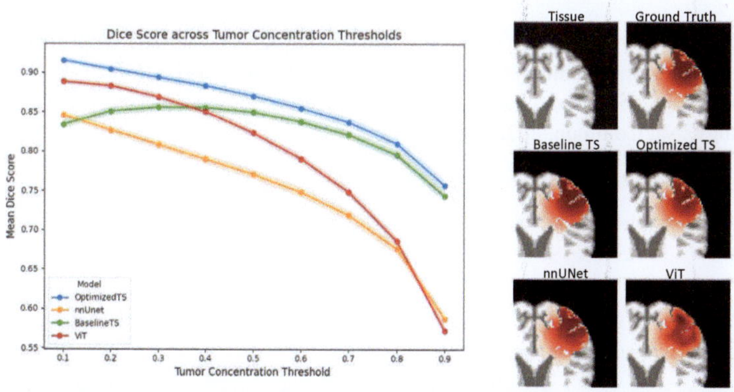

Fig. 2. (left) Comparison of Dice overlap for the different network architectures across varying tumor concentration thresholds. We plot the mean Dice score and standard error on the test set. (right) Example images of tumor concentration prediction.

The ViT model showed promise at lower tumor cell concentrations but performed worse at higher thresholds, likely due to its coarse patch-based tokenization. Future work will improve tokenization and explore conditional diffusion models. A crucial next step is translating these findings to real patient data and extending to more complex tumor growth models, including mass effect or necrosis. While this work uses solely a synthetic dataset, the focus must shift to validating the developed models on real patient datasets. We propose training the models on synthetic data derived from diffusion model-generated MRI segmentations as simulation geometries, followed by fine-tuning on a fraction of real patient data. This transfer learning approach leverages the extensive knowledge gained from synthetic data while adapting to real patient characteristics.

References

1. Weller M, Bent M van den, Preusser M et al. EANO guidelines on the diagnosis and treatment of diffuse gliomas of adulthood. Nat Rev Clin Oncol. 2021;18(3):170–86.
2. Niyazi M, Andratschke N, Bendszus M et al. ESTRO-EANO guideline on target delineation and radiotherapy details for glioblastoma. Radiother Oncol. 2023;184:109663.
3. Lipková J, Angelikopoulos P, Wu S et al. Personalized radiotherapy design for glioblastoma: integrating mathematical tumor models, multimodal scans, and Bayesian inference. IEEE Trans Med Imaging. 2019;38(8):1875–84.
4. Ezhov I, Scibilia K, Franitza K et al. Learn-Morph-Infer: a new way of solving the inverse problem for brain tumor modeling. Med Image Anal. 2023;83:102672.
5. Pati S, Sharma V, Aslam H et al. Estimating glioblastoma biophysical growth parameters using deep learning regression. Proc MICCAI. 2021:157–67.
6. Weidner J, Ezhov I, Balcerak M et al. Rapid personalization of PDE-based tumor growth using a differentiable forward model. Proc MIDL. 2024.
7. Ezhov I, Mot T, Shit S et al. Geometry-aware neural solver for fast Bayesian calibration of brain tumor models. IEEE Trans Med Imaging. 2021;41(5):1269–78.
8. Isensee F, Jaeger PF, Kohl S et al. nnU-Net: a self-configuring method for deep learning-based biomedical image segmentation. Nat Methods. 2021;18(2):203–11.
9. Lin K, Heckel R. Vision transformers enable fast and robust accelerated MRI. Proc MIDL. 2022.
10. Balcerak M, Amiranashvili T, Wagner A et al. Physics-regularized multi-modal image assimilation for brain tumor localization. arXiv: 2409.20409. 2024.
11. Yeh FC. Population-based tract-to-region connectome of the human brain and its hierarchical topology. Nat Commun. 2022;13(1):4933.

Is Self-supervision Enough?
Benchmarking Foundation Models Against End-to-end Training for Mitotic Figure Classification

Jonathan Ganz[1], Jonas Ammeling[1], Emely Rosbach[1], Ludwig Lausser[1], Christof A. Bertram[2], Katharina Breininger[3,4], Marc Aubreville[5,1]

[1]Technische Hochschule Ingolstadt, Ingolstadt, Germany
[2]University of Veterinary Medicine, Vienna, Austria
[3]Center for AI and Data Science, Julius-Maximilians-Universität Würzburg, Würzburg, Germany
[4]Department of Artificial Intelligence in Biomedical Engineering, Friedrich-Alexander-Universität Erlangen-Nürnberg, Erlangen, Germany
[5]Flensburg University of Applied Sciences, Flensburg, Germany
jonathan.ganz@thi.de

Abstract. Foundation models (FMs), i.e., models trained on a vast amount of typically unlabeled data, have become popular and available recently for the domain of histopathology. The key idea is to extract semantically rich vectors from any input patch, allowing for the use of simple subsequent classification networks potentially reducing the required amounts of labeled data, and increasing domain robustness. In this work, we investigate to which degree this also holds for mitotic figure classification. Utilizing two popular public mitotic figure datasets, we compared linear probing of five publicly available FMs against models trained on ImageNet and a simple ResNet50 end-to-end-trained baseline. We found that the end-to-end-trained baseline outperformed all FM-based classifiers, regardless of the amount of data provided. Additionally, we did not observe the FM-based classifiers to be more robust against domain shifts, rendering both of the above assumptions incorrect.

1 Introduction

Mitotic figures (MFs) in histologic images represent cells undergoing division, and their frequency within a standardized area is a key biomarker for assessing tumor patient survival in both veterinary and human medicine [1]. However, manual detection of MFs presents a number of challenges, including the tedious nature of the counting process and the low inter-rater agreement [2]. Consequently, there is a high level of interest in deep learning-driven detection and classification methods.

Recently, foundation models (FMs) have attracted significant interest in the digital pathology community and there is a rapid development of new models [3–7]. These models, which are typically large vision transformers (ViTs), are trained in an unsupervised manner on extensive collections of histopathology images. As a result of their comprehensive training, they are capable of generating image embeddings with high semantic value, which enables them to perform well in tasks such as few-shot learning and to serve as a robust foundation for a multitude of downstream applications [3–7].

C. Palm et al. (Hrsg.), *Bildverarbeitung für die Medizin 2025*, Informatik aktuell,
https://doi.org/10.1007/978-3-658-47422-5_15

Tab. 1. Foundation models compared in this study, ordered by the size of the respective model.

Name	Pretraining Algorithm	Dataset size WSI	Tiles	Model Type	Size
Prov-GigaPath [7]	DINOv2	170K	1.3B	ViT-G	1.1B
H-optimus-0[1]	DINOv2	500K	-	ViT-G	1.1B
Virchow [4]	DINOv2	1.5M	2B	ViT-H	632M
Virchow2 [5]	DINOv2	3.4M	1.7B	ViT-H	632M
UNI [3]	DINOv2	100K	100M	ViT-L	307M
Phikon [6]	iBOT	6K	43M	ViT-B	86M

In recent work, Vorontsov et al. [4] have shown that the patch embeddings of FMs can be utilized effectively for MF classification. They have reported promising performance by training linear classifiers directly on these patch embeddings, which is of particular interest given that MF classification is often used as a second stage in modern detection pipelines [8]. As a result, FMs could be employed to further enhance performance of such pipelines or to reduce the need for large amounts of annotated data. However, there has been no in-depth analysis of how the performance of such classifiers depends on training set sizes or how much it is influenced by domain shifts (i.e., performance degradation due to source-target domain differences). This study aims to shed light on these questions by comparing the embeddings of several state-of-the-art histopathology FMs for MF classification. To provide a comprehensive evaluation, we compare the FM-based classifiers against several baselines across two publicly available MF datasets.

2 Materials

In this study, we used two publicly available MF datasets. The first is the training set from the second edition of the Mitosis Domain Generalization Challenge (MIDOG) [1], which consists of 11,051 MFs and 9,501 MF look-alikes on 354 regions of interests from five different domains, including human breast cancer (domain 1), canine lung cancer (domain 2), canine lymphoma (domain 3), canine cutaneous mast cell tumor (CCMCT) (domain 4), and human neuroendocrine tumor (domain 5). The second dataset comprises 32 whole slide images (WSIs) of CCMCTs and originally contains 262,481 annotations of different cell types [9]. In this study, we only used 44,880 annotations representing MFs and 27,965 annotations belonging to MF look-alikes.

3 Methods

We compared six different models in this work, with detailed information provided in Tab. 1. All of the models are Vision Transformers (ViTs) of varying sizes. Most of the compared models were trained using DINOv2, a self-supervised learning algorithm that trains vision models by contrasting differently augmented views of the same image, allowing them to learn high-level features without the need for labeled data [10].

For MF classification, we used the linear probing implementation by Chen et al. [3], which trains a linear classifier on top of pre-extracted embeddings. To generate embeddings, we extracted patches of size 224×224 pixels for the MFs and look-alikes at a resolution of 0.25 microns per pixel. For Virchow and Virchow2, these embeddings were created by concatenating the class token and the mean across all 256 patch tokens, as described in [4]. For all other models, only the class token was used [4]. During image extraction, the patches were normalized according to the means and standard deviations provided in the respective works. No additional data augmentation was applied.

We compared the embeddings of the FMs to three different baselines. First, we used two feature extractors (ResNet50 with 25M and ViT-H 632M parameters) pretrained on ImageNet. As with the FMs, these models were used to generate embeddings for linear probing. Additionally, we compared the models to an end-to-end-trained baseline. For this, we used a classifier based on a ResNet50 stem pretrained on ImageNet. Unlike the embedding generation process, we applied a standard image augmentation pipeline during the training, which included random color jitter, Gaussian blurring, flipping, and random rotations. Besides this, the patches were extracted as for the FMs. We used the one-cycle learning rate policy with a maximum learning rate of 10^{-4} [11], and the best-performing model was selected retrospectively based on its validation loss.

To examine performance as a function of training set size, we trained the models using different subsets of the two datasets. To increase the statistical informativeness of our results, we applied five-fold Monte Carlo cross-validation for each model and dataset size. With four different training set sizes (0.1%, 1%, 10%, and 100%) a total of 20 trainings were performed per model. During each training, 20% of all annotations of the respective dataset were randomly selected as test set, while 20% of the respective training annotations were selected for validation. To ensure comparability, all models were trained and evaluated using the same training and test sets. Please note that the percentages refer to the size of each dataset, meaning substantially less data was available for the respective training set sizes in the MIDOG dataset compared to the CCMCT dataset. In a second experiment to assess cross-domain performance, we split the MIDOG dataset into training and test sets across different domains. For each evaluation, one domain served as the training set, while the remaining domains were used for testing. To assess in-domain performance, 20% of the in-domain data was separated from the training set and included in the test set. At the end of the experiment, performance was measured separately for each domain. As in the previous experiment, five training sessions were conducted per domain and per model, resulting in a total of 25 training sessions per model.

4 Results

The results of the analysis on the influence of dataset size on model performance are shown in Fig. 1. We observed that, for all models, performance improved significantly as the size of the available training data increased. On the CCMCT dataset, the performance increase in relation to the amount of training data was similar across all FM-based classifiers. However, on the MIDOG dataset, classifiers using embeddings from Phikon and UNI lagged behind the other FM-based approaches. The two ImageNet baselines were significantly outperformed by both the end-to-end trained ResNet50 and the FM-based classifiers on both datasets. Across data set sizes, the end-to-end trained baseline model outperformed all other models across both datasets. With 100% of the respective dataset available, it achieved a mean AUROC of 0.87 ± 0.01 on the CCMCT dataset and 0.89 ± 0.01 on the MIDOG dataset. Among the classifiers based on FM embeddings, the H-optimus-0[1], Prov-GigaPath, Virchow, and Virchow2 models demonstrated similar performance. With 100% of the data available, on the CCMCT dataset, Virchow2 embeddings had a slight advantage over the other FMs, while on the MIDOG dataset, H-optimus-0 embeddings delivered the best performance among the FMs.

The mean in-domain and out-of-domain performances over the different domains for all models are given in Tab. 2. As embeddings of the the H-optimus-0 model gave the best results in the first experiment, we choose to compare it to the end-to-end baseline in more detail in Fig. 2.

Like in the first experiment, the end-to-end baseline clearly outperforms all other models, both in terms of in-domain performance but also in terms of out-of-domain performance (Tab. 2). Among the FMs, the classifiers using the embeddings of the H-optimus-0[1], Prov-GigaPath, Virchow, and Virchow2 models performed slightly bet-

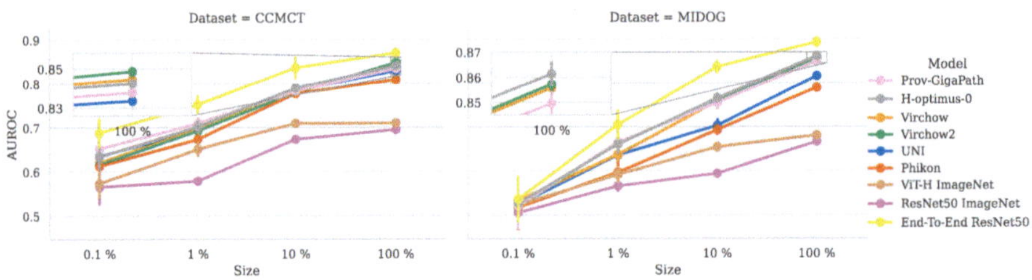

Fig. 1. Results of the investigation of the influence of training set size on model performance. The percentages refer to the total size of the data set.

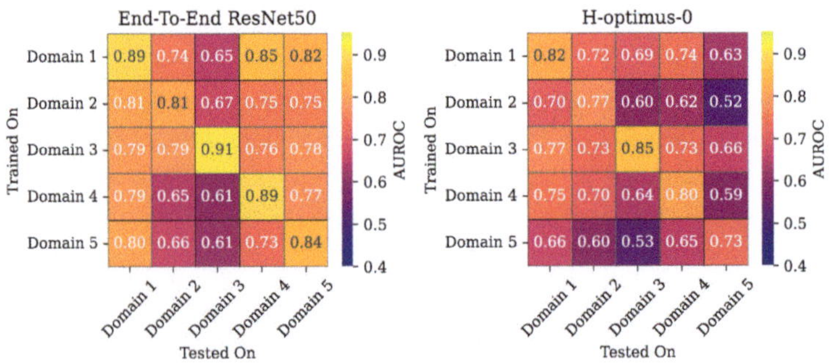

Fig. 2. Cross-domain AUROC results for the end-to-end trained ResNet50 baseline model and the classifier based on H-optimus-0 embeddings.

[1] https://huggingface.co/bioptimus/H-optimus-0

Model	AUROC	
	In domain	Out of domain
Prov-GigaPath	0.79 ± 0.04	0.66 ± 0.07
H-optimus-0	0.79 ± 0.04	0.66 ± 0.07
Virchow	0.79 ± 0.04	0.66 ± 0.06
Virchow2	0.79 ± 0.04	0.66 ± 0.06
UNI	0.76 ± 0.03	0.64 ± 0.05
Phikon	0.76 ± 0.03	0.61 ± 0.05
ViT-H ImageNet	0.68 ± 0.05	0.56 ± 0.04
ResNet50 ImageNet	0.63 ± 0.04	0.53 ± 0.03
End-To-End ResNet50	**0.87 ± 0.04**	**0.74 ± 0.07**

Tab. 2. In-domain and out-of-domain AUROC results for different models on the MIDOG dataset (mean ± standard deviation of five-fold Monte Carlo cross-validation).

ter then those using the UNI and Phikon embeddings. However, given the standard deviations, the performance were relatively similar.

Both the FM-based classifiers and the end-to-end baseline experienced substantial performance drops when the in-domain trained models were applied to different domains, as shown in Tab. 2. Additionally, Fig. 2 demonstrates that, for both the end-to-end trained ResNet50 and the H-optimus-0 models, this drop in performance was not evenly distributed across the external domains. This observation aligns with the findings of [1], which highlight that domain shift is not a symmetrical phenomena.

5 Discussion

In this study, we compared classifiers based on FM embeddings to different baseline models. In both experiments, the end-to-end-trained ResNet50 baseline outperformed the FM-based classifiers. Thus we conclude that there is no benefit in employing the embeddings generated by those models directly for MF classification. It should be noted that the FM-based classifiers consisted of only a single linear layer trained with pre-extracted features, whereas the end-to-end model was fully trainable. Nevertheless, the FMs underwent extensive pretraining on large histopathology datasets, while the ResNet baseline, despite being pretrained on ImageNet, was only trained on the data available for each experiment. This suggests that extensive pretraining is no substitute for task-specific supervision, at least for the given task. However, better results might be achievable if the FMs were fine-tuned for the specific task, though this would require significantly more computational resources and might be inefficient given the strong performance of the standard CNN baseline. The positive impact of the FMs' pretraining- on the given tasks suggests a comparison with the ViT-H based classifier, which, despite having a comparable number of parameters, achieved lower performance (Fig. 1).

The FM-based classifiers didn't turn out to be more data-efficient in comparison to our end-to-end trained ResNet50 model. However, the performance on both datasets in Fig. 1 does not seem to have converged yet. Hence, it might be interesting to see how the performance scales with even more data being available.

We also did not find the FM-based classifiers to be more robust to domain shifts than one of our baselines. This suggests that the pretraining of the FMs did not result in entirely domain-agnostic embeddings. Interestingly, the in-domain results of the FM-based classifiers in Tab. 2 show that all models performed quite similarly, whereas in the first experiment, the Uni and Phikon-based models performed slightly worse on the MIDOG dataset compared to the other FMs. Indeed, the results in Tab. 2 resemble those on the CCMCT dataset, where all FM-based classifiers performed similarly. This may indicate that the Uni and Phikon embeddings are marginally less generalizable than those of the other FMs, as the latter were able to perform better when trained on the mixed MIDOG domains in the first experiment.

Acknowledgement. M.A. and C.A.B. acknowledge support by the DFG and FWF, respectively (project numbers 520330054, I 6555). K.B. acknowledges support of the DFG, project 460333672 CRC1540 EBM.

References

1. Aubreville M, Stathonikos N, Donovan TA et al. Domain generalization across tumor types, laboratories, and species—Insights from the 2022 edition of the Mitosis Domain Generalization Challenge. Med Image Anal. 2024;94:103155.
2. Ganz J, Marzahl C, Ammeling J et al. Information mismatch in PHH3-assisted mitosis annotation leads to interpretation shifts in H&E slide analysis. Sci Rep. 2024;14(1):26273.
3. Chen RJ, Ding T, Lu MY et al. Towards a general-purpose foundation model for computational pathology. Nat Med. 2024;30(3):850–62.
4. Vorontsov E, Bozkurt A, Casson A et al. A foundation model for clinical-grade computational pathology and rare cancers detection. Nat Med. 2024:1–12.
5. Zimmermann E, Vorontsov E, Viret J et al. Virchow 2: scaling self-supervised mixed magnification models in pathology. arXiv: 2408.00738. 2024.
6. Filiot A, Ghermi R, Olivier A et al. Scaling self-supervised learning for histopathology with masked image modeling. medRxiv. 2023:2023–7.
7. Xu H, Usuyama N, Bagga J et al. A whole-slide foundation model for digital pathology from real-world data. Nature. 2024.
8. Aubreville M, Bertram CA, Marzahl C et al. Deep learning algorithms out-perform veterinary pathologists in detecting the mitotically most active tumor region. Sci Rep. 2020;10(1):16447.
9. Bertram CA, Aubreville M, Marzahl C et al. A large-scale dataset for mitotic figure assessment on whole slide images of canine cutaneous mast cell tumor. Sci Data. 2019;6(1):274.
10. Oquab M, Darcet T, Moutakanni T et al. Dinov2: learning robust visual features without supervision. arXiv: 2304.07193. 2023.
11. Smith LN, Topin N. Super-convergence: very fast training of neural networks using large learning rates. arXiv: 1708.07120. 2017.

Look, No Convs! Permutation- and Rotation-invariance for MetaFormers

Mattias P. Heinrich

Institute of Medical Informatics, University of Luebeck, Lübeck, Germany
mattias.heinrich@uni-luebeck.de

Abstract. Despite their success for numerous medical image analysis tasks the use of convolutional neural networks and vision transformers (ViT) have an important limitation of permutation- and rotation-dependency. By design the convolutional filter and positional encoding in ViTs impacts the performance with oftentimes severe robustness issues when using scans with a different input orientation. For biomedical images of tissue samples the orientation is arbitrary and ultrasound scans can be flipped depending on usage. The successful roto-translation equivariant networks tackle the problems at the expense of probing multiple versions of the same filter within each layer, resulting in many times higher computational demand. We revisit and expand this concept by implementing it into MetaFormers that are already partially equivariant and have very few layers which require extra computations. Our experimental validation on several MedMNIST datasets demonstrate the advantages of rotational- and permutation-invariance for the replicated Roto-ResNet18 and our novel Roto-MetaFormer-S12.

1 Introduction

Convolutional neural networks (CNNs) and vision transformers (ViTs) are ubiquitously used for state-of-the-art vision and medical image analysis applications. Their key working principal relies on learning spatial relations and visual patterns that are either realised as convolutional filters or data-adaptive self-attention patterns. CNNs are translational invariant - when ignoring boundary effects - but yield different outputs for rotated or transposed inputs. ViTs invariances depend on whether or not positional encodings are employed and their convolutional stems, but generally speaking virtually all state-of-the-art approaches are not rotational invariant. Nevertheless, rotational- and permutation-invariance are desirable properties that should be considered to address the robustness and high reliance on large labelled datasets in particular in the biomedical domain. Here, we build upon the recent MetaFormers framework that demonstrated an unexpectedly high performance of transformer-like architectures with very few spatially dependent self-attention layers and nearly no convolutions. We replace its remaining non-invariant blocks, the convolutional patch embeddings, with rotational invariant kernels to create a fully invariant framework.

For biomedical data in particular the relevance of rotational invariance has been previously studied. Many imaging modalities, in particular microscopy but also to some degree MRI and ultrasound, do not fully restrict the spatial orientation of images to be the same for each acquisition of the same patient or specimen. Hence, the effect that the output of most of the currently used deep learning models is different depending on

C. Palm et al. (Hrsg.), *Bildverarbeitung für die Medizin 2025*, Informatik aktuell,
https://doi.org/10.1007/978-3-658-47422-5_16

input rotation and permutation (flips) is undesirable and leads to a loss in robustness. The common work-around to use heavy data augmentation is neither theoretically well founded nor does it guarantee predictable and robust results for differently oriented inputs. We here restrict our discussion on two complementary approaches that showed to address this challenge in CNN frameworks

1. roto-translation equivariant networks [1] aim to implement a specific operation that established equivariance for the SE(2) group.
2. XEdgeConv replaces traditional convolutions with message passing operations known from geometric deep learning [2].

Both approaches predate the widespread vision transformer adoption in medical image analysis and still require a large number of convolutional layers to be replaced.

In parallel to the developments of rotational invariant networks there has been a recent trend in computer vision to question the common belief of importance of learnable operators that directly employ spatial relations across image regions and/or pixels. While self-attention layers themselves are invariant to permutations of the input sequence and would on their own yield rotation- and permutation-invariant networks they are commonly combined with positional embeddings, patch embedding [3] and convolutional patch merging, when employing a hierarchical architecture as e.g. done in SegFormer [4].

The MetaFormer framework published at CVPR 2022 [5] highlights the fact that self-attention is not necessarily the key ingredient for high performance vision models - but rather the spatially invariant MLP in the transformer block is contributing most to the successes of ViTs. They propose a very strong baseline called PoolFormer that nearly removes all learnable spatial operations and only retains four patch embeddings blocks (in the smallest version) along with untrainable, equivariant spatial pooling operators. In the more general MetaFormer, few layers in preferably deep blocks are implemented using spatial self-attention, which can be realised without positional encodings.

While deep learning model designs without convolutions have been explored for small datasets, such as CIFAR10 [6] and further alternatives of rotational equivariance was investigated for histological images in [7], we are not aware of any comprehensive study of modern vision transformers with rotation- and permutation-invariance that is focussed on biomedical data.

We hence present a first evaluation on four complementary 2D medical imaging modalities and classification tasks that compares Roto-CNNs in traditional fully-convolutional ResNets with our novel formulation of Roto-MetaFormers. Fig. 1 highlights the blocks of CNNs in particular ResNets [8], and MetaFormers that break our desired invariance and would require Roto-CNNs as a replacement, along with their computational load. Whereas, Roto-CNNs have an eightfold increased run time Roto-MetaFormers less than double the computations of the original model.

2 Materials and methods

We will now discuss the employed datasets and methodological concepts explored in our study on rotation and permutation invariance.

To ensure reproducibility and ease of comparison, we consider four 2D tasks of the enhanced MedMNIST+ dataset [9] with a common resolution of 128×128 pixels focussing on classification tasks. This covers different types of permutation and rotation that are common causes of error and require robustness in clinical practice. Namely we include breast ultrasound for lesion detection, where the probe could be flipped; blood cell microscopy and the Path histopathology dataset, where the output should not depend on the input orientation or flipped axes; and pneumonia detection in X-ray, which may in practice occasionally yield rotated scans due to misplacement of mobile scanners. Those tasks do not necessarily represent the most challenging research problems, but should rather highlight the practical problems that may occur when inputs are unexpectedly rotated or flipped.

As a baseline we trained a ResNet-18 and achieved an average accuracy of 92.2% and F1 scores of 90.1% for those tasks when there is no discrepancy between the orientation during training and testing. This is slightly better than the published accuracy of 89.1%[1], hence we are able to reproduce the state-of-the-art. Next, we explored a 90 degree rotation and horizontal flip during testing without adapting the model or training routine. This leads to a substantial drop in F1 scores to 72.3%, clearly highlighting the need for more robustness.

Since our present work builds upon the concept of roto-equivariant convolutions, we will elaborate the concept in the following. *Roto-translation equivariant networks* replace a normal convolution with the following three steps:

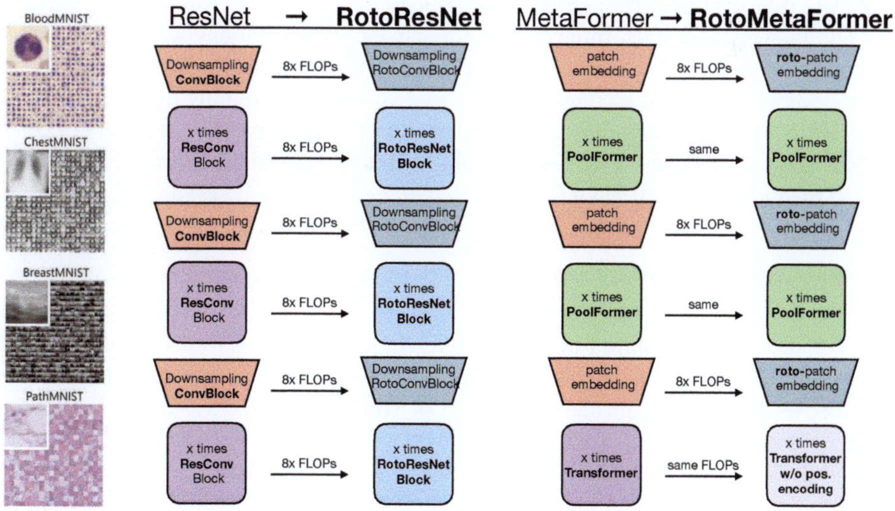

Fig. 1. Left: MedMNIST 2D datasets which commonly face challenges in clinical robustness due to misorientation of scans. Right: Methodological concept of Roto-ResNets (similar to [1]) and our new Roto-MetaFormers, in which permutation and rotation invariance is achieved by removing positional encoding and replacing all convolutions with their invariant version.

[1] https://medmnist.com/

1. lifting the inputs from $\mathbb{R}^2$ into $SE(2)$, i.e. adding an additional dimension to the tensors and replicating the input or filter kernels for all considered rotations;
2. applying the filter operation for each copy; and
3. projecting the outputs back to $\mathbb{R}^2$ e.g. by using a max-operation over the additional dimension

While the original paper focused on rotations we here also add mirroring flips (dimension permutations) and restrict ourselves to 90 degree angles. This leads to eight possible versions of filter kernels (or equivalently input images) that yield an eightfold increase in computational complexity while keeping the trainable parameters the same. For notational clarity: a whole classification network is considered rotationally and permutationally invariant if the output does not depend on the input orientation (including mirroring), whereas each layer should be rotation- and permutation-equivarent meaning their result of a e.g. 90 degree rotated image is equivalent to a 90 degree rotated output of the non-rotated input.

We replace all 18 or 34 convolutional layers in a ResNet-18 or ResNet-34 respectively with Roto-CNNs to achieve intrinsic invariance. For the MetaFormers we focus on the S12 and M36 model with three blocks of PoolFormers (only average pooling and MLPs) and the fourth deepest block with normal transformer layers (using self-attention). The two models comprise 12 and 36 million trainable parameters and thus approximately match the aforementioned CNNs. At the beginning and in-between each block of MetaFormers there is a convolution patch merging. We replace only those by Roto-CNNs and remove the positional encoding of the transformer block to achieve complete rotation and permutation equivariance.

The networks are each trained from scratch for 3000 iterations with Adam, using a mini-batch size of 96, a learning rate of 5×10^{-4}, cosine annealing with a warm-start after 1000 iterations and an unweighted cross-entropy loss. We only employ moderate augmentation by applying a random affine transform with a standard deviation of 0.05. All trainings are repeated with new random seeds for three and five times respectively for the medium and small models. Our code will be made openly available[2].

3 Results

Our key results are displayed in Fig. 2. Here we compare the F1 classification scores along with the robustness against unexpected misorientation for the two smaller models: ResNet-18 and Metaformer-S12 - with or without Roto-Convs. It can be seen in lighter colours that when presenting the networks with input images that are flipped and rotated the accuracy is much reduced for the baseline variants for BreastMNIST and PneumoniaMNIST, while this influence is small for BloodMNIST and PathMNIST.

For the experiments with larger models (ResNet-34 and Metaformer-M36) we can see a similar trend. The CNN performance drops when adding Roto-Convs by about 4% points for microscopy data and ultrasound/X-ray for correctly oriented test data, but improves substantially (38% points) for the latter data in case of flipping and rotation.

[2] `https://github.com/mattiaspaul/RotoMetaFormer`

Metaformer models always benefit from the added invariance, 4% points for the easier data and 22% points for misoriented X-ray and ultrasound.

Finally, we explored also the DermaMNIST dataset, where the orientation of skin photographs is largely arbitrary. Here the benefits within the MetaFormer architecture were most striking. For both unexpected and normal input the Roto-MetaFormer-S12 variant outperformed the baseline by at least 10% points F1 score (achieved score is 54%), highlighting the benefit of our approach as a useful inductive bias even without the robustness concern.

The ResNet model comprises 99% of its multiply-add operations (MADs) without convolutional layers, that means a Roto-ResNet octuples the computational complexity. For MetaFormers only 12.7% of MADs are used for convolutional patch merging, wheras the majority of 87% is found in the MLPs of the PoolFormer or Transformer blocks without need to adapt them for invariance. Hence the new models require less than double the computation.

4 Discussion

In this work, we demonstrated convincing first experimental results for the reconsideration of spatial convolutions and positional encodings that break inherent invariance against rotation and flipping of deep learning models for biomedical images. In particular for transformer models replacing convolutional patch merging with Roto-CNNs is always recommendable based on our findings and could lead to the avoidance of misinterpretation of unexpected input images. Future work should consider extending the concepts to 3D and explore further tasks besides classification. A limitation of our study is that we did not consider test-time augmentation as e.g. done within the nnU-

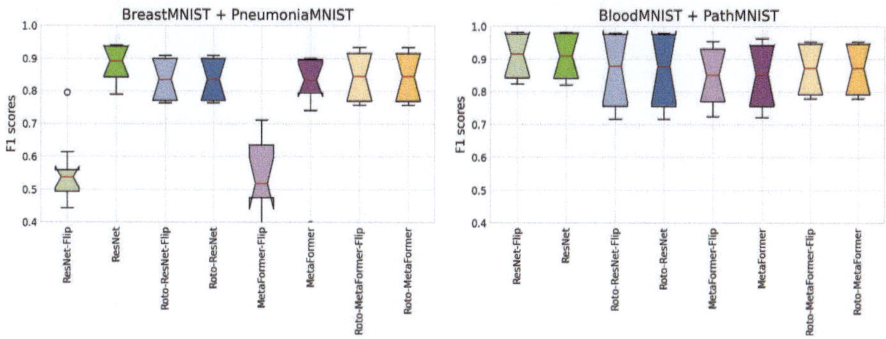

Fig. 2. Statistics over 5 runs each for two pooled datasets comparing the following methods: ■ ResNet-18, ■ Roto-ResNet-18, ■ MetaFormer-S12, ■ Roto-MetaFormer-S12. Lighter colors identify experiments where the input orientation differs during testing. For BreastMNIST and PneumoniaMNIST the advantages of invariance of the models are very clear. Whereas the improvement for Roto-MetaFormer on the microscopy domains is more subtle (+2% F1 score) and the Roto-ResNet deteriorates compared to its baseline.

Net segmentation framework [10]. This could provide a complementary path for more robustness at the expense of prolonged inference.

References

1. Lafarge MW, Bekkers EJ, Pluim JP et al. Roto-translation equivariant convolutional networks: application to histopathology image analysis. Med Image Anal. 2021;68:101849.
2. Weihsbach C, Hansen L, Heinrich M. XEdgeConv: leveraging graph convolutions for efficient, permutation-and rotation-invariant dense 3D medical image segmentation. Proc Geom Deep Learn Med Image Anal. 2022;194:61–71.
3. Dosovitskiy A, Beyer L, Kolesnikov A et al. An image is worth 16x16 words: transformers for image recognition at scale. Proc ICLR. 2020.
4. Xie E, Wang W, Yu Z et al. SegFormer: simple and efficient design for semantic segmentation with transformers. Adv Neural Inf Process Syst. 2021;34:12077–90.
5. Yu W, Luo M, Zhou P et al. Metaformer is actually what you need for vision. Proc IEEE CVF CVPR. 2022:10819–29.
6. Urban G, Geras KJ, Kahou SE et al. Do deep convolutional nets really need to be deep and convolutional? Proc ICLR. 2022.
7. Graham S, Epstein D, Rajpoot N. Dense steerable filter cnns for exploiting rotational symmetry in histology images. IEEE Trans Med Imaging. 2020;39(12):4124–36.
8. He K, Zhang X, Ren S et al. Deep residual learning for image recognition. Proc IEEE CVPR. 2016:770–8.
9. Yang J, Shi R, Wei D et al. Medmnist v2-a large-scale lightweight benchmark for 2d and 3d biomedical image classification. Sci Data. 2023;10(1):41.
10. Isensee F, Jaeger PF, Kohl SA et al. nnU-Net: a self-configuring method for deep learning-based biomedical image segmentation. Nat Methods. 2021;18(2):203–11.

Abstract: Evaluating the Explainability of Attributes and Prototypes for a Medical Classification Model

Luisa Gallée[1], Catharina S. Lisson[2], Christoph G. Lisson[2], Daniela Drees[2], Felix Weig[2], Daniel Vogele[2], Meinrad Beer[2,3], Michael Götz[1,3]

[1]Experimental Radiology, Ulm University Medical Center, Germany
[2]Department of Diagnostic and Interventional Radiology, Ulm University Medical Center, Germany
[3]i2SouI - Innovative Imaging in Surgical Oncology Ulm, Ulm University Medical Center, Germany

luisa.gallee@uni-ulm.de

Due to the sensitive nature of medicine, it is particularly important and highly demanded that AI methods are explainable. This need has been recognised and there is great research interest in xAI solutions with medical applications. However, there is a lack of user-centred evaluation regarding the actual impact of the explanations. We evaluate attribute- and prototype-based explanations with the Proto-Caps model [1]. This xAI model reasons the target classification with human-defined visual features of the target object in the form of scores and attribute-specific prototypes. The model thus provides a multimodal explanation that is intuitively understandable to humans thanks to predefined attributes. A user study [2] involving six radiologists shows that the explanations are subjectivly perceived as helpful, as they reflect their decision-making process. The results of the model are considered a second opinion that radiologists can discuss using the model's explanations. It was shown that the inclusion and increased magnitude of model explanations objectively can increase confidence in the model's predictions when the model is incorrect. In terms of diagnostic performance, this led to increased acceptance of the model prediction. When the model prediction was correct, this had a positive effect, whereas overconfidence in the model led to a decrease in diagnostic performance when the model was incorrect. We can conclude that attribute scores and visual prototypes enhance confidence in the model. Nevertheless, further developments of the explainable models and user studies are necessary to adapt the explanation to the specific use case, thereby ensuring that the model predictions and explanations are genuinely beneficial.

References

1. Gallée L, Beer M, Götz M. Interpretable medical image classification using prototype learning and privileged information. Proc MICCAI. 2023:435–45.
2. Gallée L, Lisson CS, Lisson CG et al. Evaluating the explainability of attributes and prototypes for a medical classification model. Proc XAI. 2024:43–56.

C. Palm et al. (Hrsg.), *Bildverarbeitung für die Medizin 2025*, Informatik aktuell,
https://doi.org/10.1007/978-3-658-47422-5_17

Evaluating the Fidelity of Explanations for Convolutional Neural Networks in Alzheimer's Disease Detection

Bjarne C. Hiller[1], Sebastian Bader[1], Devesh Singh[2], Thomas Kirste[1], Martin Becker[1], Martin Dyrba[2]

[1]Institute of Visual and Analytic Computing, University of Rostock, Germany
[2]German Center for Neurodegenerative Diseases (DZNE), Rostock, Germany
bjarne.hiller@uni-rostock.de

Abstract. The black-box nature of deep learning still prevents its widespread clinical use due to the high risk of hidden biases and prediction errors. Over the last decade, various explanation methods have been proposed to reveal the latent mechanisms of neural networks and support their decisions. However, interpreting the explanations themselves can be challenging, and there is still little consensus on how to evaluate the quality of explanations. To investigate the fidelity of explanations provided by prominent feature attribution methods for Convolutional Neural Networks in Alzheimer's Disease (AD) detection, this paper applies relevance-guided perturbation to the Magnetic Resonance Imaging (MRI) input images. According to the fidelity metric, the AD class probability showed the steepest decline when the perturbation was guided by Integrated Gradients or DeepLift. We conclude by highlighting the role of the reference image in feature attribution with regard to AD detection from MRI images. The source code for the experiments is publicly available on GitHub at `https://github.com/bckrlab/ad-fidelity`.

1 Introduction

Deep learning methods achieved accuracy levels comparable to human experts in many image analysis tasks and therefore possess the potential to support physicians in the evaluation of medical images. However, due to their vast number of parameters, neural networks are considered to be black boxes and reliability concerns prevent their use in high-risk environments such as clinical settings. For instance, Tinauer et al. showed that deep learning models for detecting Alzheimer's Disease (AD) from Magnetic Resonance Imaging (MRI) scans relied on artifacts outside the brain parenchyma that have been introduced by the skull-stripping preprocessing step [1]. To reveal and verify how deep neural networks arrive at decisions, *post hoc explanation methods* have been proposed in the field of eXplainable Artificial Intelligence (XAI). Many of the available post hoc explanation methods rely on so-called *local feature attribution*: given an input, the model and the corresponding model output, the explanation method assigns a distinct relevance score to each input feature that describes its contribution to the output. For example, when considering a convolutional neural network (CNN) for AD detection, each voxel in the volumetric MRI input image would receive a relevance score, resulting in a 3-dimensional heatmap that highlights brain structures deemed relevant for the classification.

C. Palm et al. (Hrsg.), *Bildverarbeitung für die Medizin 2025*, Informatik aktuell,
https://doi.org/10.1007/978-3-658-47422-5_18

However, different attribution-based explanation methods generate different explanations, and there is still little consensus within the eXplainable Artificial Intelligence (XAI) community on what constitutes a good explanation. Arun et al. compared popular feature attribution methods on radiology datasets regarding four main criteria, of which each considered method failed at least one [2]. In the context of detecting AD from MRI, Eitel, Ritter investigated the robustness of relevance maps across several identically trained classifiers, showing varying degrees of coherence depending on the selected feature attribution method [3]. Dyrba et al. provided a visual comparison of popular feature attribution methods [4]. Differences in the quality of relevance maps were pointed out but mostly evaluated based on the perceived concentration of relevance matching a priori known brain regions from the literature such as the hippocampus. Leonardsen et al. validated the relevance maps by comparing them against a ground truth reference map and performing a perturbation test, where parts of the image were iteratively occluded according to their importance [5]. However, only one feature attribution method, i.e., layerwise relevance propagation (LRP), was considered.

In this study, we use relevance-guided perturbation to compare the fidelity of prominent feature attribution methods regarding their explanations of a CNN classifier for detecting AD from MRI images.

2 Materials and methods

We used data provided by the Alzheimer's Disease Neuro-Iniative (ADNI), containing $N = 443$ T1-weighted images from subjects diagnosed with Alzheimer's Disease (AD = 189) and Cognitively Normal controls (CN = 254). MRI preprocessing was carried out using the CAT12 toolbox in MATLAB and included skull stripping, tissue segmentation to yield the gray matter maps, as well as high-dimensional non-linear registration to the MNI reference space. To reduce dimensionality, gray matter images were cropped to $100 \times 120 \times 100$ voxels. Additionally, intensities have been standardized regarding the mean and variance of all voxels in the training dataset. During training, data augmentation methods have been applied to compensate for the small size of the dataset, including random translations as well as reflections along the sagittal plane.

The architecture of the CNN with three 3D convolutional blocks and three fully connected layers as displayed in Fig. 1 was adapted from Dyrba et al. [6] and implemented in PyTorch. A stratified 5-fold cross-validation scheme was used to estimate generalization ability and evaluate the robustness of feature attribution maps. Models

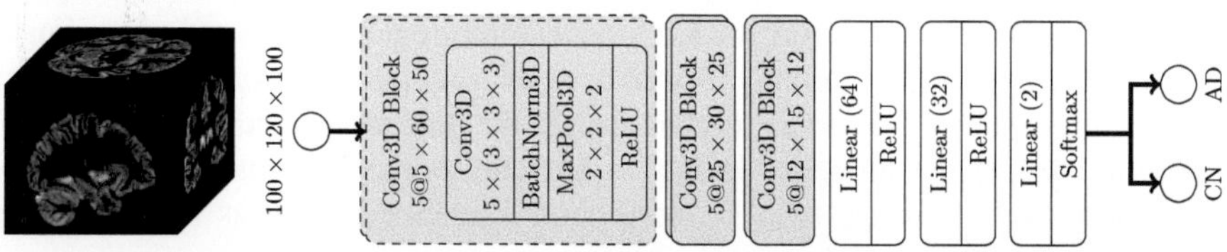

Fig. 1. Architecture of the CNN classifier.

have been trained for 30 epochs each with a batch size of 16. As optimizer, Adam was selected using a learning rate of 10^{-3} and a weight decay of 10^{-3}. The best-performing model from the 5-fold cross-validation was selected for further investigation.

We considered the feature attribution methods occlusion, deconvolution, Saliency Maps, guided backpropagation, Grad-CAM, Input∗Gradient, LRP, Integrated Gradients (IG), DeepLIFT, and DeepSHAP. Since attributions are often generally referred to as saliency maps, we will use the term *relevance maps* to avoid confusion with the original method. For comparison, we also included a random baseline, sampling relevance maps from $\mathcal{N}(0, 1)$. Implementations of the explanation methods have been provided by *Captum* (version 0.6). For an overview of feature attribution algorithms and corresponding references, we refer to captum's documentation [1]. Relevance maps have been computed for all AD instances in the test data set regarding the output probability of target class AD. Some of the feature attribution methods allow the user to provide a *reference image*, resulting in explanations of the relative change in model output with regard to input and reference. For methods that allowed the use of a reference image, the *null image* (all intensities set to 0) as well as the mean of all CN instances was used. Only DeepSHAP received 20 random reference images sampled from the standard normal distribution $\mathcal{N}(0, 1)$ since the method approximates Shapley values by averaging over multiple baselines. For Occlusion, a relatively large window of $20\times20\times20$ voxels and a step size of 10 voxels were selected. This compromise between the resolution of Occlusion's relevance maps and computation time was necessary since the algorithm's time complexity is cubic in step size for 3D images. Regarding Saliency Maps, the signed gradient instead of the absolute gradient was used, allowing a more detailed interpretation. As usual, Grad-CAM was applied to the model's third and final convolutional layer and configured to keep negative attributions.

In the absence of ground truth explanations, perturbation-based metrics present an objective, model-agnostic, and straightforward option to evaluate the performance of feature attribution methods: Input features are perturbed in order of their attributed relevance to observe the change in model output. Intuitively, when comparing two relevance maps, the one with a more rapid change in model output appears to more accurately capture the model's underlying logic, since the model reacts more sensitive to the features with high attribution. Petsiuk, Das, Saenko presented two formalized fidelity metrics referred to as *deletion* and *insertion*, which represent the area under the class probability curve obtained by iteratively masking or revealing parts of the image according to their relevance [7]. To compare popular feature attribution methods, we performed a perturbation test similar to the deletion metric: For all AD instances in the test data set, voxel intensities were iteratively replaced with a constant value in descending order of their relevance, until 5% (60,000 voxels) of the MRI image was masked in total – for illustration, the left hippocampus region consists of approximately 1,000 voxels in the data. Initially, 0 was used as a replacement value, aligning with the null image that was used as a reference for the attribution methods. For methods supporting an explicit reference image for attribution, the perturbation was repeated using the mean CN image both for attribution reference as well as for perturbation replacement.

[1] `https://captum.ai/docs/attribution_algorithms`

3 Results

During the 5-fold cross-validation, the CNN models achieved a mean Area under the Operator Receiver Curve (AUROC) score of 0.95 ± 0.02 on the test datasets for the binary AD vs CN classification task. The best-performing model achieved an AUROC of 0.97 and an accuracy of 87% on the respective test dataset. Therefore, it was selected to compute the feature attribution.

Fig. 2 shows the mean relevance maps regarding the target class AD and a null reference for all AD instances in the test dataset. From visual inspection of the generated relevance maps, the feature attribution methods seem to generally agree on the brain structures that are utilized by the model for AD detection. Most methods highlighted the hippocampal area, which is especially affected by AD and the most utilized neuroimaging marker in AD diagnosis. Other brain regions highlighted by the feature attribution methods included the amygdala and thalamus, as well as the temporal and frontal lobe, and to a smaller degree the cerebellum. Therefore, the model appears to have learned reasonable disease patterns for classification. The gradient- and backpropagation-based approaches like IG, LRP, and DeepLIFT produce visually similar mean relevance maps. However, like previous work, we also notice differences regarding the resolution and focus of the attribution. Most noticeable for Saliency Maps, the attribution appears to have noise-like characteristics. The low resolution of Occlusion and Grad-CAM might explain their non-zero relevance attribution to locations outside the brain.

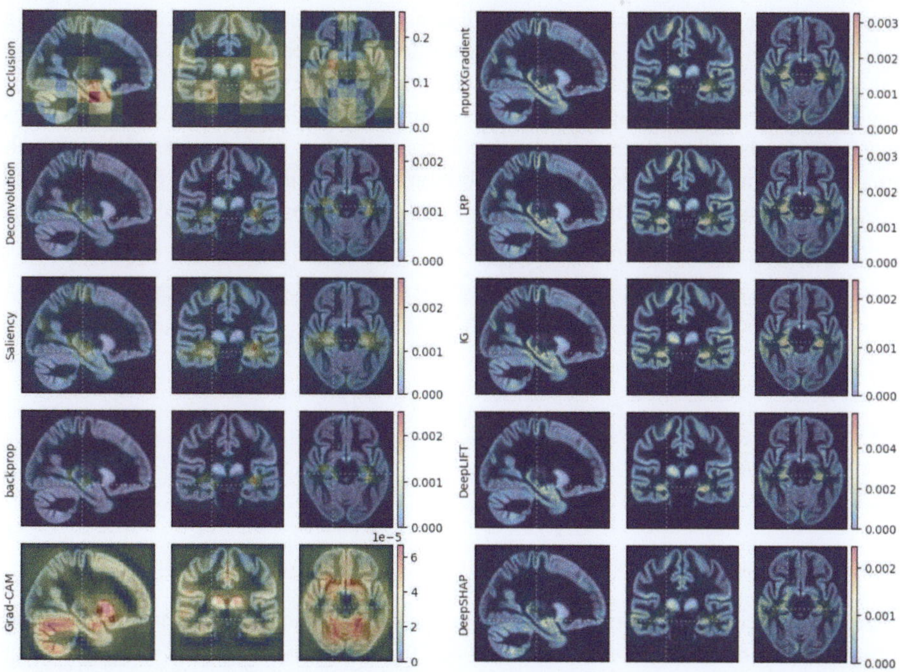

Fig. 2. Mean absolute AD relevance maps for all AD instances in the test set using a null reference.

The result of the relevance-guided perturbation is displayed in Fig. 3. As expected, random perturbation did not alter the class probabilities. However, when using a null reference for attribution and perturbation (Fig. 3a), most methods also fail to decrease the AD class probability. A possible explanation might be that the model learned to associate AD with atrophy patterns. Since perturbing the input image with the null reference artificially introduces more atrophy, flipping the predicted class label from AD to CN by perturbation might be challenging. Just DeepSHAP manages to rapidly decrease class probability, probably due to being the only attribution method to average over multiple random baselines. More meaningful attributions can be achieved using the CN mean image for attribution and perturbation (Fig. 3b). Although the relevance maps visually appear quite similar, the perturbation test shows that there are differences in the fidelity of each method regarding the considered model. Occlusion appears to result in a linear decay of class probability. Notably, for the other investigated methods, we observed an exponential decay with the predicted class label starting to flip from AD to CN when approximately 2% of the voxels were perturbed.

4 Discussion

Although feature attribution methods are intended to enable the interpretation of black-box models, the interpretation of the relevance maps themselves can be challenging. One of the most important aspects to consider is the choice of an appropriate reference image. While some methods, such as Occlusion or IG, explicitly allow the selection of a reference image, others, such as Input$*$Gradient, can be interpreted as implicitly using a null image as a baseline. Relevance scores must always be interpreted with respect to the selected reference image, as it allows an almost arbitrary manipulation of relevance scores. In particular, taking the reference image into account can explain attributions that would otherwise appear confusing or contradictory. For example, when a null image is used as a reference, feature attribution methods such as occlusion may assign a negative contribution to the AD class to the hippocampal region even for AD data,

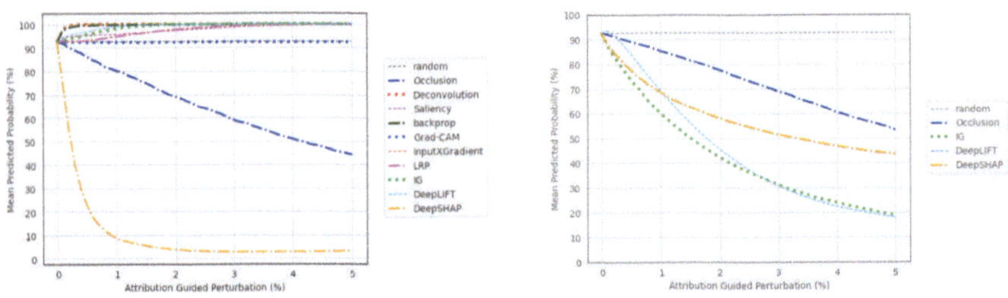

(**a**) Null reference. (**b**) Mean CN reference.

Fig. 3. Relevance-guided perturbation for AD instances in the test dataset for different reference images. 3a: Notably, for the null reference image, most methods fail to decrease the AD class probability. 3b: When using the mean CN image for reference and/or replacement, AD class probability decreases.

even though the hippocampus is used as a (positive) AD marker. This happens because in the null reference, all signals in the hippocampus are zeroed out, so it corresponds to maximizing atrophy patterns in an unnatural way, and thus receives an even higher AD class probability prediction than the original input, as visible in the upper part of Fig. 3a. Therefore, we found the mean image of all CN instances to be a more helpful reference for generating explanations, since it asks the question: „Why was this sample classified as AD compared to a control sample?“

In conclusion, we compared popular feature attribution methods by performing a relevance-guided perturbation, showing differences in fidelity for attributions that otherwise appear to be visually similar and highlighting the same brain regions. From the considered methods, IG and DeepLIFT were found most suited to reflect the regions that influenced the model's decision to predict AD over CN. Finally, we highlighted the need for careful selection of a reference image to align the generated explanation with the intended question. With the correct interpretation, relevance maps can provide key insights to improve Deep Learning classifiers for MRI images. However, without critical reception, relevance maps might create a false sense of transparency.

Acknowledgement. Funding was provided by the BMBF (01IS22077) and DFG (DY151/2-1). Data was provided by the Alzheimer's Disease Neuroimaging Initiative (ADNI)[2].

References

1. Tinauer C, Heber S, Pirpamer L et al. Interpretable brain disease classification and relevance-guided deep learning. Sci Rep. 2022;12(1):20254.
2. Arun N, Gaw N, Singh P et al. Assessing the trustworthiness of saliency maps for localizing abnormalities in medica imaging. Radiol: Artif Intell. 2021;3(6):e200267.
3. Eitel F, Ritter K. Testing the robustness of attribution methods for CNNs in MRI-based Alzheimer's disease classification. Proc MICCAI. 2019;11797:3–11.
4. Dyrba M, Pallath AH, Marzban EN. Comparison of CNN visualization methods to aid model interpretability for detecting Alzheimer's disease. Proc BVM. 2020:307–12.
5. Leonardsen EH, Persson K, Grødem E et al. Constructing personalized characterizations of structural brain aberrations in patients with dementia using explainable artificial intelligence. NPJ Digit Med. 2024;7(1):1–14.
6. Dyrba M, Hanzig M, Altenstein S et al. Improving 3D convolutional neural network comprehensibility via interactive visualization of relevance maps: evaluation in Alzheimer's disease. Alzheimers Res Ther. 2021;13(1):191.
7. Petsiuk V, Das A, Saenko K. RISE: randomized input sampling for explanation of black-box models. arXiv: 1806.07421. 2018.

[2] `https://adni.loni.usc.edu/`

Abstract: Metrics Reloaded

Recommendations and Online Toolkit for Image Analysis Validation

Emre Kavur[1,2], Metrics Reloaded Consortium[3], Lena Maier-Hein[‡1,4], Annika Reinke[‡1]

[1]German Cancer Research Center (DKFZ) Heidelberg, Division of Intelligent Medical Systems & Helmholtz Imaging, Germany
[2]DKFZ Heidelberg, Division Medical Image Computing, Germany
[3]Full author list and affiliations can be found in [1]
[4]National Center for Tumor Diseases (NCT), NCT Heidelberg, Germany
a.reinke@dkfz-heidelberg.de

Increasing evidence shows that flaws in machine learning (ML) algorithm validation are an underestimated global problem. Particularly in automatic biomedical image analysis, chosen performance metrics often do not reflect the domain of interest, thus failing to adequately measure scientific progress and hindering translation of ML techniques into practice. To overcome this, we created Metrics Reloaded, a comprehensive framework guiding researchers in the problem-aware selection of metrics. It was developed by a large international consortium in a multi-stage Delphi process and is based on the novel concept of a problem fingerprint – a structured representation of the given problem that captures all aspects that are relevant for metric selection, from the domain interest to the properties of the target structure(s), data set and algorithm output. Based on the problem fingerprint, users are guided through the process of choosing and applying appropriate validation metrics, while being made aware of potential pitfalls. Metrics Reloaded targets image analysis problems that can be interpreted as a classification task at image, object or pixel level, namely image-level classification, object detection, semantic segmentation, and instance segmentation tasks. The selection of appropriate validation metrics with consideration of all potential pitfalls can be complex. The complexity partly arises from the need to capture all possibilities at once in the figures and decision trees. Many figures could, e.g., be greatly simplified for two-class problems. To leverage this potential and to improve the general user experience with our framework, we developed the Metrics Reloaded online tool[1]. The tool captures our framework in a user-centric manner and can serve as a trustworthy common access point for image analysis validation. Following the convergence of ML methodology across application domains, Metrics Reloaded fosters the convergence of validation methodology. Its applicability is demonstrated for various biomedical use cases [1].

References

1. Maier-Hein L, Reinke A, Godau P et al. Metrics reloaded: recommendations for image analysis validation. Nat Methods. 2024;21(2):195–212.

[‡]These authors contributed equally the least to this work.
[1]https://metrics-reloaded.dkfz.de/

C. Palm et al. (Hrsg.), *Bildverarbeitung für die Medizin 2025*, Informatik aktuell,
https://doi.org/10.1007/978-3-658-47422-5_19

Real-time Landmark Guidance for Radial Head Localization in Ultrasound Imaging

Lennart Meyling[1,2], Christoph Großbröhmer[2], Jürgen Lichtenstein[3], Mattias P. Heinrich[2], Lasse Hansen[1]

[1]EchoScout GmbH, Lübeck
[2]Institute of Medical Informatics, University of Lübeck
[3]Clinic of Oral and Maxillofacial Surgery, UKSH, Kiel, Germany
lennart@meyling.com

Abstract. This work presents a method to enhance radial head localization in ultrasound imaging through landmark-based guidance. We created a dataset of ultrasound images containing three anatomical classes: radius, radial head, and humerus, recorded by an examiner. Using this dataset, we trained an nnU-Net model to perform real-time landmark detection, generating predictions at a rate of 20 frames per second. In two studies, participants without medical training were asked to locate their own radial head using a handheld ultrasound probe, first without guidance and then with visual and textual cues based on the model's real-time segmentation. With this landmark-based guidance, 11 out of 12 participants successfully located the radial head, compared to 6 out of 12 without guidance. These results highlight the potential of landmark guidance to improve accuracy and usability in ultrasound interpretation, making it more accessible to users without medical training.

1 Introduction

Ultrasound imaging offers numerous advantages compared to other medical imaging methods. It exposes neither the subject nor the examiner to ionizing radiation, is cost-effective, can be used in real time, and is highly portable. These attributes make ultrasound an invaluable tool in various clinical settings, from emergency rooms to remote healthcare facilities. However, major drawbacks include low image quality, limited penetration depth, and difficulty in interpretation. Addressing the latter, our research aims to enhance the ability of users to acquire and analyze of ultrasound images, making this technology accessible and easy to use for individuals without specialized medical expertise.

1.1 Related work

Numerous studies have focused on landmark detection in ultrasound images, employing various deep learning architectures, data dimensions, and anatomical targets. Some, such as [1, 2], demonstrate performance on par with medical experts. However, most existing methods lack real-time capability.

For instance, [3] uses a Transformer-Based U-Net to detect landmarks in infant hip ultrasound, leveraging transformer models' ability to capture long-range dependencies

C. Palm et al. (Hrsg.), *Bildverarbeitung für die Medizin 2025*, Informatik aktuell,
https://doi.org/10.1007/978-3-658-47422-5_20

for improved localization accuracy. Similarly, [4] explores lamina landmark detection, demonstrating the feasibility of real-time application, though without evaluating its practical clinical effectiveness. This gap underscores the need for further research on real-time performance in ultrasound landmark detection.

There has also been growing interest in real-time guidance for ultrasound imaging. [5] presents a CNN-based approach for detecting fetal standard views and locating fetal structures with bounding boxes, highlighting the potential for real-time application in clinical ultrasound. [6] addresses anatomical region detection and localization in fetal ultrasound, aiming to provide guidance with image-level labels only. In the field of real-time probe guidance, [7] introduces US-GuideNet, a neural network that offers real-time movement guidance for standard plane acquisition in obstetric ultrasound, evaluated on clinical data from expert sonographers.

While significant advancements have been made, real-time performance in ultrasound-based landmark detection remains a challenge that our work seeks to address.

1.2 Contribution

Our contributions are twofold. First, we conduct a study in which participants are tasked with identifying their own radial head using a handheld ultrasound probe. During this study, we create a dataset recorded by the examiner, specifically focusing on three anatomical classes: the radius, radial head, and humerus (Fig. 2). Second, we utilize this dataset to train a deep learning-based landmark detection model and subsequently evaluate the accuracy improvements in a second study (Fig. 1), where participants are again asked to locate their radial head, this time with the assistance of visual landmark guidance.

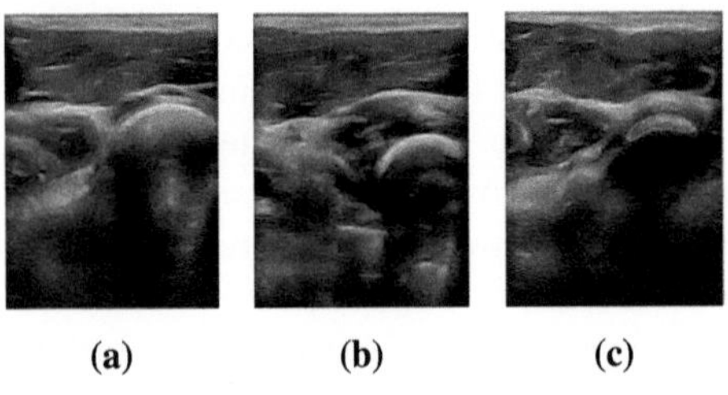

Fig. 1. Examples of the three anatomical classes in the dataset: (a) radial head, (b) radius, and (c) humerus.

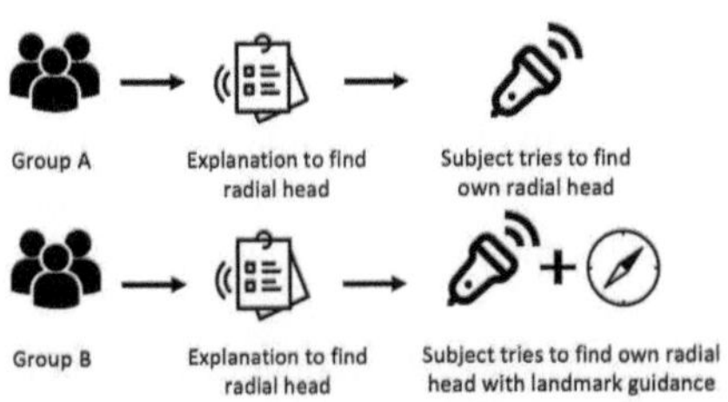

Fig. 2. Study design: Group A follows an unguided approach after receiving an explanation, while Group B uses landmark-based guidance.

2 Materials and methods

For landmark detection, we use the nnU-Net architecture [8], a robust neural network for medical image segmentation. The network is trained to produce segmentation masks that classify each frame into three anatomical classes: radius, radial head, and humerus. Including the humerus as a separate class in training improves the model's ability to distinguish it from the radial head, as they appear visually similar in ultrasound images. We opted for a 2D version of the nnU-Net with ultrasound images downsampled to half-resolution, balancing segmentation accuracy with computational efficiency.

The nnU-Net model was trained on manually annotated ultrasound images, with normalization applied to scale pixel values to a range of [0,1]. During inference, each image is horizontally flipped to create a mirrored pair for each frame. Both the original and flipped image are input to the model, and the final class is determined by applying an argmax over the combined predictions. Model performance during training was monitored using the Dice score.

To improve detection of the radial head, we balanced class distributions in the dataset and adjusted class weights in the Generalized Dice Loss (GDL) function to reduce class imbalance.

To capture temporal context, we experimented with 3D configurations of UNet, testing stacks of 8, 12, and 16 slices. While the 3D models showed potential for improved accuracy, they required significantly higher computational resources, limiting their suitability for real-time guidance. For a balance between performance and real-time capability, we ultimately selected a 2D UNet model, achieving temporal consistency by averaging predictions over the last 25 frames. With each new frame, the average is updated, and the system assigns the most frequently predicted class to provide stable positional feedback.

The guidance workflow begins with the user positioning their arm flat on a table and placing the probe on the radius. The system captures 25 frames per second, generating predictions for 20 frames per second, and displays a segmentation overlay along with text prompts. The user is instructed to move the probe upward, receiving cues to start recording (on the radius), stop (just beyond the radial head), or start again at the radius if the humerus is detected. The guidance process is illustrated in Fig. 3.

2.1 Data

Our dataset comprises ultrasound images of three manually labeled anatomical classes: the radius, radial head, and humerus, collected from 12 subjects. Each image was captured at a resolution of 800×611 pixels and a frame rate of 25 fps using a handheld ultrasound probe. Frames were annotated by medical experts with over three years of experience. On average, each subject contributed approximately 400 frames, yielding a total of 4800 frames, with 400 frames of the radial head, 300 frames of the humerus, and 3000 frames of the radius. The models were trained using 5-fold cross-validation, and two recordings were designated as a test set for performance evaluation.

2.2 Implementation details

For landmark detection, multiple configurations of the nnU-Net model were trained, including 2D slices at the original resolution of 800×611 pixels, a downsampled version at 384×320, and a 3D version using stacks of 8 to 16 slices to capture temporal information. Training was conducted in PyTorch, and models were subsequently converted to Swift for deployment on Apple devices with ARM processors. The entire guidance software, including model inference, was implemented in Swift to enhance performance across devices, with optimization for tablets to improve visualization and user interaction. The downsampled 2D model was selected for real-time applications, balancing computational efficiency with detection accuracy.

3 Results

In the unguided study, non-medical students were instructed to perform self-recordings by locating their own radial head using the ultrasound probe on their own arm. After viewing a video tutorial, they were directed to position the probe on the radius, move it slowly upwards, and stop the recording once the radial head was just out of view. No assistance was provided by the examiner, and the self-recorded images were later evaluated by a medical professional to assess accuracy.

In the guided study, non-medical students followed a protocol with real-time assistance provided by the trained landmark detection model (Fig. 2). After locating the radius, subjects received on-screen prompts to adjust the probe's position based on model guidance, facilitating accurate localization of the radial head. The effectiveness of both the self-directed and guided approaches were evaluated by a medical professional to compare accuracy, usability, and consistency across participants.

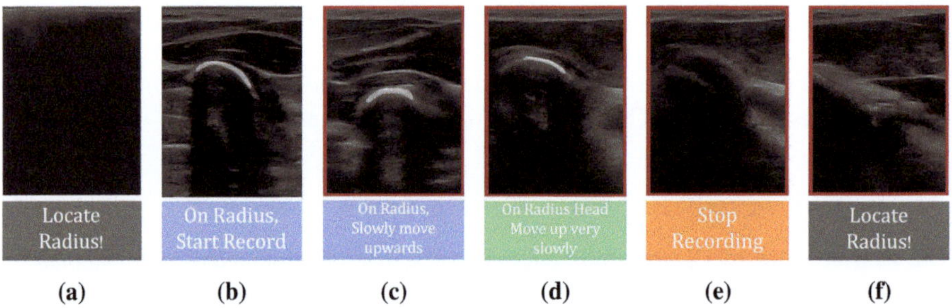

Fig. 3. Step-by-step guidance for locating the radial head during ultrasound imaging. The sequence begins with locating the radius (a), initiating recording (b), and gradually moving the probe upward (c). Upon reaching the radial head, the probe movement is slowed (d), and recording stops once the radial head is no longer visible (e). If the probe moves too far, the user is prompted to re-locate the radius (f). During the process, the user sees the live ultrasound image with a textual cue displayed at the bottom to assist with each step.

3.1 Study

Landmark guidance improved participants' ability to locate and pause at the radial head, while reducing task time. We evaluated performance using three metrics:

- *Time Taken*, defined as the duration of each recording in seconds, measured the time participants needed to locate the radial head and correctly complete the task.
- *Radius Head Found* indicates whether participants successfully located the radial head at least once during the recording, confirming its visibility in the ultrasound.
- *Correctly Paused* represents whether participants accurately paused the recording at the precise moment when the radial head was just out of view, assessing their adherence to the task instructions.

The results for these metrics are illustrated in Fig. 4, which shows that guided participants had higher success rates in locating and pausing at the radial head while also completing the task in less time.

3.2 Model performance

Tab. 1 presents the macro and radial head Dice scores across different nnU-Net configurations, with the 3D nnU-Net 12 slices achieving the highest overall scores. Meanwhile, Fig. 5 illustrates the trade-off between accuracy (detection rate of the radial head) and inference time. Notably, the 2D small configuration achieves an inference time of 0.045 seconds, making it well-suited for real-time applications despite its slightly lower accuracy compared to the 3D configurations. This combination of accuracy and speed highlights the balance between configurations based on application needs.

4 Discussion

Our results demonstrate the significant potential of ultrasound imaging when combined with landmark-based guidance, particularly in addressing challenges related to its interpretability from unexperienced users. By improving the accuracy and efficiency with

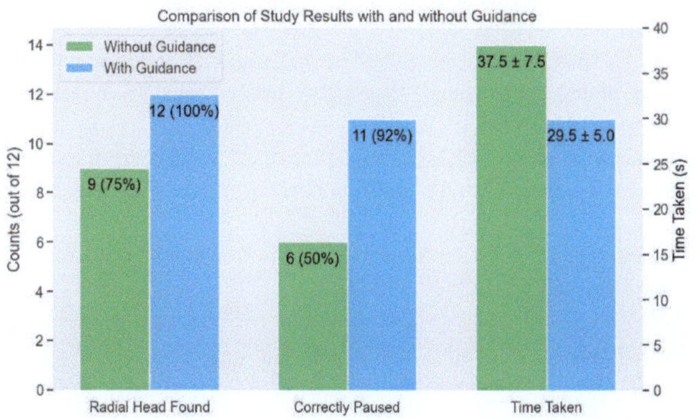

Fig. 4. Comparison of study results with and without guidance, showing the number of participants who located the radial head, paused correctly, and the average time taken (± standard deviation).

Config	Dice	$Dice_{R Head}$
2D small	0.64±0.049	0.76±0.031
2D original	0.68±0.041	0.78±0.026
3D 8 slices	0.69±0.028	0.79±0.022
3D 12 slices	0.71±0.023	0.81±0.022
3D 16 slices	0.68±0.062	0.78±0.032

Tab. 1. Dice scores across different configurations.

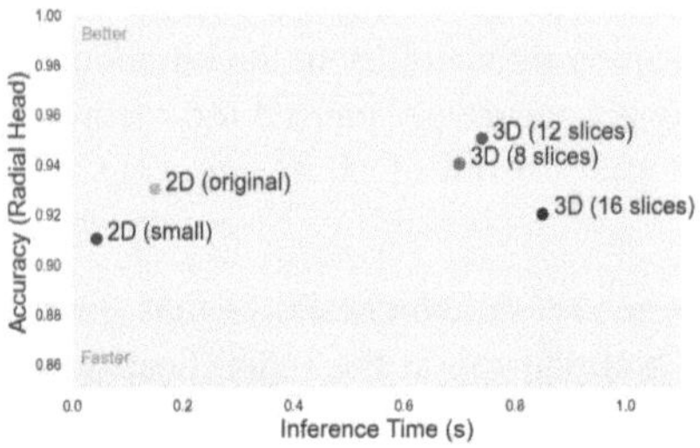

Fig. 5. Performance vs. inference time for various configurations, highlighting the trade-off between accuracy and speed.

which users can locate anatomical structures, our approach shows that the inherent complexities of ultrasound interpretation can be mitigated. This study highlights the feasibility of enhancing user guidance in real-time, making ultrasound more accessible and effective even for individuals without medical training. Future work will focus on refining model accuracy and expanding guidance systems to additional anatomical targets.

References

1. Xu Z, Huo Y, Park J et al. Less is more: simultaneous view classification and landmark detection for abdominal ultrasound images. Proc MICCAI. 2018:711–9.
2. Tuysuzoglu A, Tan J, Eissa K et al. Deep adversarial context-aware landmark detection for ultrasound imaging. Proc MICCAI. 2018:151–8.
3. Huang T, Shi J, Li J et al. Involution transformer based U-Net for landmark detection in ultrasound images for diagnosis of infantile DDH. IEEE J Biomed Health Inform. 2024;28(8):4797–809.
4. Li S, Gauthier L, Cheriet F et al. Lamina landmark detection in ultrasound images: a preliminary study. Proc SPIE. 2023:10.
5. Baumgartner CF, Kamnitsas K, Matthew J et al. SonoNet: real-time detection and localisation of fetal standard scan planes in freehand ultrasound. IEEE Trans Med Imaging. 2017;36(11):2204–15.
6. Toussaint N, Khanal B, Sinclair M et al. Weakly supervised localisation for fetal ultrasound images. Deep learning in medical image analysis and multimodal learning for clinical decision support. 2018:192–200.
7. Droste R, Drukker L, Papageorghiou AT et al. Automatic probe movement guidance for freehand obstetric ultrasound. Proc MICCAI. 2020:583–92.
8. Isensee F, Jaeger PF, Kohl SAA et al. nnU-Net: a self-configuring method for deep learning-based biomedical image segmentation. Nat Methods. 2020;18(2):203–11.

Ultrasound-based 3D Reconstruction of Residual Limbs using Electromagnetic Tracking

Pauline Heine[1], Luise Robra[1], Jan Komposch[2], Janis Börsig[2], Jonas Bornmann[3], Andreas Leiniger[3], Rainer Brucher[1], Alfred M. Franz[1,2,4]

[1]Institute for Medical Engineering and Mechatronics, Ulm University of Applied Sciences
[2]Institute for Computer Science, Ulm University of Applied Sciences, Germany
[3]Ottobock SE & Co. KGaA, Duderstadt
[4]Division of Intelligent Medical Systems, German Cancer Research Center (DKFZ), Heidelberg
paulineheine@gmx.de

Abstract. When manufacturing leg prostheses, accurate measurement of the geometry of residual limbs is essential. Conventionally, this is done using plaster casts or optical scanners. Ultrasound (US) appears to be a promising complementary method, as it can be used to scan internal structures such as bone and muscle tissue. In this paper, we demonstrate the feasibility of 3D reconstruction of skin surface and bone of an residual limb phantom using a US probe placed on the skin and localized by electromagnetic tracking. Different movement trajectories were investigated in order to capture as much of the limb as possible. Compared to a computed tomography (CT) reference image, a mean error of 2.3 mm was measured at 23 points distributed on the skin surface, while a mean error of 4.7 mm (n=20) was determined for the bone geometry.

1 Introduction

Approximately 150,000 amputees in Germany live with a leg prosthesis, restoring their mobility, gaining independence and increasing self-esteem [1]. Proper socket design is crucial to establish an optimal connection between prosthesis and body. Therefore, a 3D-model is required and the limb's anatomical characteristics must also be taken into account [2]. Conventional methods include plaster casting, manual measurements and optical 3D scanning [3]. While plaster casting is manual and subjective, optical scanning requires free line of sight and patient movements can disrupt image capture [4]. Both methods exclusively measure the surface geometry of the limb. Research is therefore investigating new quantitative and reproducible procedures capable of capturing the geometry as well as the limb musculature and tissue inhomogeneity [1].

Related work to create a 3D-model visualizing external and internal structures typically involves computed tomography (CT) or magnetic resonance imaging (MRI). Despite their advantages in depicting bones and soft tissues, these methods have drawbacks, including high costs, ionizing radiation and are not available throughout different healthcare systems [5]. In addition, the examination is performed with the patient lying down, which changes the natural shape of the residual limb [1, 4]. The detection of limb geometry using ultrasound (US) has been researched as well. For example, the skin surface was scanned, although from the outside through the air [6], and the geometry was measured [4, 7]. In another related study, US was used in a water bath [1]. However,

C. Palm et al. (Hrsg.), *Bildverarbeitung für die Medizin 2025*, Informatik aktuell,
https://doi.org/10.1007/978-3-658-47422-5_21

disadvantages are a complex and bulky setup of water bath and US probe as well as decreased image quality caused by signal attenuation and limb movements. It would be simpler than the setups mentioned to place the US probe directly on the skin as is usual with other US examinations. Compared to conventional methods, this approach could simplify, standardize and make the measurement process more objective while also allowing for the detection of internal structures. Additionally, the use of US is much cheaper than CT or MRI, is radiation-free and commonly available. [5]

In a previous study [8], we showed feasibility of detecting skin surface and bone of a limb phantom using an US probe placed on the skin. The probe was rotated using a mechanical device and only part of the limb was inspected. Free movement of the US probe on the skin would be necessary to maintain the flexibility of classic US examinations on the one hand and to collect information from several insonation points to reconstruct the entire residual limb on the other. A well-researched option for 3D reconstruction using a freely movable US probe is the use of a tracking system to localize the US probe, also known as tracked US [9]. Electromagnetic (EM) tracking is particularly suitable as it enables probe localization without requiring a line of sight and offers compact sensor integration. Note at this point that there are also other approaches for 3D US scans such as motorized probes or matrix array transducers. However, in these cases, only a partial reconstruction from a single insonation position is performed. For a complete scene, scans from several insonation positions would have to be combined, for example again with tracked US. While promising, artificial intelligence (AI) based approaches that attempt to do this (e.g., [10]) face challenges such as variability in data quality and generalizability, which may limit their current application for residual limbs.

Therefore, the objective of this study is to use tracked US to reconstruct skin and bone in an residual limb phantom in 3D. The goal is to find the best possible way to 3D reconstruct and then compare the final reconstruction with reference measurements in terms of its accuracy.

2 Methods

2.1 System setup and calibration

The tracked US system for 3D reconstruction, systematically shown in Fig. 1, integrates a GE Logiq P5 US device (GE HealthCare Technologies, Chicago, USA) with a GE 3S phased array transducer to capture the US images of the residual limb's geometry. It uses the NDI (Northern Digital Inc., Waterloo, Canada) Aurora EM tracking system to track the probe in real-time, with a 6 degrees-of-freedom sensor ("Aurora 6DOF Reference", NDI part no.: 610066) attached to the US probe.

The used software includes the Public software Library for Ultrasound Toolkit (PLUS, version 2.8.0.2019-11-05), 3D Slicer (version 5.0.3) and the Medical Imaging Interaction Toolkit (MITK, version v2022.10). The PlusServer application, part of PLUS, acts as the central hub for data flow and synchronization between US device, tracking system and software, handling coordinate transformations and calibration settings. 3D Slicer is used for point-based calibration and allows real-time visualization of US images and tracking data. The Freehand tracked US calibration application (fCal), part of PLUS, captures the US images together with their positional data. PLUS also provides tools for creating a 3D reconstruction from the collected data, while MITK is used to visualize and analyze the final 3D reconstruction.

Before tracking the US probe, calibration is required to determine the ImageToProbe transformation (see Fig. 1b). Point calibration was preferred over N-wire and wall-based methods due to its superior accuracy in our setup. For calibration, the US probe is dipped into a water bath to capture the tip of a tracked pointer, which is also held in the water bath within the imaging area of the probe. The needle tip is manually selected on the US image and its position is recorded in both image and tracking coordinates relative to the sensor attached to the probe. To calculate the ImageToProbe transformation by means of a landmark-based transformation, at least 3 corresponding positions in both coordinate systems are needed. To include redundancy, we selected 9 points evenly distributed over the US image for calibration. The mean Euclidean distance between the pairs of corresponding points after transformation, also referred to as Fiducial Registration Error (FRE), was 3.2 mm in our experiments.

2.2 Residual limb phantom

To simulate residual limb anatomy, a phantom shown in Fig. 2a was used. It was manufactured based on individual specifications by CIRS (Computerized Imaging Reference Systems, Inc., Norfolk, VA, US). The tissue in this phantom is simulated by ATS Urethane with a speed of sound of 1450 m/s. The bone is 3D printed, made from Acrylonitrile Butadiene Styrene (ABS) to provide high sound reflection similar to real bone in tissue. ATS urethane was chosen for its high robustness and durability.

To evaluate the 3D reconstruction, two different references were created. First, a tracked pointer was used to capture points on the skin evenly distributed across the limb by drawing four lines, each with six points, except for one missing point due to the hip bone ($n = 3 \cdot 6 + 1 \cdot 5 = 23$), as shown in Fig. 2b. This allows direct comparison of the 3D reconstructed surface with the skin positions in the same coordinate space. Second, as shown in Fig. 2c and d, a CT reference was used to create 3D models of skin and bone. CT was chosen for its ability to capture internal structures as well.

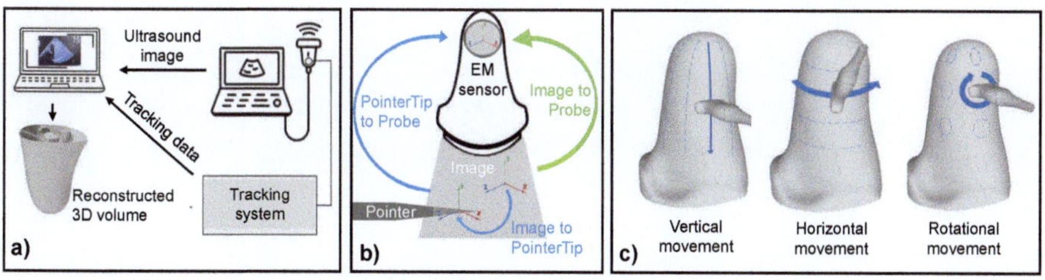

Fig. 1. (a) System setup for 3D reconstruction. (b) Coordinate transformations for point-based calibration. (c) Possible movement types for tracked ultrasound recording of residual limbs. Rotating movements were excluded due to poor results in preliminary tests.

2.3 Reconstruction approach

The proposed approach for 3D reconstruction of a residual limb using tracked US integrates a series of recorded 2D B-mode US images including their pose, recorded by a EM sensor. To create a 3D volume from these 2D US images, we used a volume reconstruction algorithm implemented in PLUS. The following parameters were set to achieve the best reconstruction: *Interpolation* was set to linear, estimating values between the samples data points, providing smoother transitions between slices; *compounding mode* was set to maximum to select the highest value from multiple US images of the same point, improving surface detail accuracy by reducing inconsistencies; *optimization* was set to partial to refine the reconstruction by focusing on the most relevant areas and *hole filling* was enabled to fill holes in the reconstruction. To capture the complete geometry of the residual limb with a freehand-moved US probe, various types of movement were considered. As shown in Fig. 1c, we examined vertical and horizontal movement as well as rotation of the probe. The best results were obtained with a combination of horizontal and vertical movement. For the final reconstruction, we performed 8 vertical movements evenly distributed around the residual limb, from the tip to the hip, and 4 horizontal movements distributed along the length of the limb.

2.4 Evaluation

To evaluate our 3D reconstruction we compared it with both, the tracking reference (just skin) and the CT reference (skin and bone). To account for the difference in speed of sound of the phantom compared to human tissue, the 3D US model was first scaled with a factor of 1450 [m/s] divided by 1540 [m/s] = 0.94156. Afterwards, the skin and bone surface extracted from the CT reference was registered to the US volume by means of a point-based registration, using the three reference fiducials F1-F3 (see Fig. 2). F4 and F5 were not used since only the region below the hip was imaged in US. Beside a 3D visualization of the scene, the average Euclidean distance between the 23 reference points and the US volumes was used as a quantitative measure. Therefore, 23 points

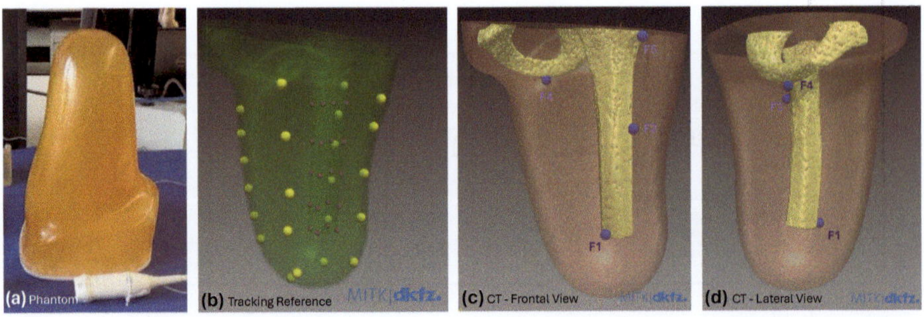

Fig. 2. (a) Residual limb phantom with US probe. (b) Tracking reference acquired in the tracking coordinate space using a tracked pointer. For better overview, the CT reference (transparent green) and the 20 bone reference points (small purple points) are shown as well. (c,d) CT reference including bone and 5 fiducials (F1-F5) visible in CT and US images.

near to the tracking reference were selected on the CT skin surface. In CT, additional 20 reference points were selected on the bone surface. All 23 + 20 = 43 corresponding points were manually selected in the US volume. This leads to 23 distances between tracking reference and US volume as well as 43 distances between CT reference and US volume.

3 Results

Different views on the final scene showing the reconstructed US volume and the registered CT reference are shown in Fig. 3. The average distance of 23 points on skin between CT reference and 3D reconstruction was 2.3 ± 2.3 mm ($\mu \pm \sigma$). Using the tracking reference, we achieved an error of 5.7 ± 3.2 mm. In case of the bone, the distance between 20 points in CT reference and 3D reconstruction was 4.7 ± 4.1 mm. In the spirit of Open Science, we provide the raw US images with XML configurations for reconstruction with PLUS, the 3D reconstructions with registered references and the distance measurements in the Open Science Framework.

4 Discussion and conclusion

In our study we demonstrated 3D reconstruction of a residual limb phantom using US. As shown in Fig. 3, skin and bone are visible in good contrast and the geometry matches the CT reference. An average error of 2.3 ± 2.3 mm (n=23 points) on the skin compared to the CT reference seems promising. When comparing the bone surface from the CT image, the average error is 4.7 ± 4.1 mm (n=20). The higher error of the tracking reference (5.7 ± 3.2 mm, n=23) is possibly caused by the difference in the speed of sound in the phantom (1450 m/s) compared to human tissue (1540 m/s). We therefore had to scale the image (starting from the center of the image), which changed the reference coordinate system. This did not affect the CT reference, as it still had to be registered to the reconstructed 3D volume anyway. We had previously expected the tracking reference to work better, not least because we considered the difference in the speed of sound (approx. 6%) to be negligible. It, however, became apparent that we reached a level of accuracy at which this did have an effect, which is why we corrected the factor after all.

The 3D reconstruction looks promising in most areas of the phantom. Only at the lower, proximal end of the limb phantom the surface could partially not be reconstructed.

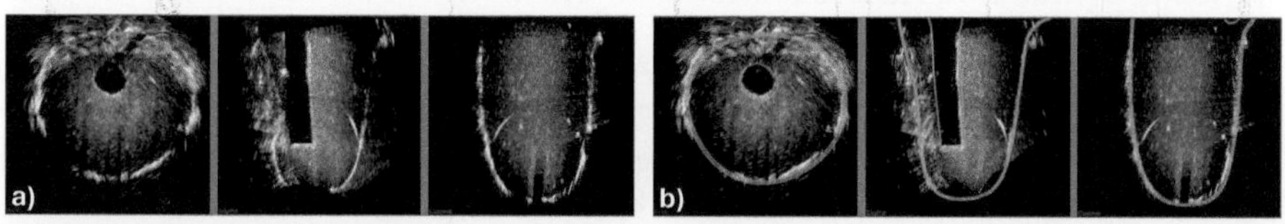

Fig. 3. Axial, sagittal and coronal view of (a) the reconstructed US volume and (b) the same views with overlaid CT reference which is colored green.

In this context, it is worth mentioning that we had originally planned additional reference points in this area, but had to remove them due to lack of correspondence (see Fig. 2b bottom). The next step after reconstruction of the 3D volume might be extraction of surfaces, e.g. of the skin or of the bone from that volume. Advanced methods, such as model-based or AI-based segmentation, can possibly be used for this task. However, future work must first clarify whether 3D volumes or surface data are more helpful for fabricating a socket.

It should be noted that the additional tracking hardware is a disadvantage of our approach, as it makes the setup more complex compared to conventional US and causes additional costs. The costs for the US device and tracking hardware are in the mid five-digit range, which is cheaper than CT or MRI, but could still hinder practical use. In future, we therefore aim to enable a purely image-based 3D reconstruction, e.g. with the AI-based approaches already mentioned (e.g., [10]). The final step towards real residual limbs with anatomical variation is also still pending and will be a challenge. However, we believe that the intermediate step of reconstruction on a phantom presented here is an important milestone and provides important insights for the next steps.

In conclusion, 3D reconstruction of residual limbs using US seems feasible. The reconstructed skin surface with an error of 2.3 ± 2.3 mm (n=23) compared to the CT reference demonstrated a high possible accuracy. However, the scanning approach must be simplified and optimized to cover all parts of limbs, especially the proximal end.

References

1. Douglas T, Solomonidis S, Sandham W et al. Ultrasound imaging in lower limb prosthetics. IEEE Trans Neural Syst Rehabil Eng. 2002;10(1):11–21.
2. Olsen J, Turner S, Chadwell A et al. The impact of limited prosthetic socket documentation: a researcher perspective. Front Rehabil Sci. 2022;3:853414.
3. Cutti AG, Santi MG, Hansen AH et al. Accuracy, repeatability, and reproducibility of a hand-held structured-light 3D scanner across multi-site settings in lower limb prosthetics. Sensors. 2024;24(7):2350.
4. Ranger BJ, Feigin M, Zhang X et al. 3D ultrasound imaging of residual limbs with camera-based motion compensation. IEEE Trans Neural Syst Rehabil Eng. 2019;27(2):207–17.
5. Lohmann CH, Rampal S, Lohrengel M et al. Imaging in peri-prosthetic assessment: an orthopaedic perspective. EFORT Open Rev. 2017;2(5):117–25.
6. Feng Y, Allison R, Hu XH et al. An ultrasonic device for source to skin surface distance measurement in patient setup. Int J Radiat Oncol Biol Phys. 2005;61(5):1587–9.
7. He P, Xue K, Chen Q et al. A PC-based ultrasonic data acquisition system for computer-aided prosthetic socket design. IEEE Trans Rehabil Eng. 1996;4(2):114–9.
8. Krosse C, Brucher R, Franz A. Ermittlung der Geometrie von Amputationsstümpfen mittels Ultraschall. Proc BVM. 2022:101–6.
9. Mercier L, Langø T, Lindseth F et al. A review of calibration techniques for freehand 3-D ultrasound systems. Ultrasound Med Biol. 2005;31(2):143–65.
10. Prevost R, Salehi M, Jagoda S et al. 3D freehand ultrasound without external tracking using deep learning. Med Image Anal. 2018;48:187–202.

Autocalibration for 3D Ultrasound Reconstruction in Infant Hip Dysplasia Screening

Wiebke Heyer[1], Christian Weihsbach[2], Christoph Otte[1,2], Jürgen Lichtenstein[3], Sebastian Lippross[4,5], Mattias P. Heinrich[1], Lasse Hansen[2]

[1]Institute of Medical Informatics, University of Luebeck
[2]EchoScout GmbH, Luebeck
[3]Clinic of Oral and Maxillofacial Surgery, UKSH Kiel
[4]Department of Orthopedics and Traumatology, UKSH Kiel
[5]Department of Surgical Sciences, University of Otago
w.heyer@uni-luebeck.de

Abstract. Hip dysplasia, a prevalent skeletal anomaly, necessitates accurate and early diagnosis to ensure effective treatment. This study presents a novel phantom-free autocalibration technique for 3D reconstruction of 2D ultrasound sweeps, evaluated for infant hip anatomy. By refining the probe-to-image transformation directly on anatomical structures, our approach eliminates the reliance on calibration phantoms, enhancing accessibility and accuracy in clinical settings. We demonstrate that our method improves alignment accuracy compared to traditional calibration methods as well as an existing autocalibration approach. By optimising the alignment of extracted surface keypoints from automatic segmentations, our results demonstrate superior performance, as evidenced by reduced Hausdorff (1.76 mm) and average surface distances (0.38 mm) between sweep reconstructions.

1 Introduction

Hip dysplasia, a malformation of the hip joint, is the most common skeletal anomaly globally, with an incidence of approximately 2–4%. Early diagnosis in the neonatal period using ultrasound and the scientifically validated Graf standard method [1] is essential to achieve complete normalisation of the hip joint during infancy. Early intervention reduces the orthopaedic and surgical demands later in life, compared to corrective surgeries in adulthood. However, reliable diagnosis is only achievable when the three-dimensional (3D) anatomical structures of the hip joint are accurately identified and displayed in the two-dimensional (2D) ultrasound (US) cross-sectional image, making the examination highly user-dependent and requiring a high level of expertise.

Despite advancements in 3D imaging, 2D ultrasound remains the primary method for clinical diagnosis. Its affordability and portability make it widely accessible to clinicians. Nevertheless, interpreting 2D ultrasound images can be challenging due to the limited field of view and a lower signal-to-noise ratio compared to other imaging modalities. While 3D ultrasound probes offer a three-dimensional field of view, they are not as readily available. Another option is to continuously track the precise position of a 2D ultrasound probe during freehand acquisition, enabling 3D volume reconstruction by spatially transforming each 2D image based on the tracking information.

C. Palm et al. (Hrsg.), *Bildverarbeitung für die Medizin 2025*, Informatik aktuell,
https://doi.org/10.1007/978-3-658-47422-5_22

Tracking systems, typically marker-based optical or electromagnetic, are essential for monitoring the probe's position during freehand acquisition. Accurate 3D reconstruction relies on the precise calibration of the probe's spatial position relative to the 2D image plane. Traditional calibration methods often require specialised phantoms, which add complexity to clinical workflows and necessitate repeated recalibrations when probe setups change, potentially slowing procedures. In contrast, autocalibration optimises the probe-to-image transformation directly from anatomical ultrasound data, removing the need for separate calibration devices and streamlining clinical workflows. Although recalibration may still be required after setup adjustments, autocalibration significantly accelerates the process, enhancing realignment speed and reducing interruptions. This method could be particularly beneficial in hip dysplasia screening, where accurate 3D reconstructions may improve diagnostic reliability and minimise operator dependence.

Calibration is essential for reconstructing 3D volumes from freehand 2D ultrasound sweeps, as it aligns the image plane with the probe's 3D spatial context. This process involves two main transformations: (1) mapping the ultrasound image plane to the probe's orientation and (2) mapping the probe's orientation to the world coordinate system defined by the external tracker. While the tracking system handles the second transformation reliably, the first, linking image coordinates to the probe, requires precise calibration. Traditional calibration methods use specialised phantoms, like single-point, cross-wire, or N-wire phantoms [2], which offer defined geometrical properties. However, phantom-based calibration has drawbacks, adding steps to workflows, requiring specialised equipment, and needing frequent recalibration that can disrupt clinical efficiency. Alternative self-calibration methods have been developed to optimise calibration directly from image data, aligning data across different probe positions. In 2006, Boctor et al. proposed an image-based approach for self-calibration [3] which encounters difficulties with out-of-plane calibration parameters in 2D US data. Similarly, Wein et al. introduced an image-based calibration method [4] that requires two perpendicular ultrasound sweeps at a fixed point. In clinical practice, this special acquisition protocol is often impractical, for instance, due to patient positioning constraints. Barratt et al. [5] proposed an alternative approach that registers segmented bone surfaces in ultrasound images to preoperative models. Yet this method relies on precise manual surface segmentation, which is both time-consuming and prone to error, and on the availability of the preoperative model. The most recent development in autocalibration, introduced by Toews and Wells in 2018 [6], employs a generative model of local scale-invariant features that calculates the posterior probability of calibration parameters based on features observed across multiple sweeps. Again, the method is image-based, making it susceptible to challenges in US imaging, such as tissue deformations, bone shadows, and other artifacts. In contrast, our approach avoids these limitations by relying on surface keypoint alignment rather than full image data, enhancing robustness to artifacts and irregularities. This work presents a phantom-free autocalibration technique for reconstructing three-dimensional volumes from two-dimensional ultrasound sweeps, specifically targeting infant hip anatomy for hip dysplasia screening. The proposed method refines an initially estimated probe-to-image transformation matrix directly on the target anatomy, eliminating the need for external calibration phantoms by incorporating optimisation-based alignment of surface keypoints from multiple ultrasound sweeps.

2 Materials and methods

An overview of our setup and method can be seen in Fig. 1. A 2D ultrasound probe[1], equipped with optical markers, is tracked in real time using a camera-based optical tracking system[2], allowing continuous monitoring of the probe's position during freehand sweeps. The transformation T between the optical markers and the tracking camera is known, but the relationship between the markers and the ultrasound image plane T_{calib} is initially a rough estimate based on probe geometry. This transformation is refined through the autocalibration process. We validate our proposed method on a calibration phantom, as described in [7], and an infant hip phantom[3]. While this phantom effectively replicates echogenic characteristics of real infant hip anatomy, the method has yet to be tested on real clinical data. From the calibration phantom, we recorded five sweeps, each containing between 221 and 464 frames, while for the infant hip phantom, we captured four sweeps with 79 to 162 frames per sweep. Each image is sized at 800 by 611 pixels with a spacing of 0.0625 mm.

Initially, the acquired ultrasound sweeps are segmented to delineate echogenic structures using an nnU-Net model [9]. This segmentation identifies anatomical and high-gradient structures critical for surface extraction. Keypoints are then randomly sampled from these regions. Autocalibration is achieved by parameterising the calibration matrix as a nine-degree-of-freedom transformation matrix that encodes both rotational and translational adjustments. An AdamW optimiser iteratively adjusts this matrix to minimise alignment errors, employing a smooth L1 distance loss function to measure discrepancies in reconstructed keypoints between sweeps. For reconstruction, we employ DiVRoC (Differentiable Volumetric Rasterisation of Point Clouds) [8], which rasterises

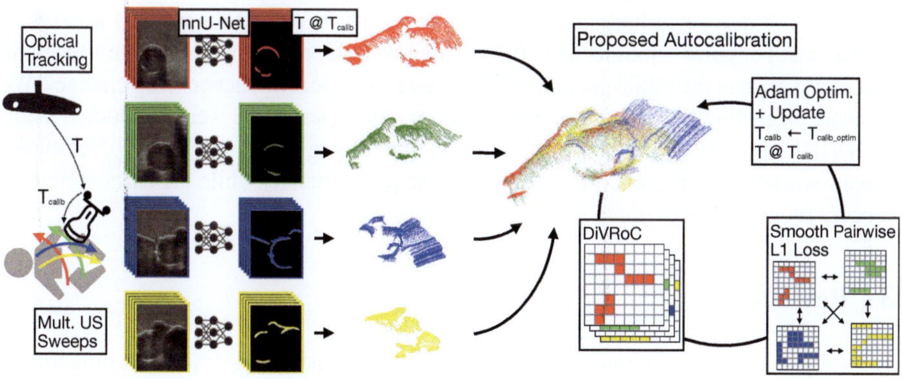

Fig. 1. Overview of our method from data acquisition (left) to sweep segmentation and keypoint extraction (middle) followed by alignment between sweeps with Adam optimiser and smooth pairwise L1 Loss. For 3D reconstruction we employ DiVRoC [8].

[1] Clarius L7HD3

[2] NDI Polaris Spectra

[3] Kyoto Kagaku US-13 Infant Hip Sonography Training Phantom

Tab. 1. Evaluation of calibration accuracy through surface distance metrics, comparing alignment across individual reconstructed US sweeps of the hip phantom.

	Phantom	HD 95 in mm	FASD in mm	BASD in mm
Initial	-	2.71 ± 0.94	0.84 ± 0.28	0.80 ± 0.29
Baseline	Calib.	2.15 ± 0.64	0.50 ± 0.08	0.46 ± 0.16
Toews and Wells [6]	Hip	2.16 ± 0.61	0.53 ± 0.08	0.51 ± 0.21
Ours	Calib.	1.73 ± 0.56	0.40 ± 0.04	0.42 ± 0.17
Ours	Hip	1.76 ± 0.54	0.36 ± 0.07	0.40 ± 0.16

each surface point cloud into a single volume for subsequent efficient metric computation. The optimised calibration matrix is combined with the initial estimate and the marker-to-camera transformation to facilitate the 3D reconstruction.

To evaluate the robustness and accuracy of the proposed autocalibration method, a series of experiments were conducted on both the acquired sweeps of the calibration phantom and the infant hip phantom. Initially, the 3D reconstruction was evaluated using only the estimated transformation without any calibration. Using our surface keypoint alignment-based method, the calibration matrix was derived either from the calibration phantom or directly from the hip phantom as autocalibration. Additionally, a simple baseline approach was applied, relying on the detection of a spherical structure in the calibration phantom, identifying extreme points on the sphere's surface, and using these points to compute a rigid transformation matrix to achieve alignment between the sweeps. This matrix was subsequently applied for reconstruction on the hip phantom. To further benchmark our approach, we applied the autocalibration by Toews and Wells[4] [6] to our hip phantom data for comparison. To assess the robustness of our method, we conduct an ablation experiment by introducing controlled perturbations to the initial estimation. These perturbations include translation shifts up to 10 mm along all axes as well as small angular rotations up to 0.1 rad applied independently to simulate variations that might arise in the initial estimate introduced by physical impact or setup changes. We evaluate all methods on the infant hip phantom. All experiments were conducted using an NVIDIA L4 GPU with 24 GB of memory. The inference time of the nnU-Net model is approximately 40 ms, enabling near real-time performance, while the autocalibration process requires approximately 2 seconds.

3 Results

To evaluate the proposed autocalibration method alongside baseline and comparative techniques, we compute masked pairwise surface distances between the segmentations of individually reconstructed sweeps of the hip phantom, focusing on the 95th percentile Hausdorff distance (HD 95) and average surface distance, calculated in both forward (FASD) and backward (BASD) directions. Each ultrasound sweep is reconstructed independently, and a binary mask is generated from the reconstructed images to define regions where image data is present within the overall reconstruction volume.

[4] `https://github.com/mt3000/TMI-2017-Ultrasound-Toews`

The results are presented in Tab. 1. The method by Toews and Wells achieves alignment similar to the baseline approach, which uses landmark detection on the calibration phantom's sphere, but both methods fall short of our approach. Calibration on the calibration phantom, evaluated on the hip phantom, yields results comparable to those of direct autocalibration on the hip phantom. The ablation study shows that our method is robust against perturbation of the initial calibration matrix with only a slightly worse HD 95 of 2.09 mm with the initial transformation translated by 10 mm and an HD 95 of 1.98 mm with a rotation of 0.1 rad.

Fig. 2 illustrates the comparison of 3D reconstructed surface keypoints between the initial alignment and the alignment achieved with our autocalibration method, for both the calibration phantom and the infant hip phantom. Improved alignment is particularly visible in the sphere of the calibration phantom and in the femoral head imitation of the infant hip phantom.

4 Discussion

We show that our method effectively addresses the limitations of traditional calibration techniques that rely on dedicated phantoms. By refining the probe-to-image transformation directly on anatomical structures, we enhance both the accessibility and accuracy of 3D ultrasound imaging in clinical practice. Our results show that our autocalibration achieves improved alignment accuracy, as evidenced by the lowest surface distances compared to baseline methods. Notably, our method's performance is also superior to the approach by Toews and Wells, which in our experiments, despite its innovative use of generative models, does not achieve the same level of alignment accuracy as our technique. With the advancements in deep learning that allow for automatic segmentation of echogenic structures in real time and radiologist-level quality, we also effectively address the limitations encountered by Barratt et al.

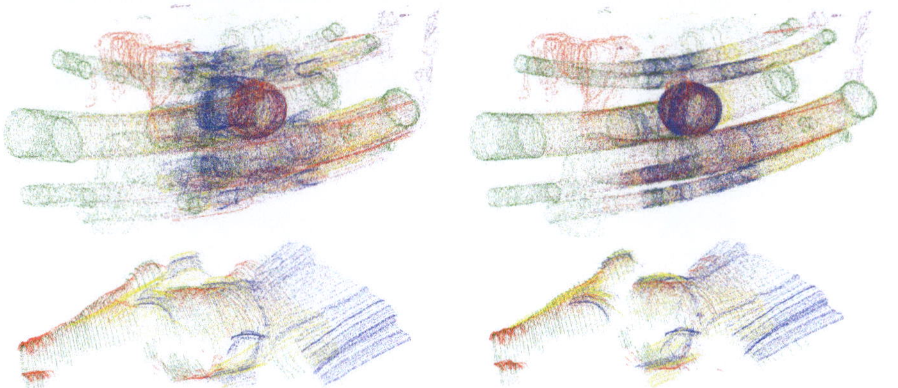

Fig. 2. 3D reconstruction of surface keypoints extracted from individual colour-coded freehand ultrasound sweeps before (left) and after autocalibration (right). Top: Calibration phantom. Bottom: Infant hip phantom.

Nonetheless, our study has limitations, primarily the remaining need for validation on real clinical datasets, which would, however, be directly feasible as we confirmed in first experiments. Future work will focus on assessing the robustness and generalisability of our autocalibration technique in practical scenarios and exploring its application in other anatomical regions and medical conditions.

Acknowledgement. This study was partly funded by the German Federal Ministry of Education and Research (BMBF) (grant number 16SV9254).

References

1. Kolovos S, Sioutis S, Papakonstantinou ME et al. Ultrasonographic screening for developmental dysplasia of the hip: the Graf method revisited. Eur J Orthop Surg Traumatol. 2024;34(2):723–34.
2. Lu W, Chen J, Wang Y et al. Coplanarity constrained ultrasound probe calibration based on N-wire phantom. Ultrasound Med Biol. 2023;49(10):2316–24.
3. Boctor E, Iordachita I, Fichtinger G et al. Ultrasound self-calibration. Proc SPIE. 2006.
4. Wein W, Khamene A. Image-based method for in-vivo freehand ultrasound calibration. Proc SPIE. 2008.
5. Barratt D, Penney G, Chan C et al. Self-calibrating 3D-ultrasound-based bone registration for minimally invasive orthopedic surgery. IEEE Trans Med Imaging. 2006;25(3):312–23.
6. Toews M, Wells W. Phantomless auto-calibration and online calibration assessment for a tracked freehand 2-D ultrasound probe. IEEE Trans Med Imaging. 2018;37(1):262–72.
7. von Haxthausen F, Ipsen S, Schwegmann H et al. A 3D slicer module for calibration of spatially tracked 3D ultrasound probes. Int J Comput Assist Radiol Surg. 2020;15:14–6.
8. Heinrich MP, Bigalke A, Großbröhmer C et al. Chasing clouds: differentiable volumetric rasterisation of point clouds as a highly efficient and accurate loss for large-scale deformable 3D registration. Proc IEEE CVF ICCV. 2023:8026–36.
9. Isensee F, Jaeger PF, Kohl SA et al. nnU-Net: a self-configuring method for deep learning-based biomedical image segmentation. Nat Methods. 2021;18(2):203–11.

[4]Department of Ophthalmology, University Medical Center Mannheim, Heidelberg University
[3]Lamarr Institute for Machine Learning and Artificial Intelligence

Weakly Supervised Segmentation of Hyper-reflective Foci with Compact Convolutional Transformers and SAM 2

Olivier Morelle[1,2], Justus Bisten[1], Maximilian WM. Wintergerst[2,3], Robert P. Finger[2,4], Thomas Schultz[1,5]

[1]B-IT and Department of Computer Science, University of Bonn
[2]Department of Ophthalmology, University Hospital Bonn
[5]Augenzentrum Grischun, Chur, Switzerland
schultz@cs.uni-bonn.de

Abstract. Weakly supervised segmentation has the potential to greatly reduce the annotation effort for training segmentation models for small structures such as hyper-reflective foci (HRF) in optical coherence tomography (OCT). However, most weakly supervised methods either involve a strong downsampling of input images, or only achieve localization at a coarse resolution, both of which are unsatisfactory for small structures. We propose a novel framework that increases the spatial resolution of a traditional attention-based multiple instance learning (MIL) approach by using layer-wise relevance propagation (LRP) to prompt the segment anything model (SAM 2), and increases recall with iterative inference. Moreover, we demonstrate that replacing MIL with a compact convolutional transformer (CCT), which adds a positional encoding, and permits an exchange of information between different regions of the OCT image, leads to a further and substantial increase in segmentation accuracy.

1 Introduction

Age-related macular degeneration (AMD) is a leading cause of vision loss with age, characterized by the deterioration of the central retina [1]. Optical coherence tomography (OCT) provides high-resolution cross-sectional images of the retina. Within these images, hyper-reflective foci (HRF) appear as small, bright spots whose segmentation is crucial for assessing disease severity and progression [2], and treatment efficacy.

However, manual segmentation of HRFs is a time-consuming task, particularly due to the high resolution of the images and the minute size of HRFs. Our dataset comprises images of size 496×1024 pixels, with HRFs exhibiting a median size of only 17 pixels.

This makes weak supervision, which achieves pixel-level localization based on image-level annotations, an attractive alternative. In the context of OCT data, one such method generated segmentation maps using multi-scale class activation maps [3]. Another one focused on anomalous structures, which it segmented without requiring detailed annotations [4]. The TSSK Net employed a teacher-student architecture to enhance segmentation performance under weak supervision [5]. It has been employed for the segmentation of various biomarkers in OCT, including HRFs, but involves downsampling images to 256^2 pixels. At that resolution, 16% of the annotated HRFs in our dataset are lost. RETFound, a Vision Transformer (ViT) pretrained on retinal images [6], has

C. Palm et al. (Hrsg.), *Bildverarbeitung für die Medizin 2025*, Informatik aktuell,
https://doi.org/10.1007/978-3-658-47422-5_23

an input size of 224^2 pixels, which loses 22% of our annotated HRFs. Therefore, we investigate methods for weak supervision that preserve the full resolution.

The first contribution of our work is a framework for weakly supervised HRF segmentation based on multiple instance learning (MIL), which classifies full-resolution images by treating them as a bag of patches. Attention-based MIL [7] improves accuracy, and enables a certain level of localization, by computing an attention score per patch. Since HRFs are often much smaller than patches, we combine that approach with layer-wise relevance propagation (LRP) [8], leading to relevance maps that highlight the contributions of individual pixels to the model's predictions.

We achieve a final segmentation by using the relevance map to prompt version 2 of the segment anything model (SAM 2) [9], a powerful foundation model capable of producing accurate segmentation masks based on minimal input prompts. We derive a prompt from the most relevant pixel, developing a suitable prompting strategy that compensates for the fact that SAM 2 is not well-suited for small structures such as HRFs. Since a single image can contain more than one HRF, we iteratively pass it through the pipeline, occluding all previously detected HRFs, until no further HRFs are found.

Our second contribution is to investigate the relative benefit of replacing MIL with a CCT [10], a transformer architecture that is well-suited for small datasets, and flexible with regard to input resolution. We hypothesized that the CCT model would outperform the MIL model due to its ability to capture positional information and facilitate information exchange between patches through attention mechanisms, reducing the likelihood of missing small HRFs on patch borders.

2 Materials and methods

2.1 Data

This study utilized 191 OCT volumes from the laser intervention in early stages of age-related macular degeneration (LEAD) study [11], all imaged using Heidelberg Spectralis devices and manually annoted for hyperreflective foci (HRF) by three raters [12]. Due to the poor between-rater reproduction of very small annotations (less than 5 pixels),

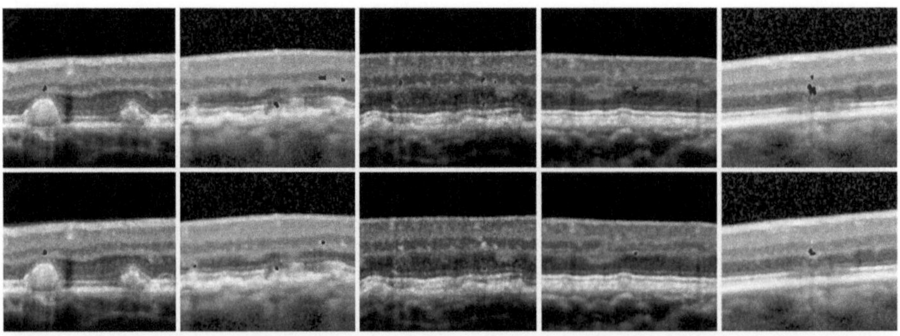

Fig. 1. Example HRF segmentations (red) from the test set. Top: Ground truth segmentation. Bottom: output of our best performing weakly supervised segmentation model.

we excluded them from the analysis. Each volume consists of multiple slice images (B-scans), leading to 962 B-scans with HRF and 8,392 B-scans without HRF. Overall 2,146 HRFs where annotated with an average of 12 per volume. To ensure robust evaluation, the dataset was divided into training and test sets using an 80/20 split, stratified by HRF count per volume to maintain similar distributions. To prevent information leakage, B-scans from the same patient were not split across the training and test sets. 20% of the training set was reserved for validation during model training.

2.2 Image-level predictions

We investigated the relative benefits of different forms of weak supervision by reducing the pixel-level annotations to three types of image-level labels which contain increasing amounts of information, at an increasing expected annotation effort: In a *binary* classification task, we only differentiated between B-scans with and without HRF. In *multi-class* classification, we categorized B-scans into no HRF, one HRF, or more than one HRF. In a *regression* approach, we trained a model to estimate the number of HRFs in a given B-scan, with labels clipped to a maximum of 10 HRFs per B-scan to focus on values with sufficient support in our data.

Two architectures that can process the B-scans at full resolution were employed for image-level predictions: a multiple instance learning (MIL) model and a CCT. The regression variant of both models used a sigmoid-activated output, scaled by a factor of 10.

The MIL model consisted of a bag of AlexNets with an input shape of 64×64 pixels. Inspired by Ilse et al. [7], instances were weighted and averaged via self-attention. The model was initialized with ImageNet weights from `torchvision` and trained using a batch size of 64 for 50,000 steps, following a OneCycle learning rate policy with a maximum learning rate of 1×10^{-6}. The optimizer used was AdamW with a weight decay of 0.01. The retinal region in the input images was localized using Otsu thresholding, and 3 rows of patches were extracted from this region.

The CCT model, based on Hassani et al. [10], is designed for small datasets and integrates convolutional layers for tokenization. This approach captures local spatial relationships and preserves high-resolution details, beneficial for tasks requiring precise localization. The model was trained from scratch with a batch size of 16 for 50,000 steps, using a OneCycle learning rate policy with a maximum learning rate of 1×10^{-5} and the AdamW optimizer with a weight decay of 0.01.

Data augmentation during training included random vertical shifts, horizontal flips, scaling, rotation, and intensity adjustments. Images were normalized using the mean and standard deviation of the training dataset.

2.3 Weakly supervised segmentation

For weakly supervised segmentation, Layer-wise Relevance Propagation (LRP) [8] was implemented for both models. For the CCT, this involved a recent extension of LRP to transformer architectures [13]. Based on the resulting relevance maps, a square, fixed-size bounding box around the most relevant pixel was used as a prompt for version 2

Tab. 1. Classification and segmentation metrics, with and without iterative inference, for CCT and MIL models. The 2-classes task is a binary classification for the presence of HRF. For the 3-classes task, the classes are no HRF, 1 HRF and more than 1 HRF. For the regression task, the target is the HRF count in the B-scan, clipped to a maximum of 10.

Model	Task	Classification			Segm. 1 iteration			Segm. 6 iterations		
		AUROC	Avg. Prec	F1	Dice	Recall	Preci	Dice	Recall	Preci
CCT	2-Classes	0.90	0.70	0.64	**0.33**	**0.35**	**0.47**	**0.33**	**0.42**	**0.37**
	3-Classes	**0.92**	**0.74**	**0.65**	0.29	0.30	0.41	0.31	0.40	0.36
	Regression	0.90	0.58	0.6	0.22	0.25	0.29	0.21	0.35	0.22
MIL	2-Classes	0.86	0.58	0.53	0.11	0.09	0.23	0.13	0.12	0.23
	3-Classes	0.86	0.58	0.51	0.08	0.06	0.19	0.08	0.07	0.18
	Regression	0.85	0.42	0.41	0.05	0.04	0.13	0.07	0.07	0.13

of the Segment Anything Model (SAM 2) [9]. Since we found that SAM 2 is not well-suited for the segmentation of small objects such as HRFs at the native resolution, we crop the B-scan, centered on the position of the prompt, and subsequently upsample the resulting patch to SAM's input resolution, effectively making the HRF sufficiently large for reliable segmentation. The most suitable crop and bounding box sizes were established using a grid search over all HRFs from the training data. A box size of 4 pixels and crop sizes between 50 and 100 pixels yielded optimal results, achieving a mean Dice around 0.67 when prompting with ground truth HRF centers.

The highest scoring mask returned by SAM is selected. Optionally, an attempt is made to segment additional HRFs with an iterative procedure that inpaints the previously detected HRFs with the image mean and re-runs the model until the predicted value falls below a threshold of 0.05, or a maximum number of iterations is reached.

3 Results

We evaluated the performance of the CCT and MIL models as binary classifiers and weakly supervised segmentation models. For both models, three variants where trained for binary classification, multi-class classification, or regression.

The resulting metrics are presented in Tab. 1. For classification, the CCT model consistently outperforms the MIL model across all metrics and for all training regimes. The CCT model that was trained with three classes achieved the highest classification scores, slightly better than the one trained with two classes. It achieves an AUROC of 0.92, an Average Precision of 0.74 and an F1 score of 0.65. For the MIL model there is also not much difference between training with two or three classes. For both models, the regression task performs worst.

For the weakly supervised segmentation task, the CCT trained with two classes yields the best results. The difference in performance between the MIL model and the CCT is even more pronounced. Iterative inference increases the (pixel-level) recall, but also reduces precision, and therefore does not yield a substantial benefit in terms of Dice. This is mostly due to the fact that averages in Tab. 1 include a large number of B-scans with only one HRF. Images that contain more than one HRF are more challenging to

Tab. 2. Average Dice score when post-processing the relevance maps differently. Threshold (Val) is a global threshold, calibrated on the validation set. Applying this threshold to the relevance maps from the validation and test set result in the Val Dice and Test Dice columns. The Oracle Test Dice is the highest Dice from varying the threshold per HRF, thus represents an upper bound of what could be achieved with adaptive thresholding.

Model	Task	Threshold (Val)	Val Dice	Test Dice	Oracle Test Dice	SAM Dice
CCT	2-Classes	0.0037	0.16	0.16	0.35	0.33
	3-Classes	0.0065	0.14	0.11	0.31	0.31
	Regression	0.0001	0.06	0.06	0.21	0.21
MIL	2-classes	0.0025	0.11	0.11	0.19	0.13
	3-Classes	0.0013	0.10	0.03	0.15	0.08
	Regression	0.0007	0.05	0.01	0.08	0.07

segment (average Dice with the 2-class CCT after the first iteration is only 0.22), but benefit more clearly from the iteration (Dice increases to 0.28 after three iterations).

Tab. 2 evaluates multiple approaches to obtain segmentation masks from the relevance maps. A global threshold calibrated on the validation data is straight forward but results in a Dice of only 0.16 for the best model. Our approach to generate prompts for SAM from the relevance maps clearly outperforms this with a Dice of 0.33 after 6 iterations. This is close to what we call "Oracle Test Dice", an upper bound for adaptive thresholding approaches which sets the threshold per HRF, using its ground truth segmentation as a guide. Notably, the MIL models showed less pronounced gains from postprocessing with SAM.

Fig. 1 shows several example segmentations from the test set. One can see that our model successfully localizes several HRFs despite their small size.

4 Discussion

Regarding annotation style, it was our original hypothesis that training a model to predict image-level labels that merely indicate the presence of HRF might only be sufficient to detect a single (most prominent) HRF, while training with more information-rich labels that provide a more nuanced measure of HRF load might enable a more complete detection of all HRFs.

Our experiments, in which additional HRFs are segmented by masking out the ones that have already been found, indicate that a simple binary annotation, labeling B-scans as HRF positive/negative, is sufficient, and no additional benefit is gained from more time-consuming weak annotation styles.

Our strategy for prompting SAM 2 based on the most relevant pixel proved effective for obtaining final segmentation masks, achieving much better results than a simple thresholding of the relevance maps. Comparing Dice scores to those from an oracle-based thresholding that makes use of the ground truth suggests that we cannot expect to outperform SAM 2 even with sophisticated threshold adaptation.

Overall, our study highlights the effectiveness of CCT in conjunction with LRP and SAM 2 for the weakly supervised segmentation of HRFs in OCT, and we expect that it might be similarly effective for other segmentation problems that involve small structures. In the future, we plan to further refine our iterative inference, with the goal of achieving an even more favorable balance of recall and precision.

Acknowledgement. We would like to express our sincere gratitude to our collaborators, Zhichao Wu and Robyn Guymer, whose expertise and time were invaluable in assembling the dataset. We also thank our annotators, Gabriela Guzmann, Simon Janzen, and Kai Lyn Goh, for their meticulous efforts.

References

1. Li JQ, Welchowski T, Schmid M et al. Prevalence and incidence of age-related macular degeneration in Europe: a systematic review and meta-analysis. Br J Ophthalmol. 2020;104(8):1077–84.
2. Verma A, Corradetti G, He Y et al. Relationship between the distribution of intra-retinal hyper-reflective foci and the progression of intermediate age-related macular degeneration. Graefes Archi Clin Exp Ophthalmol. 2023;261(12):3437–47.
3. Ma X, Ji Z, Niu S et al. MS-CAM: multi-scale class activation maps for weakly-supervised segmentation of geographic atrophy lesions in SD-OCT images. IEEE J Biomed Health Inform. 2020;24(12):3443–55.
4. Wang J, Li W, Chen Y et al. Weakly supervised anomaly segmentation in retinal OCT images using an adversarial learning approach. Biomed Opt Express. 2021;12(8):4713.
5. Liu X, Liu Q, Zhang Y et al. TSSK-Net: weakly supervised biomarker localization and segmentation with image-level annotation in retinal OCT images. Comput Biol Med. 2023:106467.
6. Zhou Y, Chia MA, Wagner SK et al. A foundation model for generalizable disease detection from retinal images. Nature. 2023;622(7981):156–63.
7. Ilse M, Tomczak J, Welling M. Attention-based deep multiple instance learning. Proc ICML. 2018:2127–36.
8. Bach S, Binder A, Montavon G et al. On pixel-wise explanations for non-linear classifier decisions by layer-wise relevance propagation. PLoS One. 2015;10(7):e0130140.
9. Ravi N, Gabeur V, Hu Y et al. SAM 2: segment anything in images and videos. arXiv: 2408.00714. 2024.
10. Hassani A, Walton S, Shah N et al. Escaping the big data paradigm with compact transformers. arXiv: 2104.05704. 2021.
11. Guymer RH, Wu Z, Hodgson LAB et al. Subthreshold nanosecond laser intervention in age-related macular degeneration: the LEAD randomized controlled clinical trial. Ophthalmology. 126(6):829–38.
12. Goh KL, Wintergerst MWM, Abbott CJ et al. Hyperreflective foci not seen as hyperpigmentary abnormalities on color fundus photographs in age-related macular degeneration. Retina. 44(2):214–21.
13. Ali A, Schnake T, Eberle O et al. XAI for transformers: better explanations through conservative propagation. Proc ICML. 2022;162:435–51.

Bridging Gaps in Retinal Imaging

Fusing OCT and SLO Information with Implicit Neural Representations for Improved Interpolation and Segmentation

Timo Kepp[†1], Julia Andresen[†2], Fenja Falta[2], Heinz Handels[1,2]

[1]German Research Center for Artificial Intelligence, Luebeck, Germany
[2]Institute of Medical Informatics, University of Luebeck, Luebeck, Germany
timo.kepp@dfki.de

Abstract. Optical coherence tomography (OCT), the standard clinical imaging procedure in ophthalmology, provides high-resolution cross-sectional images of the retina, but is usually performed with large slice distances. Small structures in the sparsely scanned retina can therefore be missed, and volumetric measurements are impaired. Interpolation methods that work with single images can generate densely sampled volumes, but fail to correctly interpolate shapes and cannot generate information that is missing between the given slices. In this work, we propose to use generalized implicit neural representations (INRs) for OCT interpolation and retinal layer segmentation. By using population-based training, the shape representation is improved over baselines, while the training requires only very few annotated image slices thanks to the ability of INRs to handle highly anisotropic data. To enable the integration of inter-slice information, we use additional SLO images, demonstrating a new way to combine different eye imaging modalities. Finally, it is shown that the generalized INR can be adapted to images that were not seen during training, enabling the segmentation of new images.

1 Introduction

Optical coherence tomography (OCT) is a standard imaging modality for retinal diagnostics in ophthalmology, providing cross-sectional scans (B-scans) of the retina at near-microscopic resolution [1]. In clinical routine, acquisitions with large B-scan intervals are preferred for shorter acquisition times, resulting in a sparsely scanned retina. The anisotropic OCT scans resulting from the sparse sampling scheme present challenges for both computer-assisted and clinical evaluations. The larger B-scan intervals cause structures to appear stretched or compressed, complicating the 3D reconstruction of anatomical features as well as volumetric analysis, which is usually based on the prediction of dense 3D segmentations. While convolutional neural networks (CNNs) are state-of-the-art for the segmentation of medical 3D data, they are generally developed for isotropic data. Consequently, 2D-based approaches are often used for OCT data, e.g., for the segmentation of retinal layers [2]. However, these methods are often either unable to generate smooth surfaces or rely on parameterization techniques as post-processing, such as graph-cut approaches [3]. The sole analysis of sparsely sampled OCT data

[†]These authors contributed equally the most to this work.

C. Palm et al. (Hrsg.), *Bildverarbeitung für die Medizin 2025*, Informatik aktuell,
https://doi.org/10.1007/978-3-658-47422-5_24

bears the additional disadvantage, that diagnostic precision may be limited, as smaller anatomical structures, such as blood vessels, or pathologies could be missed [4].

Various interpolation methods exist to enhance anisotropic image data resolution. Simple intensity-based methods are unable to capture shape and localization differences between B-scans, leading to artifacts and ambiguous results. Registration-based methods [5] align structural features more accurately and reduce misalignment artifacts, but cannot infer information missing between slices, limiting reconstruction quality in sparsely sampled regions. Generative approaches for super-resolution are capable of producing realistic, detailed images by reconstructing fine textures and complex structures. However, they require a large amount of training data and carry the risk of hallucinations, which makes them precarious in a clinical context [6].

Implicit neural representations (INRs) have proven particularly suitable for the processing of highly anisotropic data [7], enabling continuous representations of the imaged objects. Different from CNNs, INRs are not limited to the resolution of the voxelized training data, but deliver continuous representations of the imaged objects. This is achieved by training a multi-layer perceptron to learn a mapping from a coordinate space to the intensity space for one single image. Recently, approaches have been proposed to extend INRs to generalize to several images by separating population-trained and instance-specific parts of the network. A popular approach for this is to use instance-specific latent vectors as additional input to the INR [8, 9]. In [9], these latent priors are learned during the training process together with the shared network parameters based on two tasks, namely the reconstruction and segmentation of the images. This makes it possible to segment unknown images after completed training by freezing the network and adapting new latent codes based only on the reconstruction task.

Generalized INRs benefit from the information from the population and can therefore produce particularly smooth surfaces and dense representations, but when subject-specific information is not covered by the input data, it would still be impossible to recover this missing information through interpolation. A special feature of eye imaging is that more than one modality is usually recorded. 2D imaging modalities, e.g., Scanning Laser Ophthalmoscopy (SLO), can capture information present in-between B-Scans. The dimensional mismatch between those modalities (Fig. 1), however, makes combining SLO and OCT information non-trivial, especially for CNN-based approaches.

Here, we propose a generalized INR for OCT interpolation that benefits from additional scanning laser ophthalmoscopy (SLO) integration to represent inter-slice blood vessel information. We compare this approach to intensity- and registration-based interpolation, as well as to INRs trained on individual images, and show improved shape representation. Image reconstruction is shown to improve when using the additional SLO information. Finally, segmentation and interpolation performance is evaluated on unseen samples.

2 Materials and methods

Our proposed framework (Fig. 1) for the interpolation and segmentation of sparse OCT scans builds on [8, 9]. A generalizable INR $f_\theta = (f_\theta^{\text{recon}}, f_\theta^{\text{seg}})$ with trainable parameters θ is used to reconstruct OCT images of n different patients and to segment 12 retinal layers based on three inputs: A 3D coordinate $(x, y, z) \in \mathbb{R}^3$, the intensity of the SLO image $\text{SLO}_i(x, z)$ from patient i at the respective en-face position (x, z) and a trainable latent prior $\boldsymbol{p}_i \in \mathbb{R}^L$, which is patient-specific.

For one forward-pass, we use the coordinates (x, y, z) of an entire OCT B-scan and the loss is then computed as

$$\mathcal{L} = \sum_{i=1}^{n} \sum_{(x,y,z)} [\mathcal{L}_{\text{recon}}(f_\theta^{\text{recon}}(x, y, z, \text{SLO}_i(x, z), \boldsymbol{p}_i), \text{OCT}_i(x, y, z)) \\ + \alpha \mathcal{L}_{\text{seg}}(f_\theta^{\text{seg}}(x, y, z, \text{SLO}_i(x, z), \boldsymbol{p}_i), \text{SEG}_i(x, y, z)) + \beta \mathcal{L}_{\text{reg}}(\boldsymbol{p}_i)]$$

where $\text{OCT}_i(x, y, z)$ and $\text{SEG}_i(x, y, z)$ are the ground truth OCT intensities and segmentation labels, respectively. A combination of MSE and SSIM loss is used as reconstruction loss $\mathcal{L}_{\text{recon}} = 0.1 \cdot \mathcal{L}_{\text{SSIM}} + \mathcal{L}_{\text{MSE}}$ and as segmentation loss $\mathcal{L}_{\text{seg}}$ the BCE loss is used. Inspired by [9], we use a L2-Loss as regularization loss $\mathcal{L}_{\text{reg}}$, which penalizes large values in the latent codes. The loss components are weighted by $\alpha = \beta = 0.2$.

After convergence, the INR can be fit to an unseen patient $n+1$ with known intensities $\text{OCT}_{n+1}(x, y, z)$ but unknown segmentation labels, by freezing the network f_θ and learning the latent prior $\boldsymbol{p}_{n+1}$. The loss is then reduced to

$$\sum_{(x,y,z)} \mathcal{L}_{\text{recon}}(f_\theta^{\text{recon}}(x, y, z, \text{SLO}_{n+1}(x, z), \boldsymbol{p}_{n+1}), \text{OCT}_{n+1}(x, y, z)) + \beta \mathcal{L}_{\text{reg}}(\boldsymbol{p}_{n+1})$$

As [9] has shown, fitting the INR this way results in plausible segmentation predictions from the segmentation output f_θ^{seg}. With the learned latent prior $\boldsymbol{p}_{n+1}$, we can interpolate intensities as well as segmentation labels for any coordinate (x, y, z) for which the SLO intensity $\text{SLO}_{n+1}(x, z)$ is known by simply calculating $f_\theta(x, y, z, \text{SLO}_{n+1}(x, z), \boldsymbol{p}_{n+1})$.

Dataset and implementation details. The network architecture of f_θ consists of a six-layer multi-layer perceptron with wavelet activation functions [10] and a layer size of 128 plus two separate linear layers as decoder heads for reconstruction output f_θ^{recon} and segmentation output f_θ^{seg}. Residual connections are used in the hidden layers, and the coordinates and SLO values are repeatedly input to each of these layers. The length L of the latent vectors is chosen empirically and set to 128. As a comparison method, we use

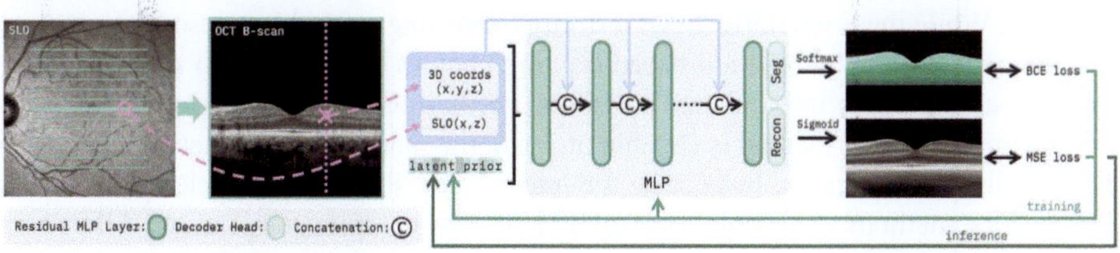

Fig. 1. Schematic overview of the proposed framework. On the left, the SLO fundus image is shown with overlaid OCT scan lines. The position marked in the SLO (pink circle) corresponds to an A-scan (dotted line) in the OCT B-scan. The input for the INR are 3D coordinates in the OCT (pink cross) and intensities at the corresponding SLO position (pink circle).

a non-generalized INR with slightly changed architecture for improved performance. It consists of three linear layers of size 512 with sinusoidal activation functions [11]. The code is publicly available at `https://github.com/tkepp/INteRp-OCT`.

For experiments, we use an in-house dataset of 100 OCT and corresponding SLO images from a Heidelberg Spectralis scanner taken from both eyes of 50 healthy probands, which are split into 80 training and 20 test cases. OCT images consist of 512 B-scans with a resolution of 496×512 pixels. The volumes cover a field of view of $2 \times 6 \times 6\,\text{mm}^3$ and were initially segmented automatically using the Iowa Reference Algorithms [3]. Subsequently, segmentation errors were corrected manually by an expert. For preprocessing, all B-scans are flattened in relation to the Bruch's membrane and cropped to 230×512 pixels so that the retina is at the center height of the image. Images of right eyes are flipped for identical orientation of all images. During training and for interpolation, only 16 B-scans per volume are known, whereas the intermediate scans are used to evaluate the accuracy. These B-scans are sampled equidistantly from the entire depth of the volumes, so that the distance between image slices is even wider than in typical clinical imaging, where usually 25 or 49 B-scans are acquired.

3 Results

The interpolation capability of our framework (GenINR) is evaluated on unseen intermediate B-scans of the 80 training images as well as on the 20 unseen test images (Tab. 1). New priors are learned for these patients, whereby the INR weights remain unchanged. We compare our method to linear as well as registration-based interpolation [5]. In the registration-based method, the interpolated slices are segmented by applying the deformations determined on the OCTs to the segmentations using nearest neighbor interpolation. In linear interpolation, the segmentations are also linearly interpolated, and the resulting continuous values are then rounded to integers to obtain segmentation labels again. Furthermore, we evaluate interpolation results when using a conventional, non-generalized INR trained for both image reconstruction and segmentation on single images (SingleINR). To evaluate the benefit of incorporating multimodal information from SLO and OCT, we train both the generalizable and non-generalizable INR with and without additional SLO intensity input.

Quantitative results (Tab. 1) show an equivalent reconstruction and improved segmentation of the interpolated slices for our GenINR compared to the instance-based methods. While the SingleINR shows a strong overfitting on the slices used for training, the generalization by population-based training enables the GenINR to achieve meaningful results even on intermediate positions. Furthermore, in contrast to the instance-specific methods, our method is capable of predicting and thus interpolating segmentations on unseen test cases. Inspecting the interpolated slices (Fig. 2), clear differences between the methods are visible. Especially in the fovea region, large shape differences between neighboring slices lead to strong interpolation artifacts in the instance-based methods, whereas our method succeeds in continuing the fovea shape (Fig. 2 left). Furthermore, the integration of SLO information into the GenINR enables correct localization of blood vessels in the outer areas of the eye (Fig. 2 right). In contrast, the highly overfitted SingleINR is not able to gain meaningful information from the ad-

Tab. 1. Image reconstruction and retinal layer segmentation performances for linear and registration-based interpolation, as well as for the INR trained for each image and the proposed generalized INR with (SingleINR$_{SLO}$ / GenINR$_{SLO}$) and without (SingleINR / GenINR) SLO guidance. Results are reported for interpolation on train and test images separately. The best results are written in bold.

		Image Reconstruction				Image Segmentation		
	Method	↓MAE$^{[\%]}$	↑PSNR	↑SSIM$^{[\%]}$	↓LPIPS	↑Dice$^{[\%]}$	↓ASSD$^{[\mu m]}$	↓HD$^{[\mu m]}$
Train	Linear	5.92±0.6	21.7±0.5	39.7±5.6	**0.12**±0.01	88.8±1.1	9.3±0.7	37.2±3.3
	Reg.	5.76±0.6	22.0±0.5	41.3±5.6	**0.12**±0.01	89.1±1.2	7.5±0.8	39.2±4.4
	SingleINR	6.65±0.6	20.6±0.5	36.7±5.9	0.26±0.02	90.8±1.1	7.7±0.7	37.6±3.6
	SingleINR$_{SLO}$	9.42±1.51	17.5±1.0	26.8±6.4	0.45±0.01	83.6±5.3	18.7±12.0	603±180
	GenINR	**5.24**±0.5	**22.6**±0.5	**48.9**±5.7	0.53±0.03	**91.9**±1.0	**7.0**±0.7	**32.5**±3.7
	GenINR$_{SLO}$	**5.24**±0.5	**22.6**±0.5	**48.9**±5.7	0.52±0.03	**91.9**±1.0	**7.0**±0.6	**32.5**±3.7
Test	GenINR	6.04±0.57	21.4±0.5	44.3±6.0	0.55±0.03	86.5±3.7	11.4±2.1	45.1±4.9
	GenINR$_{SLO}$	6.08±0.59	21.4±0.5	44.2±6.0	0.54±0.03	86.2±3.8	11.7±2.2	45.4±5.0

ditional SLO input. However, GenINR is limited in its ability to reconstruct higher frequencies, resulting in an overly smoothed appearance of the images. Consequently, small vessels (with a high-frequency appearance) around the fovea region, are also not adequately reconstructed.

4 Discussion

In this work, we demonstrated the potential of generalizable INRs for OCT interpolation. Using inter-slice distances even wider than for typical OCT images, the proposed framework manages to generate dense and smooth retinal layer segmentations. While shape representation, particularly of the fovea, surpasses both registration-based interpolation and INRs trained on individual images, image reconstruction could still be improved, as high-frequency image components are not yet fully captured.

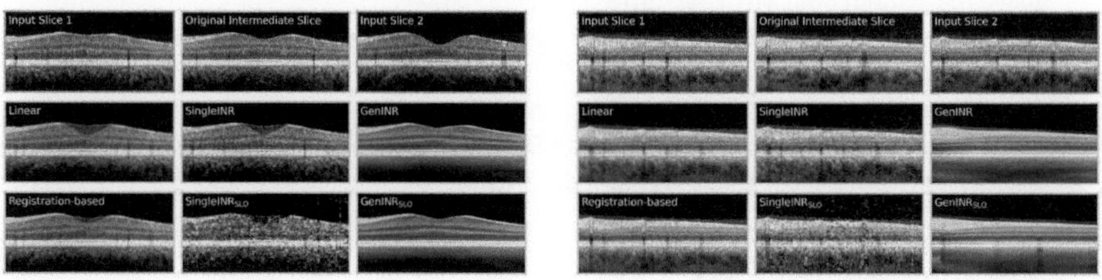

Fig. 2. Two examples of interpolated B-scans using linear, registration-based [5] and INR-based interpolation. The input slices for the different methods are shown with pink frames, while the intermediate and interpolated B-scans are shown with turquoise frames. Our GenINR enables improved shape interpolation through population-based training (example on the left) and correct localization of blood vessels through the additional SLO information (example on the right).

Manually segmenting retinal layers is a highly time-consuming task, resulting in a scarcity of sufficiently large datasets for training CNNs. Our generalized INR, however, requires only a few annotated B-scans per image and can therefore significantly reduce the annotation effort for method development. Due to the population-based training, the INR also enables the segmentation of new images, which is impossible with the comparison methods that utilize single images.

Furthermore, we showed that the integration of SLO images, which are acquired together with the OCT images and thus require no additional effort, enables the reconstruction of small blood vessels in-between B-scans. In future work, we aim to integrate additional en-face imaging modalities, e.g., fundus autofluorescence imaging or color fundus photography, to improve the interpolation of pathologies such as retinal fluid and geographic atrophy. We also plan to explore alternative network architectures and activation functions to mitigate low-frequency bias in image reconstruction.

In conclusion, generalizable INRs enable the effective interpolation of highly anisotropic OCT image data and produce smooth, densely sampled segmentations of retinal layers. By learning continuous representations, INRs improve volumetric accuracy, make OCT analysis independent of device-specific sampling, and enable the joint evaluation of different imaging modalities despite dimensional differences.

References

1. Huang D, Swanson EA, Lin CP et al. Optical coherence tomography. Science. 1991;254:1178–81.
2. Kepp T, Andresen J, Burchard C von der et al. Shape-based segmentation of retinal layers and fluids in OCT image data. Proc SPIE. 2023;12465:207–16.
3. Li K, Wu X, Chen DZ et al. Optimal surface segmentation in volumetric images-a graph-theoretic approach. IEEE Trans Pattern Anal Mach Intell. 2005;28(1):119–34.
4. von der Burchard C, Roider J, Kepp T. Analysis of OCT scanning parameters in AMD and RVO. Diagnostics. 2024;14(5):516.
5. Ehrhardt J, Säring D, Handels H. Structure-preserving interpolation of temporal and spatial image sequences using an optical flow-based method. Methods Inf Med. 2007;46(03):300–7.
6. Cohen JP, Luck M, Honari S. Distribution matching losses can hallucinate features in medical image translation. Proc MICCAI. 2018:529–36.
7. Molaei A, Aminimehr A, Tavakoli A et al. Implicit neural representation in medical imaging: a comparative survey. Proc IEEE CVF ICCV. 2023:2381–91.
8. Amiranashvili T, Lüdke D, Li HB et al. Learning shape reconstruction from sparse measurements with neural implicit functions. Proc MIDL. 2022:22–34.
9. Stolt-Ansó N, McGinnis J, Pan J et al. NISF: neural implicit segmentation functions. Proc MICCAI. 2023:734–44.
10. Saragadam V, LeJeune D, Tan J et al. WIRE: wavelet implicit neural representations. Proc IEEE CVF CVPR. 2023:18507–16.
11. Sitzmann V, Martel J, Bergman A et al. Implicit neural representations with periodic activation functions. Adv Neural Inf Process Syst. 2020;33:7462–73.

Histologic Dataset of Normal and Atypical Mitotic Figures on Human Breast Cancer (AMi-Br)

Christof A. Bertram[1], Viktoria Weiss[1], Taryn A. Donovan[2], Sweta Banerjee[3], Thomas Conrad[4], Jonas Ammeling[5], Robert Klopfleisch[4], Christopher Kaltenecker[6], Marc Aubreville[3]

[1]University of Veterinary Medicine, Vienna, Austria
[2]The Schwarzman Animal Medical Center, New York, USA
[3]Flensburg University of Applied Sciences, Flensburg, Germany
[4]Freie Universität Berlin, Berlin, Germany
[5]Technische Hochschule Ingolstadt, Ingolstadt, Germany
[6]Medical University of Vienna, Vienna, Austria
christof.bertram@vetmeduni.ac.at

Abstract. Assessment of the density of mitotic figures (MFs) in histologic tumor sections is an important prognostic marker for many tumor types, including breast cancer. Recently, it has been reported in multiple works that the quantity of MFs with an atypical morphology (atypical MFs, AMFs) might be an independent prognostic criterion for breast cancer. AMFs are an indicator of mutations in the genes regulating the cell cycle and can lead to aberrant chromosome constitution (aneuploidy) of the tumor cells. To facilitate further research on this topic using pattern recognition, we present the first ever publicly available dataset of atypical and normal MFs (AMi-Br). For this, we utilized two of the most popular MF datasets (MIDOG 2021 and TUPAC) and subclassified all MFs using a three expert majority vote. Our final dataset consists of 3,720 MFs, split into 832 AMFs (22.4%) and 2,888 normal MFs (77.6%) across all 223 tumor cases in the combined set. We provide baseline classification experiments to investigate the consistency of the dataset, using a Monte Carlo cross-validation and different strategies to combat class imbalance. We found an averaged balanced accuracy of up to 0.806 when using a patch-level data set split, and up to 0.713 when using a patient-level split.

1 Introduction

For many human and animal tumors, including human breast cancer, one of the most important tests for assessing patient prognosis is quantification of tumor cell proliferation [1, 2]. Dividing cells can be detected in standard histological tumor images (H&E stain) as mitotic figures (MFs) and are counted within a specific tumor area (mitotic count). Due to relevant inter-rater variability of pathologists in assessment of the mitotic count, deep learning models have been extensively investigated as a potential solution for assistance of the prognostication process [3–5]. For this purpose of model development, several challenge datasets have been created and made publicly available, most importantly the TUPAC dataset [4], for which an alternative ground truth label exists [6], and the datasets of the MIDOG 2021 [5] and MIDOG 2022 challenges [3]. These datasets

C. Palm et al. (Hrsg.), *Bildverarbeitung für die Medizin 2025*, Informatik aktuell,
https://doi.org/10.1007/978-3-658-47422-5_25

have fostered extensive research on this pattern recognition task and comparison of numerous deep learning approaches.

Mitosis is the process of cell division, which is highly regulated in normal cells, resulting in the histological appearance of normal/typical MFs (NMF). However, in malignant tumor cells, mutations can disrupt this regulated process. Resultant failure of equal division of the genetic material (chromosomes) between the two daughter cells can be detected in histological images as atypical MFs (AMFs, Fig. 1). Aberrant chromosome constitutions (aneuploidy) of neoplastic cells can promote tumor progression [7]. There is increasing evidence that the number of AMFs (AMF count) and the ratio of AMFs among all MFs is of high prognostic relevance in human breast cancer [8, 9] and other tumor types [10, 11]. The inter-rater agreement of classifying MFs into normal and atypical subtypes was reported as low due to the complex and highly variable morphologies [10, 12]. Deep learning models have the potential to improve reproducibility and lower time investment required for this task.

To date there are only two studies that have investigated deep learning models for AMFs [12, 13], both of which have shown that this task seems to be particularly difficult based on the overlapping morphologies of normal MFs and AMFs as well as the low frequency of AMFs (class imbalance). Open access datasets are needed to facilitate development of optimized deep learning approaches. Following common practice, a reasonable algorithmic workflow seems to be a two step process with first an object detection of all MFs within large images and a second patch classification into normal and atypical subtypes. Whereas this first step has been extensively addressed in previous research (see above), this article focuses on the patch classification task.

The aim of this dataset publication is to make the first atypical mitotic figure dataset for human breast cancer (AMi-Br) publicly available and provide baseline performance for deep learning classification models.

2 Materials and methods

2.1 Dataset creation

For this dataset we used all MFs labels from the two largest and most diverse challenge datasets in human breast cancer, namely the TUPAC challenge [4] using the improved alternative version of labels [6] and the MIDOG 2021 challenge [5]. These two datasets comprise histological sections from three pathology centers scanned with 6 different whole slide image scanners. A preliminary version of this dataset has been created for a previous study [12], whereas a third annotator was added to derive a consensus vote on the labels.

All three annotators (CAB, VW and TAD) received image patches (128×128 pixels) centered around the original MF annotations and were asked to independently (blinded to the other annotators) classify them into normal and atypical morphologies (Fig. 1). Normal MFs were defined by the characteristic morphologies of the different phases (1. prometaphase, 2. metaphase, 3. ring-shape metaphase, 4. ana- and telophase), as previously described [14]. AMFs included the following categories: 1. polar asymmetry (1A. bipolar asymmetry, 1B. tri- and multipolar asymmetry), 2. chromosome segregation abnormalities (including lagging chromosomes and bridging chromosomes) and

3. other atypical morphologies (such as dispersed chromosome fragments), based on previous definitions [8–10]. If segregation abnormalities occurred concurrently with polar asymmetry or other AMFs, the MF was assigned to the latter label class. For MF patches that lacked clear characteristics of the above mentioned label classes, annotators had to select the class with the highest resemblance. Information relating to the specific MF and AMF subtypes is available in the dataset for two pathologists, however is not considered for the technical validation as it is difficult to find a majority vote for 8 label classes.

2.2 Technical validation

To validate our dataset and assess the label consistency, we performed baseline classification experiments using a standard pipeline with DenseNet-121 and EfficientNet V2 S (both pre-trained on ImageNet) as backbones and using several strategies to combat the class imbalance. We first used weighted cross-entropy, using the class occurrences as weights. Additional strategies included testing random class prevalence-weighted sampling with replacement and using the focal loss. We trained all models for 20 epochs using the Adam optimizer with a learning rate of 10^{-3} and retrospectively selected the best model on the balanced accuracy on the validation set.

As the problem is imbalanced, we report balanced accuracy as well as area under the ROC curve (ROC AUC). We performed a five-fold Monte Carlo cross-validation for each of the conditions and report mean and standard deviation values for each metric. We employed two distinct strategies for data splitting. First, to evaluate the quality of the labels, we conducted the split at the patch level. While we acknowledge that this approach may yield overoptimistic results, we additionally performed a split at the patient level to establish a baseline for algorithmic comparisons.

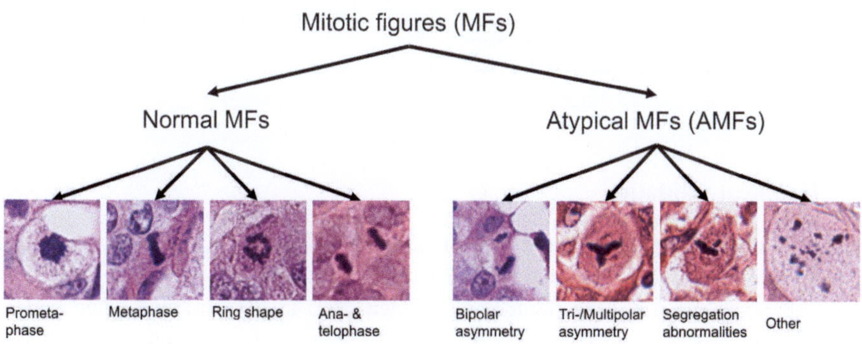

Fig. 1. Examples of the mitotic figure morphologies included in the AMi-Br dataset.

2.3 Usage notes

We make the full dataset available in our github repository[1]. The dataset is stored as CSV file, encompassing the dataset, filename, coordinates, and individual expert labels as well as the joint (majority vote) atypical label as the columns. The repository further contains the notebooks of our experiments.

3 Results

3.1 Dataset description

The dataset consists of, in total, 3,720 MFs, comprising 1,999 MFs from the TUPAC16 alternative label set and 1,721 MFs from the MIDOG21 dataset.

3.1.1 Atypical vs. typical. As the result from the majority vote between the three experts, 832 MFs were found to be atypical, while the remaining 2,888 were considered normal MFs. All experts agreed on 2,908 objects, 412 of which were atypical MFs. The agreement of individual experts can be found in Tab. 1.

3.1.2 Morphology. Overall, we found a moderate agreement ($\kappa = 0.60$) between experts 1 and 2 regarding the morphological subclassification of MFs (Tab. 1 and 2). In the mitotic phase classification of normal MFs, we found the main discrepancy between adjacent classes in the mitotic cycle (Tab. 2).

Evaluation	Experts	Agreement	Cohen's κ
	1 vs. 2	0.85	0.53
AMF/NMF	1 vs. 3	0.84	0.54
	2 vs. 3	0.87	0.66
Morphology	1 vs. 2	0.71	0.60

Tab. 1. Assessment of experts' agreement (overall agreement and Cohen's κ) on the atypical classification and the morphology classification (4 normal MF (NMF) phases and 4 AMF subtypes).

3.2 Technical validation

Using a patch-level split, we found an average balanced accuracy and ROC AUC of up to 0.806 and up to 0.899, respectively, depending on the strategy used to combat the class imbalance (Tab. 3). We found a significant drop in performance when patient-level splitting was performed, hinting towards a possible patient-specific prior that the model overfitted to. We only found a minor impact of model architecture and imbalance-countering strategy, with a slight benefit for the weighted cross-entropy loss and weighted sampling.

[1] `https://github.com/DeepMicroscopy/AMi-Br/`

Tab. 2. Confusion matrix between expert 1 and expert 2 in the assessment of MF morphology.

	AMF				NMF			
	BP	MP	O	S	A-T	M	PM	RS
AMF bipolar asym. (BP)	35	1	5	9	2	6	1	0
AMF multipolar (MP)	2	28	23	11	5	1	1	0
AMF other (O)	9	6	121	46	2	52	15	4
AMF segregation (S)	2	0	12	120	3	5	11	1
NMF anaphase-telophase (A-T)	32	0	7	32	166	14	2	0
NMF metaphase (M)	7	2	12	121	10	1175	22	0
NMF prometaphase (PM)	17	2	53	131	19	244	949	112
NMF ring shape (RS)	1	0	5	9	1	2	0	34

Tab. 3. Results of the classification experiment. We report mean ± standard deviation of five-fold Monte Carlo cross-validation for each metric on the resp. test set. WCE, weighted cross-entropy; FL, focal loss; WS, weighted sampling.

Model	Strategy	Patch-level split		Patient-level split	
		Bal. ACC	ROC AUC	Bal. ACC	ROC AUC
DenseNet-121	WCE	0.801 ± 0.019	0.879 ± 0.010	0.617 ± 0.031	0.633 ± 0.037
	FL	0.791 ± 0.018	0.899 ± 0.012	0.551 ± 0.024	0.587 ± 0.064
	WS	0.795 ± 0.030	0.877 ± 0.015	0.651 ± 0.015	0.656 ± 0.022
EfficientNet V2-S	WCE	0.806 ± 0.024	0.887 ± 0.011	0.675 ± 0.020	0.656 ± 0.025
	FL	0.785 ± 0.015	0.880 ± 0.013	0.671 ± 0.020	0.674 ± 0.012
	WS	0.789 ± 0.016	0.876 ± 0.011	0.713 ± 0.016	0.698 ± 0.026

4 Discussion

As shown by the statistics regarding expert agreement as well as the baseline experiments, AMF classification is a challenging task. The difficulty of this endeavor can be explained by 1) the high class imbalance and 2) the high morphological overlap between AMFs and normal MFs. Since erroneous cell division may occur at any phase of the cell cycle, there may be a higher resemblance between AMFs and normal MFs than within these label classes. Furthermore, some of the atypical morphologies are subtle, such as lagging chromosomes (i.e. small chromosome fragment left behind in the cytoplasm near the metaphase plate instead of being pulled apart). Algorithmic performance may be improved by annotating even larger datasets, more reproducible AMF definitions, or in regularization strategies like creating dedicated augmentation schemes for this problem. :q Future research should create an AMF dataset for additional tumor types that would allow a wider research application [3]. While there are few studies that have evaluated AMFs in tumor types other than human breast cancer [10, 11, 15], this test needs to be evaluated more extensively to gain a better understanding of its prognostic role across tumor types. Deep learning models would allow a reproducible evaluation and analysis of entire tumor sections, thereby generating an understanding of the AMF's intratumoral distribution.

Acknowledgement. CAB, VW, and CK acknowledge the support from the Austrian Research Fund (FWF, project number: I 6555). SB, TC, RK, and MA acknowledge support by the Deutsche Forschungsgemeinschaft (DFG, project number: 520330054).

References

1. Bertram CA, Donovan TA, Bartel A. Mitotic activity: a systematic literature review of the assessment methodology and prognostic value in canine tumors. Vet Pathol. 2024;61(5):752–64.
2. Van Dooijeweert C, Van Diest P, Ellis I. Grading of invasive breast carcinoma: the way forward. Virchows Archiv. 2022;480(1):33–43.
3. Aubreville M, Stathonikos N, Donovan TA et al. Domain generalization across tumor types, laboratories, and species – insights from the 2022 edition of the Mitosis Domain Generalization Challenge. Med Image Anal. 2024;94:103155.
4. Veta M, Heng YJ, Stathonikos N et al. Predicting breast tumor proliferation from whole-slide images: the TUPAC16 challenge. Med Image Anal. 2019;54:111–21.
5. Aubreville M, Stathonikos N, Bertram CA et al. Mitosis domain generalization in histopathology images – the MIDOG challenge. Med Image Anal. 2023;84:102699.
6. Bertram CA, Veta M, Marzahl C et al. Are pathologist-defined labels reproducible? Comparison of the TUPAC16 mitotic figure dataset with an alternative set of labels. Proc MICCAI. 2020:204–13.
7. Gisselsson D. Classification of chromosome segregation errors in cancer. Chromosoma. 2008;117(6):511–9.
8. Lashen A, Toss MS, Alsaleem M et al. The characteristics and clinical significance of atypical mitosis in breast cancer. Mod Pathol. 2022;35(10):1341–8.
9. Ohashi R, Namimatsu S, Sakatani T et al. Prognostic utility of atypical mitoses in patients with breast cancer: A comparative study with Ki67 and phosphohistone H3. J Surg Oncol. 2018;118(3):557–67.
10. Bertram CA, Bartel A, Donovan TA et al. Atypical mitotic figures are prognostically meaningful for canine cutaneous mast cell tumors. Vet Sci. 2023;11(1):5.
11. Matsuda Y, Yoshimura H, Ishiwata T et al. Mitotic index and multipolar mitosis in routine histologic sections as prognostic markers of pancreatic cancers: a clinicopathological study. Pancreatology. 2016;16(1):127–32.
12. Aubreville M, Ganz J, Ammeling J et al. Deep learning-based subtyping of atypical and normal mitoses using a hierarchical anchor-free object detector. Proc BVM. 2023:189–95.
13. Fick RR, Bertram C, Aubreville M. Improving CNN-based mitosis detection through rescanning annotated glass slides and atypical mitosis subtyping. Proc MIDL. 2024.
14. Donovan TA, Moore FM, Bertram CA et al. Mitotic figures—normal, atypical, and imposters: a guide to identification. Vet Pathol. 2021;58(2):243–57.
15. Travaglino A, Raffone A, Santoro A et al. Prognostic significance of atypical mitotic figures in smooth muscle tumors of uncertain malignant potential (STUMP) of the uterus and uterine adnexa. Apmis. 2021;129(4):165–9.

Preservation of Image Content in Stain-to-stain Translation for Digital Pathology

Boqiang Huang[1], Wissem Benjeddou[2], Nadine S. Schaadt[3], Johannes Lotz[4], Friedrich Feuerhake[3,5], Dorit Merhof[1,6]

[1]Institute of Image Analysis and Computer Vision, University of Regensburg, Regensburg
[2]Institute of Imaging and Computer Vision, RWTH Aachen University, Aachen
[3]Institute for Pathology, Hannover Medical School, Hannover
[4]Fraunhofer Institute for Digital Medicine MEVIS, Lübeck
[5]Institute for Neuropathology, University Clinic Freiburg, Freiburg
[6]Fraunhofer Institute for Digital Medicine MEVIS, Bremen
Dorit.Merhof@ur.de

Abstract. In digital pathology, unsupervised domain adaptation of differently stained whole-slide images (WSIs) through image-to-image translation has become increasingly important for various applications such as stain augmentation or for the stain-independent application of deep learning models. In previous work, different variants of generative adversarial networks (GANs) were proposed to translate a real WSI obtained in the staining domain A into a fake WSI in the target staining domain B. However, GANs perform unpaired image-to-image translation and do not enforce consistency with respect to image content, which limits their applicability in digital pathology settings. In this paper, we first investigate the tissue inconsistency problem in such a stain-to-stain translation scenario using a quantitative evaluation of the distortion between real and fake images in different domains. Then, we investigate two possible solutions, namely (1) stain colorization inspired by natural image colorization, and (2) a modified Cycle-GAN, where an intensity invariant loss is proposed to balance the tissue consistency across staining domains. Our results highlight the superiority of these methods compared to conventional unpaired stain translation solutions for typical staining protocols in digital pathology.

1 Introduction

The extensive digitalization of histology glass slides using slide scanners, resulting in digital whole-slide images (WSIs), along with advancements in software and hardware, collectively referred to as digital pathology, has opened new opportunities for automated, highly precise, and reproducible quantification in pathology. To observe tissue samples comprehensively from multiple perspectives, it is common practice to stain consecutive tissue slides with different staining protocols, each sensitive to various tissue components (Fig. 1).

In recent research, neural network based approaches were developed to translate a given real WSI in staining domain A (e.g., PAS) into a fake WSI in the target staining domain B (e.g., H&E), or vice versa (Fig. 3) [1]. Typical applications of those stain translation approaches in digital pathology are stain augmentation [1, 2], image segmentation [3], and cancer classification [4].

C. Palm et al. (Hrsg.), *Bildverarbeitung für die Medizin 2025*, Informatik aktuell,
https://doi.org/10.1007/978-3-658-47422-5_26

Various approaches were so far investigated to realize unpaired stain translation of WSIs and other images, that mainly rely on the concept of generative adversarial networks (GANs). Initially, image colorization [5, 6] and image translation [7, 8] approaches were proposed. Later, Cho et al. [9] constructed a "de-stain" and "re-stain" network based on style transfer learning. Lin et al. [10] adapted this concept for unpaired multi-domain stain transfer, eliminating the necessity to train multiple models for different pairs of staining protocols. Similar to the Star-GAN and its modification [11], only one generator is trained for all possible many-to-many stain translations. Other GAN-based approaches address the stain variance problem by developing stain normalization methods to translate the raw WSIs into stain normalized images [12].

Actually, both image colorization [5, 6] and image translation [8] do have their own weaknesses in stain translation problems. For example, the former has to face non-unique colorization difficulties [2] while the latter can only guarantee the cycle consistency between staining domains [1, 2]. Despite extensive exploration of various network variants and losses, e.g., deformation invariant [13], structure- and/or edge-preserving [4, 14], segmentation consistency [3], multi-scale consistency [15], and contrastive learning-based similarity loss [16], there is no straightforward solution yet to the above-mentioned difficulties. Thus, these methods cannot guarantee that the translated image in the target domain retains the same tissue texture and structural information as the image in the original domain.

In this work, we propose a novel unsupervised stain-to-stain translation based on a pixel-level tissue consistency constraint. Section 2 presents the mathematical representation of both image colorization and image translation problems. Section 3 introduces our clinically meaningful intensity invariant loss compared to the conventional identity loss, together with two incisive distortion measures from both deterministic and statistical points of view. In section 4, experiments based on two independent kidney and breast WSI datasets highlight the outstanding performance of the proposed loss in unsupervised stain translation.

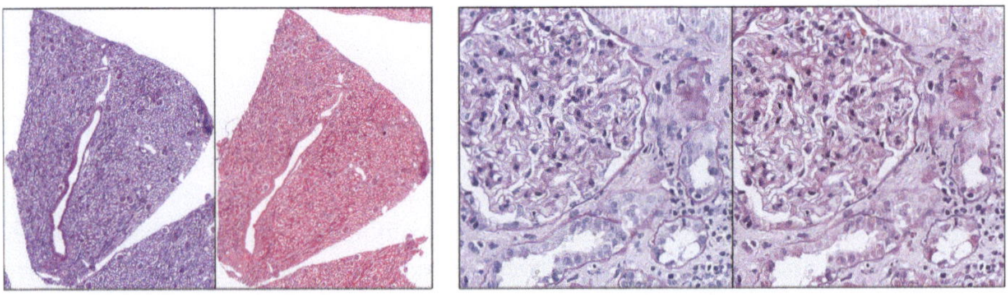

Fig. 1. Consecutive whole slide images of a kidney tissue sample stained in PAS and H&E (*left*), compared with a real image patch in PAS and its fake version in H&E (*right*) after applying the proposed stain translation method.

2 Background: stain colorization & stain translation

2.1 Color representations

A stained WSI, mathematically defined as a matrix $I \in \mathbb{R}^{H \times W \times 3}$, can be represented either in RGB space or CIE LAB space (Fig. 2). Let the nonlinear mapping relationship between these two spaces be $\mathcal{M}^{\mathrm{RGB} \leftrightarrow \mathrm{Lab}}$, both forward and inverse transforms will be

$$I^{\mathrm{Lab}} = \mathcal{M}^{\mathrm{RGB} \to \mathrm{Lab}} \left[I^{\mathrm{RGB}} \right] \tag{1}$$

$$I^{\mathrm{RGB}} = \mathcal{M}^{\mathrm{RGB} \leftarrow \mathrm{Lab}} \left[I^{\mathrm{Lab}} \right] \tag{2}$$

2.2 Supervised stain colorization

Given a staining protocol A, the colorization network C_{A} is trained for a nonlinear mapping relationship. The intensity $I_{\mathrm{T}}^{\mathrm{L}} \in \mathbb{R}^{H \times W}$ from the ground truth $I_{\mathrm{T}} \in \mathbb{R}^{H \times W \times 3}$ is the input while the colorized fake image $I_{\mathrm{F}}^{\mathrm{RGB}} \in \mathbb{R}^{H \times W \times 3}$ is the output

$$I_{\mathrm{F}}^{\mathrm{RGB}} := C_{\mathrm{A}} \left[I_{\mathrm{T}}^{\mathrm{L}} \right] \tag{3}$$

Since $\left(I^{\mathrm{a}}, I^{\mathrm{b}} \right)$ and I^{L} are paired, the training of a stain colorization network is supervised.

Moreover, the colorization can be further separated into two steps: the color estimation (from real intensity $I_{\mathrm{T}}^{\mathrm{L}}$ to fake color pair $\left(I_{\mathrm{F}}^{\mathrm{a}}, I_{\mathrm{F}}^{\mathrm{b}} \right)$ and an inverse transform (from the fake CIE LAB $\left(I_{\mathrm{T}}^{\mathrm{L}}, I_{\mathrm{F}}^{\mathrm{a}}, I_{\mathrm{F}}^{\mathrm{b}} \right)$ to the fake RGB $I_{\mathrm{F}}^{\mathrm{RGB}}$)

$$\left(I_{\mathrm{F}}^{\mathrm{a}}, I_{\mathrm{F}}^{\mathrm{b}} \right) = C_{\mathrm{A}}^{\mathrm{Lab}} \left[I_{\mathrm{T}}^{\mathrm{L}} \right] \tag{4}$$

$$I_{\mathrm{F}}^{\mathrm{RGB}} := \mathcal{M}^{\mathrm{RGB} \leftarrow \mathrm{Lab}} \left[\left(I_{\mathrm{T}}^{\mathrm{L}} I_{\mathrm{F}}^{\mathrm{a}}, I_{\mathrm{F}}^{\mathrm{b}} \right) \right] \tag{5}$$

It should be noted that $C_{\mathrm{A}}^{\mathrm{Lab}} : I^{\mathrm{L}} \to \left(I^{\mathrm{a}}, I^{\mathrm{b}} \right)$ cannot be a perfect one-to-one mapping relationship, since it is not possible to correctly estimate the color of a pixel only based on its optical intensity [5, 6]. Further, since C_{A} is trained with the knowledge in A, it would wrongly colorize a pixel from an unknown domain B with high probability, which would be uncontrollable and risky for any stain-to-stain translation.

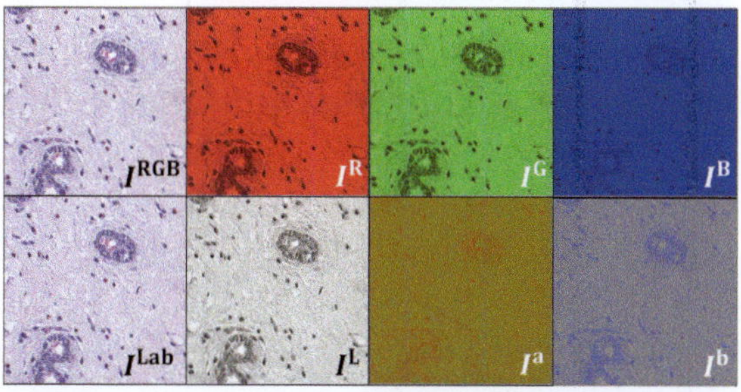

Fig. 2. WSI image $I \in \mathbb{R}^{H \times W \times 3}$ represented as I^{RGB} or I^{Lab} in RGB or a CIE LAB color space. Here, I^{R}, I^{G}, and I^{B} represent the red, green, and blue channels, while I^{L}, I^{a}, and I^{b} represent the optical intensity, green-to-red, and blue-to-yellow channels.

2.3 Unsupervised stain translation

Given two staining protocols A and B, the stain translation network $\mathcal{T}_{A\leftrightarrow B}$ is trained between unpaired WSI patches $I_{TA}, I_{TB} \in \mathbb{R}^{H\times W\times 3}$ in terms of unsupervised learning. The directional translations can be written as

$$I_{FB} := \mathcal{T}_{A\to B}\left[I_{TA}\right] \tag{6}$$

$$I_{FA} := \mathcal{T}_{A\leftarrow B}\left[I_{TB}\right] \tag{7}$$

where I_{FB} and I_{FA} denote the fake images of I_{TA} and I_{TB} in domain B and A, respectively. The so-called cycle-translation can then be written as

$$I_{RA} := \mathcal{T}_{A\leftarrow B}\left[I_{FB}\right] = \mathcal{T}_{A\leftarrow B}\left[\mathcal{T}_{A\to B}\left[I_{TA}\right]\right] \tag{8}$$

$$I_{RB} := \mathcal{T}_{A\to B}\left[I_{FA}\right] = \mathcal{T}_{A\to B}\left[\mathcal{T}_{A\leftarrow B}\left[I_{TB}\right]\right] \tag{9}$$

where I_{RA} and I_{RB} denote the reconstructed image of I_{TA} and I_{TB} in domain A and B, respectively. Since the reconstructed images should be the same as their corresponding inputs, the cycle-consistency loss is derived as follows (Fig. 3, top)

$$\mathcal{L}_{cyc}\left(\mathcal{T}_{A\leftrightarrow B}\right) := \mathbb{E}_{I\sim p_{data}}\left\{\|I_{TA} - I_{RA}\|_1\right\} + \mathbb{E}_{I\sim p_{data}}\left\{\|I_{TB} - I_{RB}\|_1\right\} \tag{10}$$

Here, the ℓ_1 norm is applied as in Cycle-GANs [1, 3, 8].

Now, by combining the standard adversarial loss functions in domain A and B

$$\mathcal{L}_{advA} := \mathbb{E}_{I\sim p_{data}}\left\{\log\left(1 - \mathcal{D}_A\left(I_{FA}\right)\right)\right\} + \mathbb{E}_{I\sim p_{data}}\left\{\log\left(\mathcal{D}_A\left(I_{TA}\right)\right)\right\} \tag{11}$$

$$\mathcal{L}_{advB} := \mathbb{E}_{I\sim p_{data}}\left\{\log\left(1 - \mathcal{D}_B\left(I_{FB}\right)\right)\right\} + \mathbb{E}_{I\sim p_{data}}\left\{\log\left(\mathcal{D}_B\left(I_{TB}\right)\right)\right\} \tag{12}$$

with the cycle-consistency loss in Eq. (10), the optimization problem of a Cycle-GAN is

$$\mathcal{T}^*_{A\leftrightarrow B} = \arg\min_{\mathcal{T}_{A\leftrightarrow B}}\max_{\mathcal{D}_A,\mathcal{D}_B}\ \mathcal{L}\left(\mathcal{T}_{A\leftrightarrow B}, \mathcal{D}_A, \mathcal{D}_B\right) \tag{13}$$

$$\mathcal{L}\left(\mathcal{T}_{A\leftrightarrow B}, \mathcal{D}_A, \mathcal{D}_B\right) = \mathcal{L}_{advA} + \mathcal{L}_{advB} + \lambda_{cyc}\cdot\mathcal{L}_{cyc}\left(\mathcal{T}_{A\leftrightarrow B}\right) \tag{14}$$

where $\mathcal{D}_A$ and $\mathcal{D}_B$ represent the discriminator in domain A and B, respectively.

3 Method: intensity invariant stain translation

3.1 Distortion measures

In order to quantitatively evaluate structural distortions between real and fake images, the peak signal-to-noise ratio (PSNR) and the similarity index measure (SSIM) are considered. Let I_t and I_f represent the target image and reference image with the same dimension, the PSNR is defined as

$$d_{PSNR}\left(I_t, I_f\right) := 10\log_{10}\left(\frac{1}{\frac{1}{\#I}\|I_t - I_f\|_2^2}\right) \tag{15}$$

where $\#I$ denotes the cardinality of the image.

Different from the Euclidean metric, the SSIM is designed based on a perception model that considers image degradation as perceived change in structural information

$$d_{\mathrm{SSIM}}(I_{\mathrm{t}}, I_{\mathrm{f}}) := \frac{(2\mu_{\mathrm{t}}\mu_{\mathrm{f}} + c_1)(2\sigma_{\mathrm{tf}} + c_2)}{(\mu_{\mathrm{t}}^2 + \mu_{\mathrm{f}}^2 + c_1)(\sigma_{\mathrm{t}}^2 + \sigma_{\mathrm{f}}^2 + c_2)} \tag{16}$$

where μ and σ represent the pixel sample mean and standard deviation, c_1 and c_2 represent two controllable constants that can stabilize the division with weak denominator.

3.2 Identity loss

Recall that the cycle-consistency is actually a very loose constraint for image translation problems. Thus, the authors in [1, 3, 8] found that it is helpful to introduce an additional loss to Eq. (14) such that the mappings $\mathcal{T}_{\mathrm{A}\leftrightarrow\mathrm{B}}$ are encouraged to preserve the color composition between the input and output

$$\mathcal{L}_{\mathrm{idt}}(\mathcal{T}_{\mathrm{A}\leftrightarrow\mathrm{B}}) := \mathbb{E}_{I\sim p_{\mathrm{data}}}\{\|I_{\mathrm{TA}} - \mathcal{T}_{\mathrm{A}\leftarrow\mathrm{B}}[I_{\mathrm{TA}}]\|_1\} + \mathbb{E}_{I\sim p_{\mathrm{data}}}\{\|I_{\mathrm{TB}} - \mathcal{T}_{\mathrm{A}\rightarrow\mathrm{B}}[I_{\mathrm{TB}}]\|_1\} \tag{17}$$

Since the input image is taken from the target domain, the presented loss is more similar to an identity loss (Fig. 3 Bottom Left). This loss is considered in comparison to our novel intensity invariant loss proposed in Section 3.3.

3.3 Intensity invariant loss

Assuming that the tissue sample is not damaged in the staining, it is reasonable to require the invariant intensity of both the input real WSI patch in the source domain and the output fake WSI patch in the target domain (Fig. 3 Bottom Right). Accordingly, we propose a novel loss function as follows

$$\mathcal{L}_{\mathrm{int}}(\mathcal{T}_{\mathrm{A}\leftrightarrow\mathrm{B}}) := \mathbb{E}_{I\sim p_{\mathrm{data}}}\{\|I_{\mathrm{TA}}^{\mathrm{L}} - I_{\mathrm{FB}}^{\mathrm{L}}\|_1\} + \mathbb{E}_{I\sim p_{\mathrm{data}}}\{\|I_{\mathrm{TB}}^{\mathrm{L}} - I_{\mathrm{FA}}^{\mathrm{L}}\|_1\} \tag{18}$$

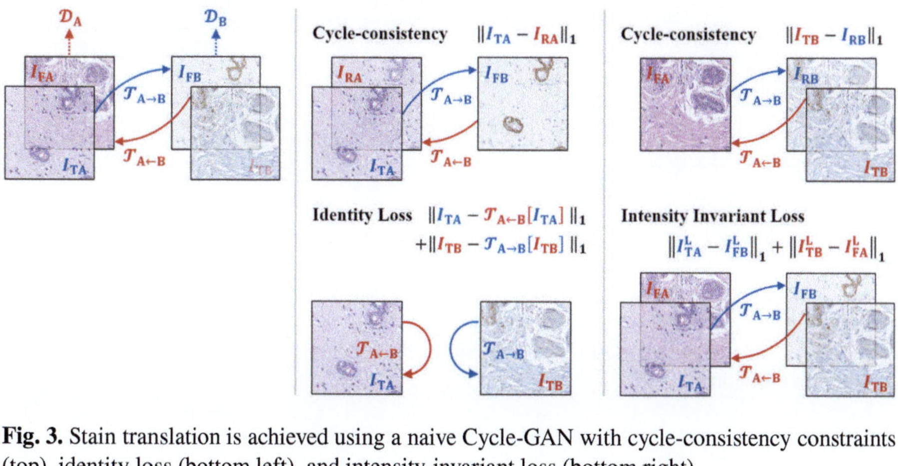

Fig. 3. Stain translation is achieved using a naive Cycle-GAN with cycle-consistency constraints (top), identity loss (bottom left), and intensity-invariant loss (bottom right).

4 Experiments and results

4.1 Datasets

Dataset D1 consists of human kidney samples stained in PAS and H&E protocols. There are five renal transplant samples stained in H&E. Another eight renal specimens were stained in PAS. The WSI image patch was tiled with 512 × 512 pixels. There were 3000 patches randomly selected for training (1500 PAS + 1500 H&E), and 500 patches randomly selected from the rest for testing (250 PAS + 250 H&E).

Dataset D2 consists of both healthy and cancerous breast samples which are stained in CK5/14 and H&E protocols. There are eight samples stained in H&E and fifteen samples stained in CK5/14. Each WSI image patch is tiled at 512 × 512 pixels, and then down-sampled to 256 × 256 pixels to reduce the computational load. There are 16000 images randomly selected for training (8000 CK5/14 + 8000 H&E), and 4000 images randomly selected for testing (2000 CK5/14 + 2000 H&E).

All WSI images were scanned with a 40X objective lens (ca. 0.25 microns per pixel (mpp)) using Aperio scanners from Leica[1].

4.2 Stain colorization results

Four stain colorization networks have been trained based on both datasets D1 and D2, which are marked by C_{PAS}, $C_{HE\text{-}1}$, C_{CK}, and $C_{HE\text{-}2}$. Here, HE-1 and HE-2 are two different

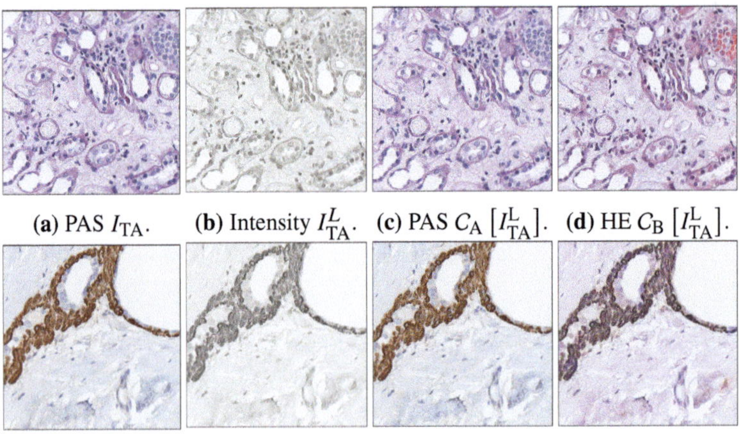

(a) PAS I_{TA}. (b) Intensity I^L_{TA}. (c) PAS $C_A\left[I^L_{TA}\right]$. (d) HE $C_B\left[I^L_{TA}\right]$.

(e) CK I_{TA}. (f) Intensity I^L_{TA}. (g) CK $C_A\left[I^L_{TA}\right]$. (h) HE $C_B\left[I^L_{TA}\right]$.

Fig. 4. Stain colorization and colorization-based stain translation. (a) and (e) are real images in PAS and CK5/14 domains, respectively. (b) and (f) are intensity images. (c) and (g) are colorized fake images. (d) and (h) are colorization-based translation results in the target H&E domain (no ground truth for comparison).

[1] www.leicabiosystems.com

datasets from D1 and D2, respectively. Network settings are the same as the ones in [8]. Visual results are shown in Fig. 4.

Tab. 1 illustrates that the colorization networks can learn the nonlinear relationship between the intensity and the color very well. Moreover, when the provided dataset is large enough, such as in D2, the immunohistochemical staining method can be learned with high accuracy.

4.3 Stain translation results

Based on the Cycle-GAN loss in Eq. (14), the identity loss in Eq. (17), and the intensity invariant loss in Eq. (18), three experiments were designed to investigate the contribution of these constrains in stain translation.

- *Scenario 1*: Cycle-GAN with neither identity loss nor intensity invariance loss
  Since the cycle-consistency loss Eq. (10) is the only constraint for the translation, the generator can certain a good reconstruction but cannot maintain a qualified translation in the target domain [8]. As shown in Fig. 5b and 5f, many unreasonable tissue components are generated in the target domain, which results in inconsistent tissue details between the original domain and the target domain. Such phenomenon can be observed in Tab. 2 as well, in which d^1_{PSNR} is the smallest one and d^1_{SSIM} values are all negative.
- *Scenario 2*: Cycle-GAN with identity loss but without intensity invariant loss
  In this case, the total loss function is updated as

$$\mathcal{L}\left(\mathcal{T}_{\text{A}\leftrightarrow\text{B}}, \mathcal{D}_{\text{A}}, \mathcal{D}_{\text{B}}\right) = \mathcal{L}_{\text{advA}} + \mathcal{L}_{\text{advB}} + \lambda_{\text{cyc}} \cdot \mathcal{L}_{\text{cyc}} + \lambda_{\text{idt}} \cdot \mathcal{L}_{\text{idt}} \tag{19}$$

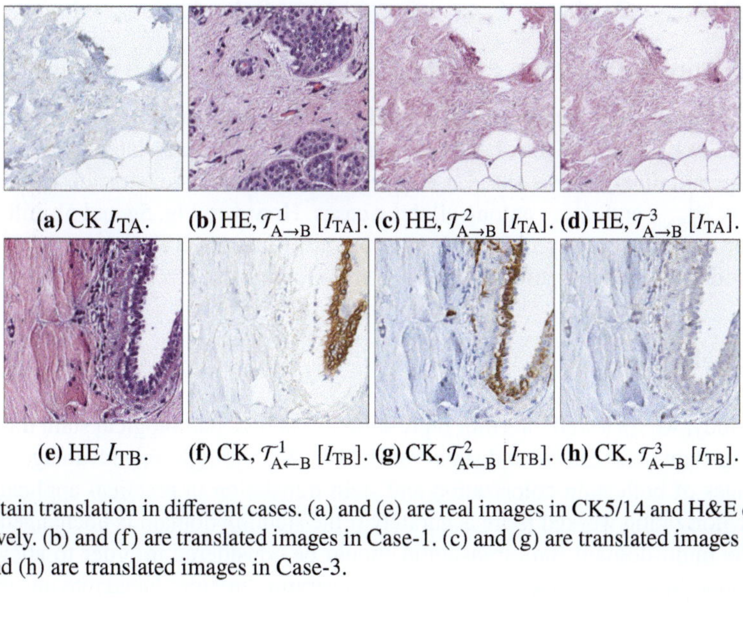

(a) CK I_{TA}. **(b)** HE, $\mathcal{T}^1_{\text{A}\to\text{B}}\left[I_{\text{TA}}\right]$. **(c)** HE, $\mathcal{T}^2_{\text{A}\to\text{B}}\left[I_{\text{TA}}\right]$. **(d)** HE, $\mathcal{T}^3_{\text{A}\to\text{B}}\left[I_{\text{TA}}\right]$.

(e) HE I_{TB}. **(f)** CK, $\mathcal{T}^1_{\text{A}\leftarrow\text{B}}\left[I_{\text{TB}}\right]$. **(g)** CK, $\mathcal{T}^2_{\text{A}\leftarrow\text{B}}\left[I_{\text{TB}}\right]$. **(h)** CK, $\mathcal{T}^3_{\text{A}\leftarrow\text{B}}\left[I_{\text{TB}}\right]$.

Fig. 5. Stain translation in different cases. (a) and (e) are real images in CK5/14 and H&E domains respectively. (b) and (f) are translated images in Case-1. (c) and (g) are translated images in Case-2. (d) and (h) are translated images in Case-3.

Tab. 1. Stain colorization performance.

$d_{(\cdot)}(I_T, I_F)$ $I_F := C_{(\cdot)}[I_T]$	C_{PAS} Train	 Test	$C_{HE\text{-}1}$ Train	 Test	C_{CK} Train	 Test	$C_{HE\text{-}2}$ Train	 Test
d_{PSNR}	33.31	33.17	30.99	30.83	38.43	38.24	36.23	36.08
d_{SSIM}	0.97	0.97	0.96	0.96	0.97	0.97	0.98	0.98

Tab. 2. Stain translation performance.

$d_{(\cdot)}(I_T^L, I_F^L)$ $I_F := \mathcal{T}_{(\cdot)}[I_T]$	$\mathcal{T}_{PAS\to HE}$ Train	 Test	$\mathcal{T}_{PAS\leftarrow HE}$ Train	 Test	$\mathcal{T}_{CK\to HE}$ Train	 Test	$\mathcal{T}_{CK\leftarrow HE}$ Train	 Test
d^1_{PSNR}	10.58	10.53	11.33	11.30	12.58	12.54	13.06	13.22
d^1_{SSIM}	−0.30	−0.30	−0.33	−0.34	−0.30	−0.30	−0.30	−0.29
d^2_{PSNR}	19.45	19.53	17.29	17.37	18.25	18.22	18.09	18.20
d^2_{SSIM}	0.80	0.80	0.77	0.78	0.81	0.81	0.82	0.82
d^3_{PSNR}	22.80	22.38	21.85	21.50	24.79	26.38	23.63	24.05
d^3_{SSIM}	0.89	0.88	0.89	0.89	0.91	0.92	0.87	0.88

Similar to the setting in [1, 3, 8], the weighting coefficients λ_{cyc} and λ_{idt} are set to 1 (i.e., equal contribution of all loss terms).
Tab. 2 shows that the identity loss can preserve the content and therefore constraint the behavior of the generator. Comparing to the Case-1, all distortion measures had been improved significantly.

- *Scenario 3*: Cycle-GAN with both identity loss and intensity invariant loss
Now, all the proposed loss terms are integrated into

$$\mathcal{L}(\mathcal{T}_{A\leftrightarrow B}, \mathcal{D}_A, \mathcal{D}_B) = \mathcal{L}_{advA} + \mathcal{L}_{advB} + \lambda_{cyc} \cdot \mathcal{L}_{cyc} + \lambda_{idt} \cdot \mathcal{L}_{idt} + \lambda_{int} \cdot \mathcal{L}_{int} \quad (20)$$

In practice, the weighting coefficients λ_{cyc}, λ_{idt}, and λ_{int} are set to 1 as well.

Fig. 5 shows that there is no substantial structural difference in the intensity image among the real image, the translated image in Case-2, and the translated image in Case-3. Tab. 2 quantitatively shows that Case-3 achieves the smallest distortion or the largest similarity d^3_{PSNR} and d^3_{SSIM} among all three cases. However, Fig. 5g and 5h still exhibits the color nonuniqueness problem, which cannot be quantitatively compared as there is no ground truth in the target domain.

5 Conclusion

In this study, we reviewed the color representation in histopathological stain translation, including stain colorization and stain translation. We highlight the advantages and disadvantages of both stain colorization and stain translation in practical applications. In detail, colorization worked more accurately if the staining domain is unchanged. Otherwise, the multi-domain stain translation should be considered in order to alleviate the color non-uniqueness problem, where more constraints are introduced into unsupervised deep learning solutions, e.g., by introducing identity loss and the proposed intensity invariant loss into the Cycle-GAN. Since we seriously consider the tissue texture distortion at the pixel level in terms of PSNR and SSIM, we avoid higher distortions between the images from the source and the target staining domains, as observed for methods based on geometry- / topology- / morphology- / statistics-induced loss functions.

Acknowledgement. This study was supported by the BMBF (Project No. FKZ 01IS21067A-C, FKZ 01ZX1608A), and the DFG (Project No. 445703531). The authors gratefully acknowledge the computational and data resources provided by the Leibniz Supercomputing Centre (`www.lrz.de`).

References

1. Gadermayr M, Gupta L, Appel V et al. Generative adversarial networks for facilitating stain-independent supervised and unsupervised segmentation: a study on kidney histology. IEEE Trans Med Imaging. 2019;38(10):2293–302.
2. Haan K de, Zhang Y, Zuckerman JE et al. Deep learning-based transformation of H&E stained tissues into special stains. Nat Commun. 2021;12(4884).
3. Bouteldja N, Klinkhammer BM, Schlaich T et al. Improving unsupervised stain-to-stain translation using self-supervision and meta-learning. J Pathol Inform. 2022;13(100107).
4. Berijanian M, Schaadt NS, Huang B et al. Unsupervised many-to-many stain translation for histological image augmentation to improve classification accuracy. J Pathol Inform. 2023;14(100195).
5. Nazeri K, Ng E, Ebrahimi M. Image colorization using generative adversarial networks. Proc AMDO. 2018:85–94.
6. Vitoria P, Raad L, Ballester C. ChromaGAN: adversarial picture colorization with semantic class distribution. Proc IEEE CVF WACV. 2020:2445–54.
7. Choi Y, Choi M, Kim M et al. StarGAN: unified generative adversarial networks for multi-domain image-to-image translation. Proc IEEE CVF CVPR. 2018:8789–97.
8. Zhu JY, Park T, Isola P et al. Unpaired image-to-image translation using cycle-consistent adversarial networks. Proc IEEE ICCV. 2017:2223–32.
9. Cho H, Lim S, Choi G et al. Neural stain-style transfer learning using GAN for histopathological images. Proc ACML. 2017.
10. Lin Y, Zeng B, Wang Y et al. Unpaired multi-domain stain transfer for kidney histopathological images. Proc AAAI. 2022:1630–7.
11. Choi Y, Uh Y, Yoo J et al. StarGAN v2: diverse image synthesis for multiple domains. Proc IEEE CVF CVPR. 2020:8188–97.
12. Bentaieb A, Hamarneh G. Adversarial stain transfer for histopathology image analysis. IEEE Trans Med Imaging. 2018;37(3):792–802.
13. Wang C, Yang G, Papanastasiou G et al. DiCyc: GAN-based deformation invariant cross-domain information fusion for medical image synthesis. Inf Fusion. 2021;67:147–60.
14. Wagner SJ, Khalili N, Sharma R et al. Structure-preserving multi-domain stain color augmentation using style-transfer with disentangled representations. Proc MICCAI. 2021:257–66.
15. Liu S, Zhu C, Xu F et al. BCI: breast cancer immunohistochemical image generation through pyramid Pix2pix. Proc IEEE CVF CVPR. 2022:1815–24.

16. Li F, Hu Z, Chen W et al. Adaptive supervised PatchNCE loss for learning H&E-to-IHC stain translation with inconsistent groundtruth image pairs. Proc MICCAI. 2023:632–41.

Automation Bias in AI-assisted Medical Decision-making under Time Pressure in Computational Pathology

Emely Rosbach[1], Jonathan Ganz[1], Jonas Ammeling[1], Andreas Riener[1], Marc Aubreville[2]

[1]Technische Hochschule Ingolstadt, Ingolstadt, Germany
[2]Flensburg University of Applied Sciences, Flensburg, Germany
emely.rosbach@thi.de

Abstract. Artificial intelligence (AI)-based clinical decision support systems (CDSS) promise to enhance diagnostic accuracy and efficiency in computational pathology. However, human-AI collaboration might introduce automation bias, where users uncritically follow automated cues. This bias may worsen when time pressure strains practitioners' cognitive resources. We quantified automation bias by measuring the adoption of negative system consultations and examined the role of time pressure in a web-based experiment, where trained pathology experts (n=28) estimated tumor cell percentages. Our results indicate that while AI integration led to a statistically significant increase in overall performance, it also resulted in a 7% automation bias rate, where initially correct evaluations were overturned by erroneous AI advice. Conversely, time pressure did not exacerbate automation bias occurrence, but appeared to increase its severity, evidenced by heightened reliance on the system's negative consultations and subsequent performance decline. These findings highlight potential risks of AI use in healthcare. The final dataset (including a table with image patch details), participant demographics, and source code are available at: `https://github.com/emelyrosbach/AB-TP.git`

1 Introduction

Driven by the success of deep learning algorithms in medical imaging, computational pathology seeks to augment practitioner capabilities in areas traditionally challenging for humans like quantitative image analysis tasks e.g., manual biomarker scoring. Given the safety-critical nature of healthcare and the complexity of legal liability for machine misjudgments, clinical decision support systems (CDSS) allow the full benefits of artificial intelligence (AI) integration, including improved diagnostic accuracy and increased efficiency, while keeping the responsibility for the final diagnosis with the medical expert. However, the necessity for practitioner oversight harbors the risk of introducing a new set of challenges, as the mere presence of AI advice could trigger or amplify cognitive biases, which are systematic patterns of deviation from rationality in judgment, such as automation bias (AB). AB refers to the tendency to treat automated cues as infallible, following them unquestioningly instead of vigilant information seeking. This leads to errors when issues go unnoticed because the system fails to detect them (omission errors) or when incorrect automation output is uncritically adopted (commission errors) [1]. Environmental factors like time pressure, ubiquitously present in routine pathology, can place strain on cognitive resources, resulting in heuristic-based

C. Palm et al. (Hrsg.), *Bildverarbeitung für die Medizin 2025*, Informatik aktuell,
https://doi.org/10.1007/978-3-658-47422-5_27

usage of decision support systems (DSS) or even automation overdependence [1]. In essence, time stress may amplify both the frequency and magnitude of AB. While most studies on CDSS highlight the overall performance gains from AI integration, there have been few studies on the effect size of AB in medical decision-making [1], with none in the field of pathology. While existing research typically evaluates overall acceptance of false AI advice, following Goddard et al. [1] we will measure AB through commission errors, where a previously correct independent evaluation is overturned by incorrect AI guidance (negative consultation), allowing us to isolate AB from other cognitive biases for more precise quantification. Research on the impact of time pressure on AB presents conflicting results, suggesting its effects may be context-dependent: some work demonstrates increased automation dependence under time constraints [2], while others report reduced system reliance in time critical situations [3].

2 Materials and methods

In this paper, for the first time, we quantify AB in human-AI collaboration within computational pathology and examine the additional influence of time pressure through a web-based experiment conducted with non-paid expert users (pathologists, pathology residents, and non-physician pathology staff) independently verified by us and recruited from our professional network, based on prior research collaborations.

2.1 Study task

Our study task focused on estimating tumor cell percentage (TCP) on hematoxylin and eosin (H&E)-stained tissue slides, defined as the ratio of neoplastic cells to the total cell count. Typically represented by a single percentage value or specified range, TCP is estimated briefly through visual assessment in clinical practice and is thus suitable to be performed under time constraints. Due to its innate complexity, stemming from the variability of clinical specimen, lack of standardized protocols and absence of formal training, TCP is widely acknowledged as being prone to substantial inter-observer variability [4], rendering it susceptible to cognitive bias manifestation. TCP estimation is commonly performed in routine pathology, as certain molecular tests require a specific level of tumor DNA to ensure robustness and proper interpretation of assay results [4]. Should samples falling below the threshold for a given molecular test be estimated to be above it, unwarranted confidence in the assay result may be fostered, leading to misguided treatment plans and compromised patient care [4].

2.2 Materials

For the TCP estimation, we provided participants with a selection of 23 tissue patches, presenting a broad spectrum of tumor cellularity and tissue types at different magnifications. Of these images, three were allocated for a training session, while the remaining 20 were designated for the main experiment. The study material was sourced from three openly available datasets, each featuring image patches and dense annotations of various cell types, including tumor cells: the BreCaHad dataset [5], the dataset from Frei et al.'s publication on tumor cell fraction scoring [6], and the BreastPathQ dataset [7]. A standard object detection approach based on the FCOS [8] architecture was utilized to detect tumor- and other cells, from which the TCP for each slide was calculated. This approach was trained on the BreCaHad dataset, reserving five patches for use in the experiment. Using an actual AI prevented bias from fabricated estimations, allowing us to observe participant reactions to realistic inaccuracies. When the AI model was applied to the study slides, about half showed highly accurate detections, while the remaining contained samples with both high positive- and negative error rates, indicating a realistic non-robustness caused by a covariant data shift between the datasets.

2.3 Experimental design

Based on the literature review the following hypotheses were established:

- H1: The introduction of AI support, compared to the baseline (no AI), will lead to the emergence of new errors in the form of measurable AB (negative consultations).
- H2: The presence of time constraints will increase both the frequency and severity of AB, as delineated in H1.

The study employed a 2 × 2 factorial, within-subject design with two independent variables (IVs): inclusion of AI (yes/no) and presence of time pressure (TP) (yes/no).

The occurrence of AB constitutes the key dependent variable (DV). For this, instances of negative consultations, where an initially correct assessment in the baseline treatment (Est_B) was altered to a false evaluation in the second round (Est_{AI}) after exposure to an incorrect AI prediction ($Pred_{AI}$), were quantified. To classify the correctness of TCP estimates (ranging from 0-100%), we applied the 25% threshold required for direct DNA sequencing [4]. Assessments were deemed correct if they aligned with the ground truth (GT) in relation to this threshold. For the AB analysis, only dataset entries, where the independent estimate matches the GT, while both the AI recommendation and subsequent AI-aided assessment are erroneous, were considered. After filtering, the remaining data tuples were compared to the total number of AI-assisted TCP assessments to derive the AB occurrence rate.

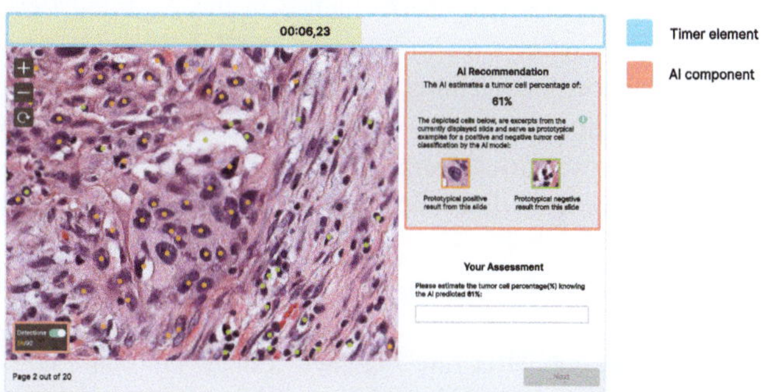

Fig. 1. Study interface as seen by participants during TCP assessment. Depending on the experimental condition, the AI component and the reverse countdown timer element were made visible.

The second DV, participant performance ($\overline{|\text{Dev}_{\text{GT}}|}$), is calculated as the mean absolute deviation of TCP estimates from the GT per condition.

Alignment with AI advice. The relative dependence on AI recommendations was also measured using the judge advisor system [9], calculated per condition as $\overline{JAS} = \frac{1}{N_{\text{slides}}}\sum_{i=1}^{N_{\text{slides}}} \frac{|\text{Est}_{\text{AI(i)}} - \text{Est}_{\text{B(i)}}|}{|\text{Est}_{\text{AI(i)}} - \text{Pred}_{\text{AI(i)}}| + |\text{Est}_{\text{AI(i)}} - \text{Est}_{\text{B(i)}}|}$. The DVs, performance and AI-alignment, were analyzed for the entire dataset and the AB-filtered subset.

After a training session to acquaint participants with the user interface (Fig. 1) and study task, the experiment unfolded as follows: subjects estimated the TCP on 20 H&E-stained slides, first independently and then with the aid of an AI. Identical image material was employed in both phases, separated by a two-week wash-out period to counteract learning effects. Half of the slides in each segment were subject to time stress, in the form of an expiring 10 second countdown. Since the TP conditions were implemented consecutively in each segment, the study material was split into two image sets, consisting of 10 different yet similar slides in terms of TCP content and AI prediction quality. A within-group approach was adopted to maximize statistical power, given the challenge of recruiting experts. We randomized which TP condition and image set participants begin both rounds with. Additionally, a balanced 10x10 Latin Square was employed to randomize the sequence of tissue slides within each image set.

3 Results

A total of 31 medical experts participated in the first round, with 28 advancing to the second phase, resulting in a final sample size of 28 subjects.

The normal distributions of all samples evaluated in this section were confirmed via Shapiro-Wilk tests. A two-way repeated measures ANOVA conducted on the mean absolute deviation from the GT revealed a statistically significant main effect of AI integration on performance (F(1, 108) = 8.32, p = <.01, $\alpha = 0.05$). However, neither the main effect of time pressure (p = 0.19) nor the interaction between AI integration and TP (p = 0.46) were statistically significant. Examining the baseline in isolation, a one-tailed paired-samples t-test revealed a statistically significant decrease in performance under time stress (no TP: M = 13.55, SD = 4.81; with TP: M = 15.29, SD = 5.00; t(27) = -1.76, p = 0.045, $\alpha = 0.05$). Comparison of performance in the AI-aided treatments, albeit not statistically significant, reflects a similar trend (no TP: M = 11.74; with TP: M = 12.23). These results suggest that AI integration contributes to an overall performance increase, evidenced by a reduced $\overline{|\text{Dev}_{\text{GT}}|}$, whereas TP seems to have the opposite effect. To evaluate the next IV, a two-tailed paired-samples t-test was conducted on the $\overline{JAS}$, revealing a statistically significant difference between the AI treatments with and without time constraints (no TP: M = 0.49, SD = 0.13; with TP: M = 0.55, SD = 0.12; t(27) = -2.80, p = <.01, $\alpha = 0.05$). This highlights that reliance on AI advice may intensify under time stress.

Due to reduced sample size after filtering (Sec. 2.3), DVs did not consistently meet normality assumptions, hence the AB analysis will be conducted using descriptive statistics. Of 560 TCP estimates made with AI aid, practitioners adopted AI recommendations contradictory to their independent assessments, pertaining to the TCP being

Tab. 1. Descriptive statistics comparing automation bias occurrence (no. negative consultations), performance ($\overline{|Dev_{GT}|}$), and dependence on AI ($\overline{JAS}$) with and without time pressure.

Frequency	All negative consultations 38/560 ≈ 7%	No TP 19/280 ≈ 7%	With TP 19/280 ≈ 7%
	M ∓ SD	M ∓ SD	M ∓ SD
Performance ($\overline{|Dev_{GT}|}$)	23.61 ∓ 19.32	19.42 ∓ 17.37	27.79 ∓ 20.71
$\overline{JAS}$	0.62 ∓ 0.29	0.58 ∓ 0.32	0.65 ∓ 0.25

below/above the 25% threshold, in only 67 cases. This included 29 positive consultations, where AI integration lead to correction of a previously erroneous decision, and 38 negative consultations, where an initially correct evaluation was overturned by incorrect AI guidance. The resulting AB rate consequently yielded approximately 7% (38/560). Regarding the influence of TP, a comparison of the descriptive statistics (Tab. 1) indicates that the AB occurrence rate remains steady at approximately 7%, irrespective of the presence of time constraints. However, time pressure appears to notably exacerbate the severity of AB, as evidenced by a decline in participant performance reflected in a heightened $\overline{|Dev_{GT}|}$ (no TP: M = 19.42; with TP: M = 27.79). Additionally, another factor that might suggest an increased magnitude of AB under time stress is the greater alignment with AI advice, reflected in the rising $\overline{JAS}$ (no TP: M = 0.58; with TP: M = 0.65), when adopting the system's negative consultations under time strain.

4 Discussion

Overall, integration of AI was found to improve participant performance. This ameliorating effect may also explain why the notable performance decline observed under time pressure in the baseline condition was less pronounced during AI-aided evaluations. Additionally, TP appeared to increase alignment with AI advice, likely due to the strain on cognitive resources under stress, which could be considered beneficial when the AI is accurate, but detrimental when the system errs. Interestingly, despite AI's potential, we recorded that pathologists were largely unwilling to adopt model recommendations, that contradicted their initial judgments, regardless of the correctness of the system's output. This suggests that AB may not be the primary cognitive bias in AI-aided medical decision-making. Nonetheless, by quantifying the number of accepted negative consultations, we determined an AB occurrence rate of approximately 7% in its "purest" form. This aligns with existing empirical research on AB [1], reporting negative consultation acceptance rates of 6% to 11%. As our findings suggest that interaction with AI can indeed induce AB, leading to errors that would not have occurred in the absence of system guidance, hypothesis 1 is fully accepted. Contrary to the expectations outlined in H2, the introduction of time pressure did not affect the occurrence frequency of AB. This could be attributed to our modest sample of AB incidents, which might not have been sufficient to capture the effect in question, as well as the nature of our TP simulation. In practice, deadlines manifest in form of volumes of specimen to be assessed rather than individual countdowns, in turn, participants' reactions may not fully reflect their responses under real clinical time constraints. Consistent with our general observations, time pressure appeared to increase dependence on negative system consultations. This heightened alignment with erroneous AI output might have exacerbated the severity of AB, mirrored in the pronounced performance decline, beyond what would be expected from the negative influence of TP on performance alone, as seen in the general analysis. In summary, while we did not observe significant effects of time strain on AB occurrence, our results indicate that its severity worsens under time stress. Thus, we partially accept hypothesis 2. It has to be acknowledged that due to the limited availability of expert participants, the study was conducted on a modest sample (n=28). Although a within-subject design was adopted to augment statistical power, the effects showcased may be under-/over-represented due to sample variability compared to the target population. Moreover, interface design choices such as the omission of clinical background information may have diminished task realism and altered participant behavior, prompting them to approach the study with less diligence as their everyday examinations, potentially impacting observable AB rates. Despite this, the findings serve as a valuable step towards a more holistic understanding of AB in AI-aided medical decision-making and its influencing factors. By highlighting the risk of cognitive biases, we aim to support the safe integration of AI in critical fields like healthcare. Future work could explore the effectiveness of debiasing strategies in minimizing AI-induced cognitive biases such as AB, specifically evaluating their utility under time stress.

Acknowledgement. This work was supported by the Bavarian Institute for Digital Transformation (bidt) through the "ReGInA" grant.

References

1. Goddard K, Roudsari A, Wyatt JC. Automation bias: a systematic review of frequency, effect mediators, and mitigators. J Am Med Inform Assn. 2012;19(1):121–7.
2. Rice S, Hughes J, McCarley JS et al. Automation dependency and performance gains under time pressure. Hum Fac Erg Soc P. 2008;52(19):1326–9.
3. Rieger T, Manzey D. Human performance consequences of automated decision aids: the impact of time pressure. Hum Factors. 2022;64(4):617–34.
4. Smits A, Kummer J, Bruin P de et al. The estimation of tumor cell percentage for molecular testing by pathologists is not accurate. Modern Pathol. 2014;27(2):168–74.
5. Aksac A, Demetrick DJ, Özyer T et al. BreCaHAD: a dataset for breast cancer histopathological annotation and diagnosis. BMC Res Notes. 2019;12(82).
6. Frei A, Oberson R, Baumann E et al. Pathologist computer-aided diagnostic scoring of tumor cell fraction: a Swiss national study. Modern Pathol. 2023;36(12):100335.
7. Martel A, Nofech-Mozes S, Salama S et al. Assessment of residual breast cancer cellularity after neoadjuvant chemotherapy using digital pathology [Data set]. 2019.
8. Tian Z, Shen C, Chen H et al. FCOS: fully convolutional one-stage object detection. arXiv: 1904.01355. 2019.
9. Sniezek JA, Buckley T. Cueing and cognitive conflict in judge-advisor decision making. Ogan Behav Hum Dec. 1995;62(2):159–74.

Abstract: Re-identification from Histopathology Images

Jonathan Ganz[1], Jonas Ammeling[1], Samir Jabari[2], Katharina Breininger[3,4], Marc Aubreville[1,5]

[1]Technische Hochschule Ingolstadt, Ingolstadt, Germany
[2]Klinikum Nuremberg, Institute of Pathology, Nuremberg, Germany
[3]Center for AI and Data Science, Julius-Maximilians-Universität Würzburg, Würzburg, Germany
[4]Department Artificial Intelligence in Biomedical Engineering, Friedrich-Alexander-Universität Erlangen-Nürnberg, Erlangen, Germany
[5]Flensburg Artificial Intelligence Research (FLAIR) and Department Information and Communication, Flensburg University of Applied Sciences, Flensburg, Germany
jonathan.ganz@thi.de

In numerous studies, deep learning algorithms have proven their potential for the analysis of histopathology images, for example, for revealing the subtypes of tumors or the primary origin of metastases. These models require large datasets for training, which must be anonymized to prevent possible patient identity leaks. Our study demonstrates that even relatively simple deep learning algorithms can re-identify patients in large histopathology datasets with substantial accuracy. Furthermore, we compared a comprehensive set of state-of-the-art whole slide image classifiers and feature extractors on two publicly available TCIA datasets including lung squamous cell carcinoma (LSCC) and lung adenocarcinoma (LUAD) for the given task. We also demonstrate the algorithm's performance on an in-house dataset of meningioma tissue. We predicted the source patient of a slide with F_1 scores of up to 80.1 % and 77.19 % on the LSCC and LUAD datasets, respectively, and with 77.09 % on our meningioma dataset. Based on our findings, we formulated a risk assessment scheme to estimate the risk to the patient's privacy prior to publication [1].

References

1. Ganz J, Ammeling J, Jabari S et al. Re-identification from histopathology images. Med Image Anal. 2025;99:103335.

C. Palm et al. (Hrsg.), *Bildverarbeitung für die Medizin 2025*, Informatik aktuell,
https://doi.org/10.1007/978-3-658-47422-5_28

Anatomy-aware Data Augmentation for Multi-organ Segmentation in CT

AnatoMix

Chang Liu, Fuxin Fan, Annette Schwarz, Andreas Maier

Pattern Recognition Lab, Friedrich-Alexander-Universität, 91058 Erlangen, Germany
chang.ch.liu@fau.de

Abstract. Multi-organ segmentation in medical images is a widely researched task and can save much manual efforts of clinicians in daily routines. Automating the organ segmentation process using deep learning (DL) is a promising solution and state-of-the-art segmentation models, such as nnUNet, are achieving promising accuracy. However, overfitting is still a critical issue for DL-based models due to the limited size of segmentation datasets especially in the medical domain. In this work, a novel data augmentation (DA) strategy is proposed to improve the over-fitting problem of multi-organ segmentation datasets, namely AnatoMix. Different from basic DA strategies based on image transformation on a single image, AnatoMix manipulates multiple images in the segmentation dataset and generates new data by mixing multiple images while maintaining human anatomy as realistic as possible. AnatoMix takes the size and location of each organ into consideration, and the corresponding segmentation ground truth is automatically obtained. The initial experiments have been done to extend the publicly available CT-ORG dataset with AnatoMix generating 1,545 new volumes from the 28 original ones. The extended dataset is then evaluated by training a U-Net on the original and the augmented dataset and tested on the same test data. In our experiments the extended dataset leads to mean dice of 76.1, compared with 74.8 on the original dataset. This shows AnatoMix can effectively improve the generalizability of a limited segmentation dataset.

1 Introduction

Multi-organ segmentation is a widely applied clinical procedure [1], i.e. for treatment planning of the radiation therapy. The organs-at-risk must be delineated for planning the radiation procedure. Then the segmentation of the radiation sensitive organs can be applied to the estimation of CT effective dose [2]. Deep learning (DL) based multi-organ segmentation models have achieved promising performance and the leading models in public challenges shows that the DL-based models can have competing performance as human annotations [3]. However, DL models are usually data-demanding and a generalizable DL model needs large-scale datasets for training.

On the one hand, large-scale organ segmentation datasets are emerging, for example AbdomenCT-1K [4], AMOS [5] and TotalSegmentator [6]. On the other hand, such researches also highlight the effort to create a large-scale segmentation dataset. Data scarcity is still a common challenge for researches on specific segmentation task and therefore over-fitting on the limited dataset remains to be an open question. Data

C. Palm et al. (Hrsg.), *Bildverarbeitung für die Medizin 2025*, Informatik aktuell,
https://doi.org/10.1007/978-3-658-47422-5_29

augmentation (DA) is the commonly used approach to extend limited segmentation datasets. Basic DA strategies include image transformation like rotation, scaling and spatial shift on the image and the segmentation mask, and they prove effective to reduce the over-fitting.

Based on the transform-based strategies, novel mixing-based strategies are proposed in recent researches for various segmentation task. Victor et al. proposed ClassMix and the two street view images are combined assisted by a pre-trained segmentation network [7]. Ying et al. proposed ComplexMix that combines ClassMix and CutMix [8] to further improve the diversity [9]. In medical imaging, Qihui et al. proposed SelfMix that extract lesions from the dataset and randomly put lesions onto other image as new images [10]. However for the multi-organ segmentation task, the intrinsic constraints of human anatomy should be respected. This inspired us to propose a novel data augmentation strategy for multi-organ segmentation dataset inspired by human anatomy, namely AnatoMix. AnatoMix combines the anatomical structures from different patients and thus leads to exponential increase of dataset, as shown in Fig. 1. AnatoMix also accounts for the correct location and size of the organs. A major difference of AnatoMix is that it will not output unlimited augmented images because the number of correct combinations is limited.

2 Methods

The pipeline of AnatoMix is shown in Fig. 2, AnatoMix contains a pipeline with two major steps: augmentation planning and object transplant. Experiments are designed to investigate AnatoMix using the publicly available CT-ORG dataset [11].

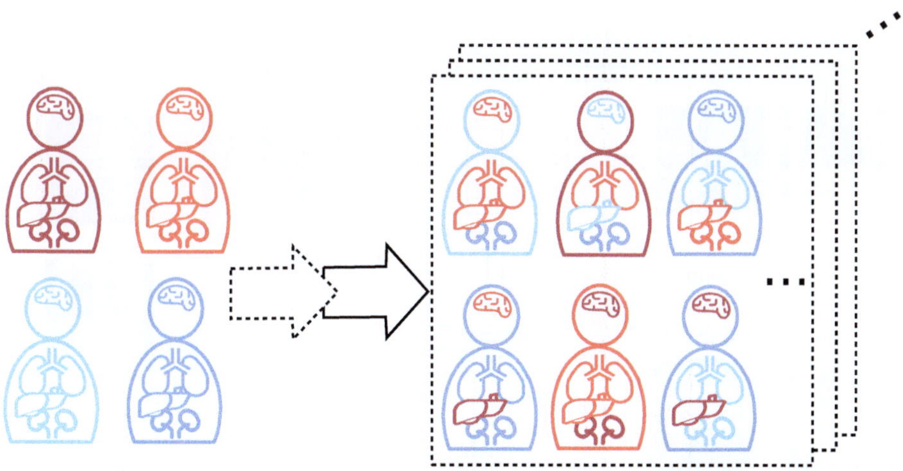

Fig. 1. Concept illustration of AnatoMix. Multi-organ segmentation datasets usually contains multiple segmentation objects and AnatoMix selects and 'transplants' the organs from different patients to generate new one.

2.1 Augmentation planning

The concept of AnatoMix is to disassemble the organs from the volumes, and recombine the organs onto the background volume as a new volume. A segmentation dataset with N_d volumes and N_t target organs can result in $N_d^{N_t+1}$ possible combinations and each combination directly corresponds to an volume with organ segmentation mask. For example in the CT-ORG dataset, where 28 CT volumes are annotated with 4 organs, in total 17,210,368 possible combinations can be generated. However, it was noted in our experiments that the different size and shape of patients can lead to incorrect combinations, for example a very large liver could be matched with a patient with a small liver and the liver region would reach outside of the body region. To avoid such bad combination, before the actual transplanting the size of each organ is extracted as a data fingerprint and a filter is applied to avoid bad combinations by the normalized size of the objects

$$r_{i,0}(M_i, M_0) = |\frac{\sum M_i - \sum M_0}{\sum M_0}| \tag{1}$$

where M_0 and M_i are the binary mask of the same object in base and mixing volume. We assume that human organs share similar shapes and thus organs with similar size will fit other patients. In our experiments, we restrain the combination by $r_i < 0.02$ and for the case of CT-ORG dataset, the number of total combinations decreases to 1,545 afterwards.

2.2 Object transplant

The filtered augmentation plan contains the base volume and N_t mixing organs from other volumes in the dataset. Usually the spatial location in the input volume will not match the mixing volume.

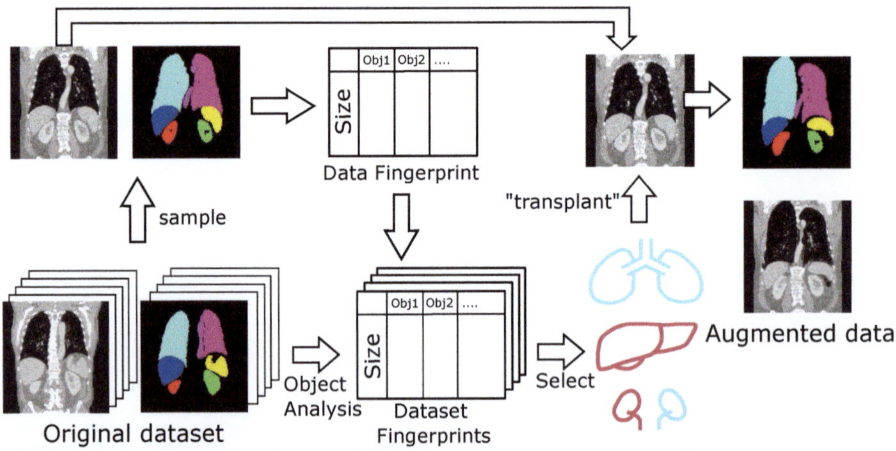

Fig. 2. The detailed pipeline of AnatoMix. Two major steps are included in AnatoMix, i.e. augmentation planning and object transplant. When one volume is sampled from the dataset, suitable organs are first selected from another volume and then transplanted.

Therefore, AnatoMix 'transplants' the mixing organs onto the background volume by a guided spatial shift. The offset (dx, dy, dz) for one object mask is calculated by

$$M_i^* = \arg\max_d \sum M_0 \cdot M_i(dx, dy, dz) \tag{2}$$

where M_i is the mixing organ mask and $M_i(dx, dy, dz)$ shifts M_i by (dx, dy, dz). After the shift, the mixing object is guaranteed to overlap with the same object in the base organ mask M_0 as much as possible. The shifted mixing organ is then pasted onto the base volume and the augmented organs mask M^* is the union region of M_i^* and M_0

$$M^* = M_i^* \cup M_0 \tag{3}$$

and the output volume I^* is

$$I^* = I_0 \cdot (1 - M^*) + I_i^* \cdot M_i^* \tag{4}$$

where I_0 is the base volume and I_i^* is the mixing volume shifted by (dx, dy, dz). Such process is then repeated to transplant all organs in the augmentation plan.

2.3 Data

AnatoMix is evaluated on the CT-ORG dataset[11]. CT-ORG contains 120 throat-abdominal CT scans with segmentation of lungs, liver, kidneys, bladder, bones and brain. After removing volumes with incorrect pixel-dimension, 108 volumes are used in the following experiments. In particular, 28 volumes are selected for training and 80 volumes for test, in order to retain maximal robustness of the test dataset. It is also noted that only few volumes contain bladder and brain in the scanning region, so we select to only the liver, lungs, kidney and bone segmentation in the data.

2.4 Experimental setting

Three experiments are designed to investigate the AnatoMix on different amount of training data, where 10, 20 and 28 volumes are used for training the network. For each experiment, we apply AnatoMix offline to augment 500 volumes from the base ones, namely the ATMX dataset. For the baseline dataset, the same base volumes are repeated to 500 volumes without any transformation. Afterwards the plain U-Net [12] is trained on ATMX dataset and baseline dataset using the same configuration. After the network training, the dice score of each organ and the average dice are used for evaluation of segmentation performance. All experiments are done on 1 Nvidia 1080 (8GB).

3 Results

Some exemplar slices from the volume by AnatoMix are shown in Fig. 3. As shown in the slices, AnatoMix can produce new CT volumes with transplanted organs. The transplanted organs are similar in size to the original organ and thus the remainder region

Tab. 1. For each experiment, AnatoMix creates 500 new volumes from N_d source training data. The dice score of each organ and the average dice are shown below.

	$N_d = 10$		$N_d = 20$		$N_d = 28$	
	Baseline	ATMX	Baseline	ATMX	Baseline	ATMX
Average	0.717	**0.740**	0.748	**0.761**	**0.793**	0.787
Liver	**0.792**	0.787	**0.809**	0.803	**0.855**	0.827
Lung	**0.948**	0.944	0.940	**0.955**	0.961	0.961
Kidney	0.502	**0.576**	0.561	**0.598**	0.617	**0.659**
Bone	0.628	**0.651**	0.681	**0.689**	**0.737**	0.703

is not deteriorated. The augmentation planning decreases the diversity of the output, but it is shown that the anatomy is preserved as much as possible.

From the segmentation results in Tab. 1, AnatoMix can lead to improvement of average dice by 3.2% and 1.7% when 10 and 20 volumes are used for image augmentation. When 28 volumes are used for training, no improvement is observed using AnatoMix.

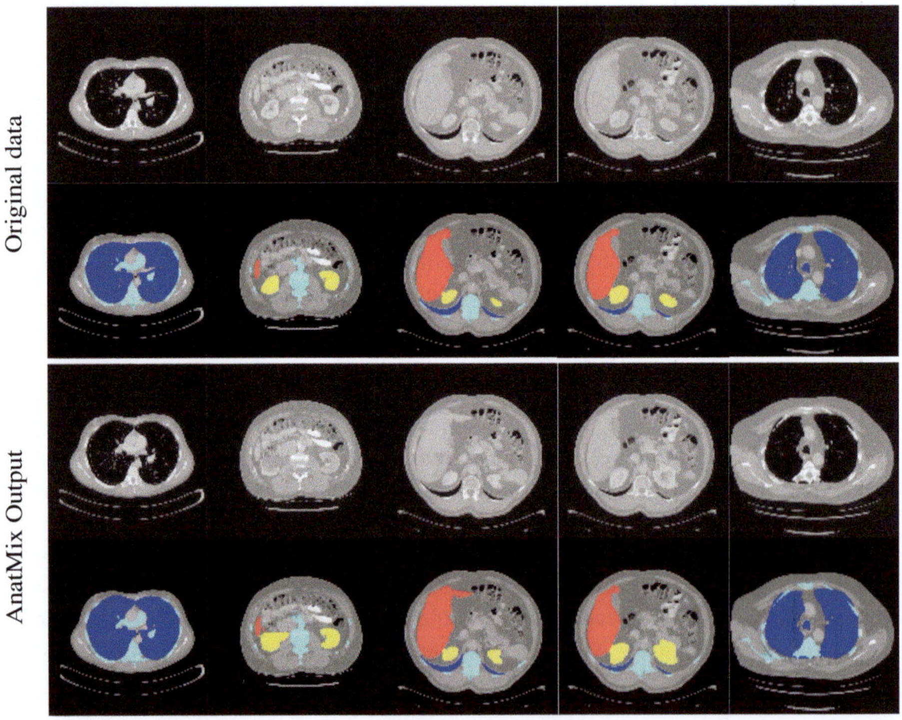

Fig. 3. Exemplar slices of the generated volumes by AnatoMix with the corresponding segmentation mask. Note that in the third and fourth column are the same base volume with mixing kidney and liver from different patients.

4 Discussion

In this work, we propose AnatoMix, an object-level DA strategy to extend multi-organ segmentation datasets, and investigate its performance on the CT-ORG dataset for initial evaluation. It is shown in our experiments, that AnatoMix is able to increase the segmentation performance in some cases.

During our experiments, it is also noticed that AnatoMix can degrade the segmentation performance when the size of the training dataset is increased. It is shown that some intrinsic annotation errors are present in the CT-ORG dataset and this can possibly lead to flaws in augmented data [13].

References

1. Maier A, Syben C, Lasser T et al. A gentle introduction to deep learning in medical image processing. Z Med Phys. 2019;29(2):86–101.
2. Klein L, Liu C, Steidel J et al. Patient-specific radiation risk-based tube current modulation for diagnostic CT. Med Phys. 2022;49(7):4391–403.
3. Isensee F, Jaeger PF, Kohl SA et al. nnU-Net: a self-configuring method for deep learning-based biomedical image segmentation. Nat Methods. 2021;18(2):203–11.
4. Ma J, Zhang Y, Gu S et al. Abdomenct-1k: is abdominal organ segmentation a solved problem? IEEE PAMI. 2021;44(10):6695–14.
5. Ji Y, Bai H, Ge C et al. Amos: a large-scale abdominal multi-organ benchmark for versatile medical image segmentation. Adv NeurIPS. 2022;35:36722–32.
6. Wasserthal J, Breit HC, Meyer MT et al. Totalsegmentator: Robust segmentation of 104 anatomic structures in ct images. Radiology: Artificial Intelligence. 2023;5(5).
7. Olsson V, Tranheden W, Pinto J et al. Classmix: segmentation-based data augmentation for semi-supervised learning. Proc IEEE CVF ACV. 2021:1369–78.
8. Yun S, Han D, Oh SJ et al. CutMix: regularization strategy to train strong classifiers with localizable features. Proc IEEE CVF ICCV. 2019.
9. Chen Y, Ouyang X, Zhu K et al. ComplexMix: semi-supervised semantic segmentation via mask-based data augmentation. Proc ICIP. 2021:2264–68.
10. Zhu Q, Wang Y, Yin L et al. Selfmix: a self-adaptive data augmentation method for lesion segmentation. Proc MICCAI. 2022:683–92.
11. Rister B, Yi D, Shivakumar K et al. CT-ORG, a new dataset for multiple organ segmentation in computed tomography. Sci Data. 2020;7(1):381.
12. Ronneberger O, Fischer P, Brox T. U-Net: convolutional networks for biomedical image segmentation. Proc MICCAI. 2015:234–41.
13. Brückner C, Liu C, Rist L et al. Influence of imperfect annotations on deep learning segmentation models. Proc BVM. 2024:226–31.

Segmentation of Spinal Necrosis Zones in MRI

Janine Hürtgen[1,2], Sylvia Saalfeld[2,3], Robert Kreher[2,4], Mathias Becker[5], Georg Rose[1,2], Georg Hille[2,4]

[1]Institute for Medical Engineering, Otto von Guericke University Magdeburg
[2]Research Campus Stimulate Magdeburg
[3]Institute for Medical Informatics and Statistics, University Hospital Schleswig-Holstein Campus Kiel
[4]Institute for Simulation and Graphics, Otto von Guericke University Magdeburg
[5]University Clinic for Radiology and Nuclear Medicine, University Hospital Magdeburg
janine.huertgen@ovgu.de

Abstract. Accurate treatment assessment for spinal metastases requires MRI-based delineation of post-ablative necrosis zones. Given the rising incidence of cancer and limited recent research in this area, there is still a need for improvements to address existing limitations and optimize outcomes. In this work, we evaluated the segmentation capabilities of four recent neural networks and explored the optimal imaging sequence combinations with regarding to their segmentation accuracy. The networks were trained using five-fold cross-validation on data from 28 patients with overall 35 necrosis zones. The segmentation performance yielded a Dice Similarity Coefficient of 83.3 ± 13.2% for nnU-Net, 83.2 ± 7.9% for TransUNet, 76.1 ± 11.6% for SwinUNETR and 75.8 ± 14.7% for SwinUNETR-V2 when utilizing a combination of contrast-enhanced T1-, native T1-, and T2-weighted sequences. The achieved results represent the current state-of-the-art in spinal necrosis zone segmentation and are on par with the inter-rater-variability of clinical experts. Therefore, this work could play an important role in the assessment of ablative interventions.

1 Introduction

Osseous metastases are the third most common site of metastases from solid tumors, following the lungs and liver, with most cases of bone metastases involving the spine, particularly the vertebrae [1]. With the rising incidence of cancer globally, the number of spinal metastasis cases is also expected to increase [2]. When radiotherapy is not feasible, surgery may be required. Ablative therapies, e.g., radiofrequency ablation (RFA), have proven to be an effective and safe option for reducing pain and disability in short-term [3]. Maximum necrosis zone coverage of metastatic tissue after the ablation is essential for a successful intervention. Currently, for assessment of treatment success pre- and post-operative images are visually compared on individual slices side-by-side, e.g., from MRI, during follow-ups, a process that is time-intensive and subjective [4]. Automated methods for highlighting and segmenting the necrosis zone could simplify image comparison [5], while also enabling efficient quantification of necrosis volume and assessment of tumor coverage. However, segmenting the necrosis zone is challenging due to its varying appearance caused by calcification, edema and diverse primary tumors in addition to possible co-pathologies like osteoporosis, fractures or previous interventions.

C. Palm et al. (Hrsg.), *Bildverarbeitung für die Medizin 2025*, Informatik aktuell,
https://doi.org/10.1007/978-3-658-47422-5_30

To the best of the authors' knowledge, only Steffen et al. [6] investigated automatic necrosis zone segmentation for vertebral metastases, using 2D and 3D U-Net models on various MRI sequences. They achieved a Dice Similarity Coefficient (DSC) of up to 77.2 ± 15.6% for the combination of contrast-enhanced T1 (ceT1) and T2 sequences. In addition, Whyne et al. [7] developed a RFA treatment planning software, estimating spinal necrosis zones from pre-operative MRIs and computed tomography images, with a DSC of 71 ± 3% and a 95th percentile Hausdorff Distance (HD95) of 2.8 ± 0.3 mm compared to manual segmentation in six porcine models.

Given the limited research on the automated segmentation of post-ablative necrosis zones within the spine, our primary contributions are: 1) The comparison of different state-of-the-art networks regarding their capability of segmenting post-ablative necrosis zones in MRI images and 2) the conduction of an ablation study to determine the optimal combination of input sequences from standard follow-up MRIs.

2 Materials and methods

We expanded the dataset provided by Steffen et al. [6], which now includes 28 different patients, resulting in 35 distinct post-ablative necrosis zones compared to the previous 26 necrosis zones. The dataset consists of three different follow-up MRI sequences from clinical routine: ceT1, native T1, and T2, acquired a few days after the RFA intervention. For pre-processing, all cases were resampled to 64 sagittal slices using cubic interpolation for the image data and shape-based interpolation for the label data. This resulted in pixel spacing ranging from 0.47 mm to 1.02 mm within sagittal slices and from 0.77 mm to 1.29 mm between slices. Considering the practical clinical scenario where a physician would select the individual necrosis zone, we applied a bounding box around the necrosis zone based on the midpoint of the segmentation mask. The default bounding box size was 128×128×64 voxels. To increase the dataset size and account for different necrosis zone sizes, nine additional bounding boxes were randomly sampled up to an image size of 256×256×64 and then resampled to a size of 128×128×64 voxels to standardize the input shape for the model resulting in 350 inputs with three sequences each as different network channels (Fig. 1).

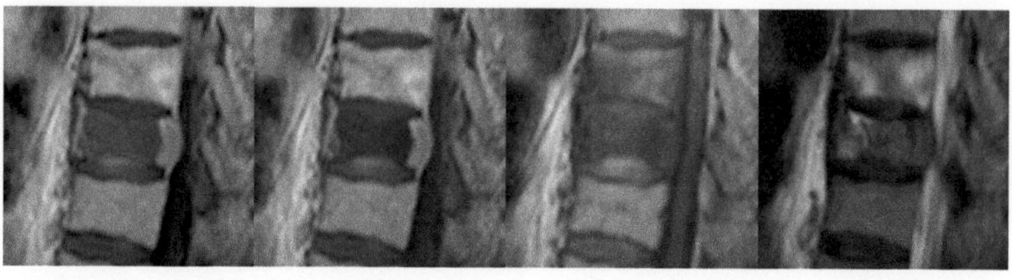

(a) ceT1 (mask) **(b)** ceT1 **(c)** T1 **(d)** T2

Fig. 1. The images display the model's input across three different sequences. In (a), the ground truth label is shown in green on the ceT1 image. Panels (b-d) show the original input sequences.

2.1 Experimental setup

Due to the constrained size of our dataset, we employed five-fold cross-validation for the experiments, ensuring each patient to be either in a validation or training set. For validation purposes, only the original image resolution was utilized, constrained within a bounding box of 128×128×64. Meanwhile, the training set encompassed images with diverse generated crop sizes. This approach yielded 280 images derived from 28 clinical cases for training, each comprising three corresponding sequences as channels, and seven distinct cases for validation for each fold. Four recent networks, selected for their robust segmentation performance across various medical tasks, were evaluated for their accuracy in segmenting post-ablative necrosis zones. The CNN-based nnU-Net model was used as the baseline [8]. In addition, three transformer-based models, integrating the U-Net architecture with attention-based transformer blocks, were also investigated [9–11]. Unless otherwise specified, the implementation follows the original design.

nnU-Net [8]: is a self-configuring U-Net architecture designed for various medical segmentation tasks. In our study, we employ its 3D full-resolution configuration with five encoder and decoder stages. The network is trained for 100 epochs using DSC and Cross Entropy loss, and a batch size of five, with images normalized to [0, 1].

TransUNet [9]: builds on a U-Net backbone, incorporating a vision transformer at the encoder's end. To mitigate the limitations of our smaller dataset, we apply additional augmentations during training, including rotations, Gaussian filtering, gamma adjustments with a 25% probability, flipping with 50%, and zooming with 75%. In contrast to other employed networks, TransUNet uses 2D inputs, dividing each [0, 1] normalized volume into 64 sagittal images, trained in batches of 24 slices over 100 epochs.

SwinUNETR & SwinUNETR-V2: In contrast to TransUNet, the encoder of SwinUNETR [10] integrates vision transformers directly, employing a shifting window strategy across all five downsampling stages in a 3D framework. A more recent iteration of the original architecture, SwinUNETR-V2 [11], introduces residual convolution before and after each swin-block. To manage memory constraints, a batch size of two with reduced patch size of 96×96×64 is chosen. We adopted a combination loss of DSC and Cross Entropy. The enhanced network complexity, coupled with the 3D approach, necessitates extended training steps of 200 epochs with the same additional but 3D augmentation techniques as mentioned above.

3 Results

The segmentation performance is evaluated using a variety of metrics to provide a comprehensive assessment. Two area-based metrics, DSC and Intersection-over-Union (IoU), are commonly employed to report segmentation results. To better differentiate between over- and undersegmentation, we also include True Positive Rate (TPR) and True Negative Rate (TNR). Additionally, a distance-based metric, HD95, provides a trade-off between a robust assessment of the segmentation accuracy and outlier consideration.

Tab. 1 shows the averaged cross-validation results for all four networks. The results indicate that the nnU-Net, serving as the baseline model, continues to excel in terms of DSC (83.3 ± 13.2%), IoU (72.8 ± 13.7%), TPR (85.1 ± 11.2%), and HD95 (4.63

Tab. 1. Cross-validation results for various network architectures. The input consists of a combination of ceT1, T1, and T2 sequences, which yielded the best performance regarding the input sequences (Tab. 2).

	DSC [%] ↑	IoU [%] ↑	TPR [%] ↑	TNR [%] ↑	HD95 [mm] ↓
nnU-Net	83.3 ± 13.2	72.8 ± 13.7	85.1 ± 11.2	99.4 ± 0.6	4.63 ± 4.61
TransUNet	83.2 ± 7.9	71.9 ± 10.5	80.0 ± 12.9	99.6 ± 0.5	5.24 ± 6.84
SwinUNTER	76.1 ± 11.6	62.6 ± 14.0	75.6 ± 15.8	99.2 ± 0.8	7.73 ± 6.00
SwinUNTER-V2	75.8 ± 14.7	62.9 ± 15.6	76.5 ± 17.3	99.2 ± 0.7	7.58 ± 6.33

± 4.61 mm) metrics. Exemplary patient cases including the predicted masks and the corresponding ground truth segmentations for the top-performing, average-performing, and outcomes below intra-rater-variability (IRV) are visualized in Fig. 2 (excluding outliers outside the range of 1.5 times the interquartile range from the first and third quartiles). The TransUNet model achieves comparable results for DSC (83.2 ± 7.9%), IoU (71.9 ± 10.5%), and TNR (99.6 ± 0.5%), with a lower standard deviation due to a more favorable segmented outlier. This finding suggests that the use of vision transformers, with their integrated attention mechanisms, better incorporates global context and is more effective at compensating for diverse appearances. For our specific use-case, both versions of SwinUNETR yield similar results, with mean DSC values of 76.1 ± 11.6% and 75.8 ± 14.7%, respectively. Nevertheless, neither of both variants was able to match the performance of nnU-Net or TransUNet.

3.1 Ablation study

Due to the variability in MRI sequences and device parameters, the optimal choice of the network input depends on the structures being visualized. Therefore, an ablation study was conducted to assess the most effective combination of available standard MRI sequences as input, using the best-performing architecture and baseline model, namely nnU-Net, while training with the same cross-validation approach outlined in section 2.1. Steffen et al. [6] demonstrated that using the ceT1 combined with the T2 sequences yielded the best segmentation results for post-ablative spinal necrosis zones. We tested the combination of ceT1 & T2, all available sequences (ceT1, T1, and T2), as well as their single channel use cases. Tab. 2 presents the results. For single input channel experiments, ceT1 achieved the highest performance (80.7 ± 16.5% DSC), while T1 and

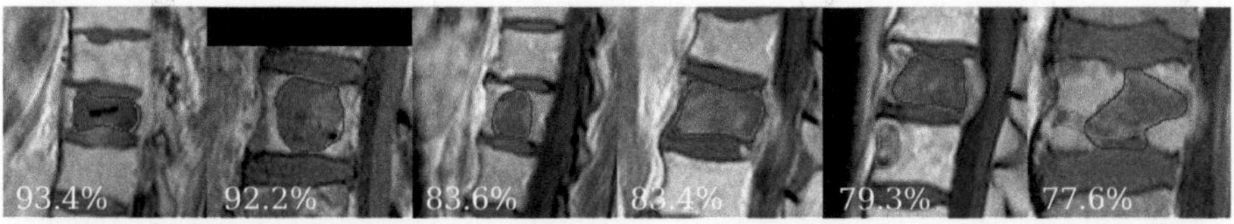

Fig. 2. Segmentation results for six exemplary patients showing high, average, and outcomes below intra-rater-variability. Predictions (red) by nnU-Net are compared to ground truth labels (green), with each patient's DSC shown in the lower left corner.

Tab. 2. nnU-Net cross-validation for various input sequence combinations.

	DSC [%] ↑	IoU [%] ↑	TPR [%] ↑	TNR [%] ↑	HD95 [mm] ↓
ceT1	80.7 ± 16.5	69.9 ± 17.4	82.4 ± 16.3	99.4 ± 0.6	5.74 ± 5.17
T1	72.2 ± 13.1	57.9 ± 13.8	76.7 ± 14.7	99.0 ± 1.3	7.27 ± 4.71
T2	68.9 ± 18.1	54.8 ± 17.3	72.1 ± 19.0	99.0 ± 1.0	7.47 ± 4.87
ceT1 & T2	81.6 ± 14.4	70.7 ± 15.3	84.3 ± 11.4	99.3 ± 0.7	5.44 ± 4.84
T1 & ceT1 & T2	83.3 ± 13.2	72.8 ± 13.7	85.1 ± 11.2	99.4 ± 0.6	4.63 ± 4.61

T2 showed inferior performance (72.2 ± 13.1% and 68.9 ± 18.1% DSC, respectively). Notably, incorporating more diverse sequences improved results, as demonstrated by the combination of ceT1 and T2, which resulted in a DSC of 81.6 ± 14.4%, and even more so by the combination of all sequences, achieving a DSC of 83.3 ± 13.2%.

4 Discussion

In the described work, we compared various high-performing networks for the segmentation of post-ablative spinal necrosis zones and exceeding the current state-of-the-art of a DSC of 77.2% [6] by 6.1 percentage points. Using the combination of ceT1, T1, and T2 MRI sequences as network input, we achieved a DSC of up to 83.3 ± 13.2% for nnU-Net and 83.2 ± 7.9% for TransUNet. SwinUNETR-based architectures produced inferior results, with DSC scores of 76.1 ± 11.6% and 75.8 ± 14.7%. These results are on par with the IRV of 82.4 ± 5.9% [4] indicating expert-level segmentation accuracy. Our ablation study demonstrated that combining all available MRI sequences yields the most accurate segmentation predictions. Moreover, we show that ceT1 sequences are crucial for segmentation, as the single-use case experiments for native T1 and T2 showed a drop in performance in comparison to ceT1. Compared to Whyne et al. [7] (71 ± 3% DSC, 2.8 ± 0.3 mm HD95), who estimated necrosis zones based on planning parameters and imaging, we achieved significantly higher DSC scores. Their lower HD95 and standard deviations likely result from a small sample size (five necrosis zones in two pigs with healthy vertebral tissue), which simplifies prediction but lacks the varied appearance of spinal metastases. However, this comparison is limited, as they used only intra-operative imaging without the necrosis zone, whereas we utilized post-operative MRIs, which could further improve segmentation accuracy.

Limitations of our proposed approach include the predefined cropping around the necrosis zone, which simplifies segmentation for the network by focusing on a smaller image patch. However, this limitation is mitigated in our context since the necrosis zone segmentation is designed for a post-operative evaluation platform for radiologists, where the physician can select a necrosis zone by clicking on the target to assess the treatment outcome rather than performing a fully automatic cohort analysis. Due to a relatively small dataset, common to this medical research area, future evaluations should assess, whether the results remain consistent when applied to an expanded dataset including cervical cases or a multi-center study. Despite this, cross-validation indicates promising results regarding robustness and accuracy for diverse appearances of necrosis zones (Fig. 2).

5 Conclusion

Segmentation of post-ablative necrosis zones in spinal metastases remains a crucial research area with few recent studies. We applied four high-performing networks (nnU-Net, TransUNet, SwinUNETR, SwinUNETR-V2), achieving up to 83.3 ± 13.2% DSC with nnU-Net and 83.2 ± 7.9% with TransUNet using ceT1, T1, and T2 MRI sequences. These results match the IRV among clinical experts, enabling accurate quantification of necrosis zones. Automated segmentation supports comparison between pre-operative metastases and post-operative necrosis zones, aiding physicians in verifying coverage and assessing treatment outcomes for informed post-interventional decisions.

Acknowledgement. This work was partially funded by the German Federal Ministry of Education and Research (within the Research Campus STIMULATE under the grant number '13GW0473A-B'). The authors declare no competing interests.

References

1. Wewel JT, O'Toole JE. Epidemiology of spinal cord and column tumors. Neurooncol Pract. 2020;7(Supplement_1):i5–i9.
2. WHO WHO. WHO report on cancer: setting priorities, investing wisely and providing care for all. World Health Organization, 2020.
3. Murali N, Turmezei T, Bhatti S et al. What is the effectiveness of radiofrequency ablation in the management of patients with spinal metastases? A systematic review and meta-analysis. J Orthop Surg Res. 2021;16:1–10.
4. Hille G. Computer-assisted approaches to support radiofrequency ablations of spinal metastases. English. PhD. Magdeburg, 2020.
5. Hille G, Saalfeld S, Serowy S et al. Multi-segmental spine image registration supporting image-guided interventions of spinal metastases. Comput Biol Med. 2018;102:16–20.
6. Steffen J, Hille G, Becker M et al. Automatic segmentation of necrosis zones after radiofrequency ablation of spinal metastases. Proc ICPRAM. 2020:96–102.
7. Whyne CM, Underwood G, Davidson SR et al. Development and validation of a radiofrequency ablation treatment planning system for vertebral metastases. Int J Comput Assist Radiol Surg. 2023;18(12):2339–47.
8. Isensee F, Jaeger PF, Kohl SA et al. nnU-Net: a self-configuring method for deep learning-based biomedical image segmentation. Nat Methods. 2021;18(2):203–11.
9. Chen J, Lu Y, Yu Q et al. TransUNet: transformers make strong encoders for medical image segmentation. arXiv: 2102.04306. 2021.
10. Hatamizadeh A, Nath V, Tang Y et al. Swin unetr: Swin transformers for semantic segmentation of brain tumors in mri images. Proc MICCAI. 2021:272–84.
11. He Y, Nath V, Yang D et al. Swinunetr-v2: Stronger swin transformers with stagewise convolutions for 3d medical image segmentation. Proc MICCAI. 2023:416–26.

Augmented Reality Prompts for Foundation Model-based Semantic Segmentation

Michael Schwimmbeck[1,2], Christopher Auer[1], Johannes Schmidt[3], Stefanie Remmele[1]

[1]Research Group Medical Technologies, University of Applied Sciences Landshut
[2]Chair for Visual Computing, Friedrich-Alexander-Universität Erlangen-Nürnberg
[3]LAKUMED Kliniken, Landshut
michael.schwimmbeck@haw-landshut.de

Abstract. Mixed reality-guided surgery may benefit from live organ segmentation and tracking, such as adapting virtual models to the deformations of target structures. The use of foundation models allows for widely applicable solutions; however, these models need to be prompted for more demanding tasks, such as surgical applications. This work investigates several user interaction concepts for prompting segmentation foundation models directly in augmented reality (AR) using the Microsoft HoloLens for AR-guided surgical applications. To achieve this, we implement eye tracking, finger tracking, ArUco marker tracking, and pointer tracking concepts and evaluate their accuracy in terms of mean absolute errors during pointing experiments at different distances and with different prompters. Furthermore, we assess their impact on segmentation performance in terms of Dice scores and include an initial user study to query the user confidence and preference. While all methods are accurate enough to perform segmentation in phantom experiments, achieving Dice scores greater than 0.96, ArUco marker tracking and eye tracking prove to be the most accurate throughout our experiments. An initial user questionnaire along with feedback from an experienced visceral surgeon indicates a preference for eye tracking and finger tracking methods. Our code is publicly available at GitHub[1].

1 Introduction

Using Augmented Reality (AR) for navigation in surgery may offer significant benefits in terms of accuracy, patient outcomes, and ergonomics. By projecting virtual organ models onto the target anatomy, the surgeon's perception of the procedure can be enhanced [1]. Some recent studies have explored this topic [1, 2]; however, most approaches rely on markers for patient registration. Automatic segmentation and tracking of structures could simplify the workflow and further enable the adaptation of models to organ deformation.

The virtual models can be registered directly to the organ surface, which can be obtained from the depth stream of commercial AR systems [2, 3]. Achieving this requires robust segmentation and tracking models that must be trained on pixel-precise annotations of all training data, which becomes cumbersome for large datasets [2, 4]. This is especially challenging for applications like open liver surgery, where training data is scarce. To contribute a task-independent solution, Kirillov et al. [5] introduced the Segment Anything Model (SAM) as the first major foundation model for semantic

[1] https://github.com/mschwimmbeck/AR-SAM

C. Palm et al. (Hrsg.), *Bildverarbeitung für die Medizin 2025*, Informatik aktuell,
https://doi.org/10.1007/978-3-658-47422-5_31

segmentation demonstrating strong zero-shot performance across a variety of applications. First works have demonstrated that SAM can aid in surgical data segmentation, however requiring user prompts such as seed points or bounding boxes [6, 7]. These prompting methods could be adapted for AR glasses e.g., using finger gestures or marker tracking, making it feasible to prompt a foundation model directly from the AR device.

But how accurate are different AR prompting methods on AR glasses such as the Microsoft HoloLens 2? How do inaccuracies impact segmentation performance? And how practical are these prompting methods on AR glasses and in clinical settings?

Our study contributes to the field of AR-guided surgery by 1) introducing a novel framework that integrates AR-based eye tracking, finger tracking, marker tracking, and pointer tracking to prompt a foundation model in Microsoft HoloLens applications, 2) systematically comparing the accuracy of these technologies w.r.t. varying distances and users, as well as their impact on SAM based segmentation in simple phantom experiments, and 3) deriving preliminary conclusions regarding user confidence and clinical applicability.

2 Materials and methods

This study expands upon the HoloLens Object Labeling (HOLa) framework, introduced by Schwimmbeck et al. [7] to integrate the foundation model SAM [5] for segmentation tasks using Microsoft HoloLens 2. For prompting SAM using seed point prompts, we supplement the AR interaction methods eye tracking, finger tracking, physical marker tracking, and pointer tracking. Furthermore, we evaluate prompting accuracy and present initial conclusions regarding user acceptance. Our system design is presented in Fig. 1.

Eye tracking was implemented using Spatial Mapping with functions provided by the HoloLens 2 Sensor Streaming framework (HL2SS) [8]. An eye calibration procedure, available through HoloLens 2 system functions, was required to adjust the eye tracking

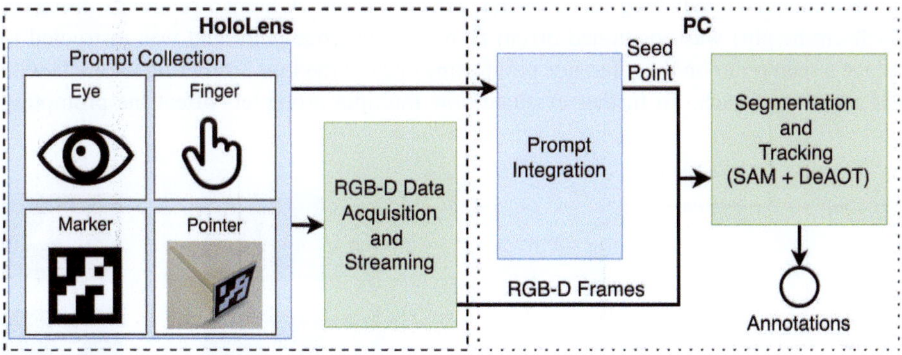

Fig. 1. This study integrates eye tracking, finger tracking, marker tracking, and pointer tracking technologies (Blue) to define seed points for foundation model based segmentation and tracking in AR apps. Therefore, we integrate the prompting methods within the HoloLens Object Labeling framework HOLa [7] (Green) based on the segmentation foundation model SAM. The resulting data (Frames + Annotations) can be utilized for data annotation tasks or live segmentation.

sensors to the user's eyes. Eye tracking data was then used to determine a point in world space based on the combined gaze ray of both user eyes.

We implemented finger tracking using the Microsoft Mixed Reality Toolkit 2 (MRTK2) finger tracking solver. The index tip of the right hand was selected for tracking. To set a point in world space, a voice command was detected by the Unity Speech KeywordRecognizer class, and corresponding 3D coordinates were then transmitted to the PC using Ultra Message Queuing (UMQ) command buffer communication.

Due to their widespread use in computer vision and high tracking accuracy, we utilize ArUco markers [9] for marker tracking that were printed in a size of 6.6 cm. To further simulate the attachment of markers to surgical tools, we designed and 3D-printed a simple pointer with a sharp tip that can be used for selecting arbitrary points. At the opposite side of the pointer, there is space to attach a 6.6-cm ArUco marker [9]. We determine the world position of the pointer tip by applying the transformation between the marker's center and the pointer tip, based on the pointer's dimensions.

As a final step for finger tracking, marker tracking, and pointer tracking, the user must move the finger/marker/pointer away from the set point to avoid occlusion in the recorded frame. For all four methods, the detected point is marked in world space using small AR spheres and projected into image coordinates using extrinsic and intrinsic sensor transforms as well as the transformations between them.

We evaluate our method with the following experiments: Fig. 2a shows our experiment setup for evaluating prompting accuracy at different distances from the object of interest and with different users. To assess seed point positioning in terms of mean absolute error (MAE) w.r.t. the distance between the HoloLens sensors and a point in the world, we established a scenario involving four different heights (+0, +12, +24, +36 cm) of a reference sheet placed on a 78 cm tall table. The reference sheet included a reference point with 1 mm diameter and five circles spanning around the reference point with radii of 1-5 cm. We utilized these circles as a scale to quantify deviations from the reference point directly from the recorded frames. To place seed points using an ArUco marker, we added a rectangle to the reference sheet, centered around the reference point, with dimensions matching those of the ArUco marker. A human reference prompter (188 cm height) was positioned 50 cm from the reference point and was instructed to place a seed point on the reference point using each of the four prompting methods with 25 repetitions each. To further evaluate how multiple prompters affect the prompting

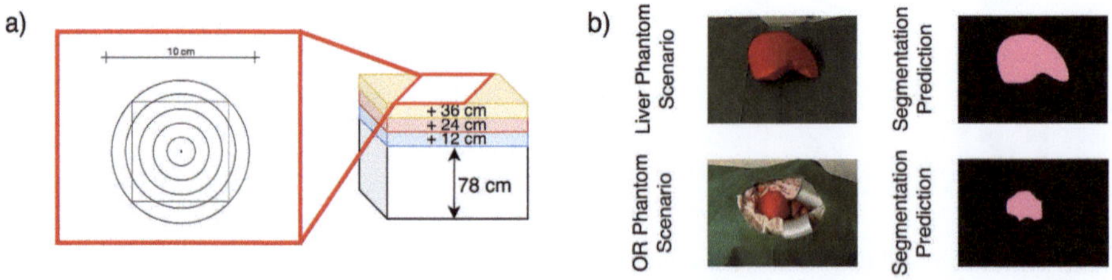

Fig. 2. (a) Our experimental setup includes varying table heights to assess the effect of object-to-sensor distances on prompting errors. (b) To evaluate the impact of the prompting methods on segmentation performance, we used two phantom scenarios with different complexity [7].

accuracy, we repeated the experiment with five prompters and five repetitions each and averaged MAEs over all test runs per method. Thereby, we utilized the table height with +24 cm offset as this height was described to be the most convenient for the prompters.

To evaluate the impact of placing seed points on SAM data annotation, the five prompters from the previous experiment were asked to place seed points with each method on two liver phantom scenarios [7] with different complexity (Fig. 2b). We obtained the first frame's annotation mask using the HOLa framework [7], which applies the SAM model to the input RGB frame based on the placed seed point. To assess segmentation accuracy, the predicted segmentation mask was compared to a manual pixel-wise reference annotation and the concordance was quantified using Dice scores. We utilized the SAM ViT-H model on an NVIDIA GeForce RTX 3090 GPU.

To obtain a preliminary impression of user acceptance for the prompting methods, the five prompters were asked to rank the methods in terms of 1) the user confidence on prompting accuracy and 2) the personal preference regarding convenience and ease of use. One prompter, a visceral surgeon with 36 years of experience, was inquired about the clinical constraints for applying the prompting methods in the operating room (OR).

3 Results

Results on prompting accuracy (25 repetitions) with respect to different table heights, and thus distances from the HoloLens, are presented in Fig. 3 (left). Mean prompting errors from the inter-prompter analysis (5 x 5 repetitions) were 3.62 ± 1.38 mm (Marker tracking), 6.90 ± 4.62 mm (Eye tracking), 7.68 ± 5.14 mm (Pointer tracking), and 10.01 ± 9.00 mm (Finger tracking). In terms of segmentation performance (1 x 5 repetitions), there were no statistically significant deviations between Dice scores for

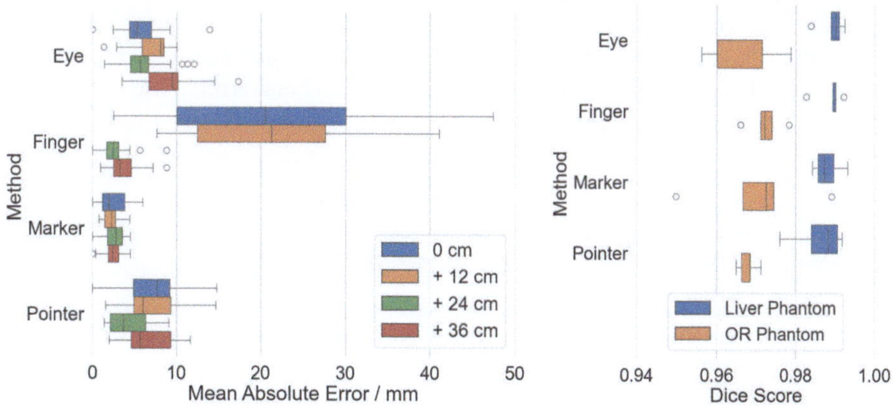

Fig. 3. (Left) Prompting errors in MAE for all prompting methods. The higher the reference sheet was placed, the closer it was to the user. Marker tracking consistently outperforms the other methods achieving the highest average accuracy across all heights, followed by pointer tracking, eye tracking, and finger tracking. (Right) Segmentation quality in terms of Dice scores w.r.t. all prompting methods (5 prompters).

both the liver phantom and the OR phantom scenario across all prompting methods (Fig. 3 (right)). An exemplary segmentation prediction for each scenario is included in Fig. 2b. We provide results from the user questionnaire in Fig. 4.

4 Discussion

While ArUco marker-based pointer tracking and marker tracking technologies show minimal deviations across different table heights, eye tracking exhibits similar errors at +0 to +24 cm but there is a performance drop at the closest distance (+36 cm), likely due to the low view angle causing distortions in spatial mapping. Finger tracking errors increase significantly at greater distances, which can be attributed to depth-sensing inaccuracies of the HoloLens Articulated Hand Tracking (AHAT) sensor if approaching its maximum sensor range. In the inter-prompter analysis, errors varied widely between prompters, particularly for pointer tracking and finger tracking. This discrepancy is also reflected in the prompters' responses regarding the user confidence on prompting accuracy. Eye tracking was generally perceived as the most accurate, despite physical marker tracking was achieving lower errors. In terms of user preference, eye and finger tracking scored significantly higher than methods involving external tools, likely due to their more intuitive usage. Regarding the scenarios used to assess the impact of prompting on segmentation, all methods were sufficiently accurate to place a seed point on the object of interest. This resulted in Dice scores greater than 0.96 in all scenarios. Future work will apply our method to more complex objects and clinical scenarios. The phantom study is certainly limited in providing absolute values for segmentation accuracy in future clinical applications, but it was meant to serve as a well-defined reference scenario to investigate the impact of all prompting methods on segmentation. Statistical significance could be increased by additional prompters in future work.

Eye tracking requires the longest preparation time, approximately 40 seconds for eye calibration, but does not require any additional steps as it does not occlude the set point unlike the other methods. One potential drawback is saccades (short-time rapid eye movements), which can cause temporary signal loss and errors. The experienced

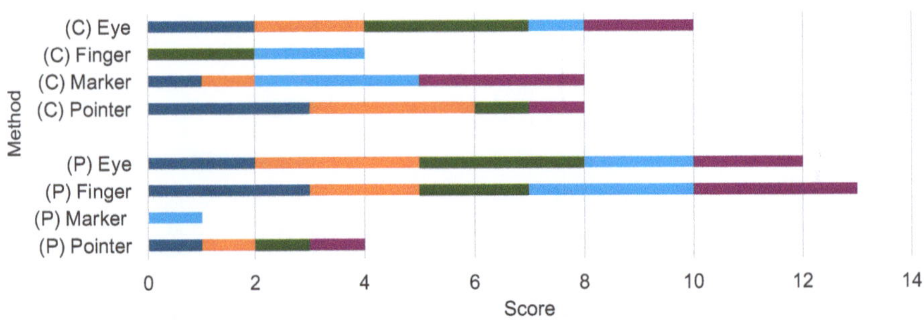

Fig. 4. Questionnaire results on the user confidence on prompting accuracy (C) and user preference (P) for all prompting methods. Five Prompters (different bar colors) were asked to rank the methods with scores from 0 (worst method) to 3 (best method).

surgeon found this method to be intuitive, although accompanying voice commands might be difficult to establish in the OR. Finger tracking is the only method that requires HoloLens AHAT depth sensing and is thus limited to close distances to the HoloLens. Comparing the higher inter-prompter errors to the errors from the experienced reference prompter, we presume that there may be a learning curve for positioning the finger for optimal tracking by the HoloLens. Future work will include a control sphere moving with the finger and evaluate different fingers or glove usage during surgery. The experienced surgeon described finger tracking as the most intuitive method during surgery. ArUco marker tracking may be challenging due to contact with human tissue. This was also noted by the experienced surgeon, who emphasized compliance with sterility, so the marker must be made from a material that is resistant to multiple sterilization sessions. Pointer tracking in this work was limited to a simple pointer. The experienced surgeon suggested that it would be beneficial to use established tools in the OR, which presents challenges for attaching markers. The orientation of the marker also affects the pointer's seed point accuracy, which needs further investigation w.r.t. optimal tracking conditions.

A general limitation of this study is the image-based measurement of seed point errors. Due to the limited resolution of the HoloLens RGB frames, errors may include inaccuracies. We measured approximately one millimeter per pixel, which might be reduced by establishing a more sophisticated measuring scenario. However, we believe that this work is of value to the community since it provides a first impression of the magnitude of prompting errors for common AR interaction methods. Presented concepts are directly adaptable to other foundation models and AR hardware as well as numerous applications involving user interaction for improved foundation model performance.

References

1. Ma L, Huang T, Wang J et al. Visualization, registration and tracking techniques for augmented reality guided surgery: a review. Phys Med Biol. 2023;68(4):04TR02.
2. Khajarian S, Remmele S, Amft O. Image-based live tracking and registration for AR-guided liver surgery using Hololens2: a phantom study. Proc IEEE EMBS. 2023:1–4.
3. Golse N, Petit A, Lewin M et al. Augmented reality during open liver surgery using a markerless non-rigid registration system. J Gastrointest Surg. 2021;25(3):662–71.
4. Pfeiffer M, Funke I, Robu MR et al. Generating large labeled data sets for laparoscopic image processing tasks using unpaired image-to-image translation. Proc MICCAI. 2019:119–27.
5. Kirillov A, Mintun E, Ravi N et al. Segment anything. Proc IEEE CVF ICCV. 2023:4015–26.
6. Huang Y, Yang X, Liu L et al. Segment anything model for medical images? Med Image Anal. 2024;92:103061.
7. Schwimmbeck M, Khajarian S, Holzapfel K et al. HOLa: HoloLens object labeling. Curr Dir Biomed Eng. 2024;10(4):571–4.
8. Dibene JC, Dunn E. Hololens 2 sensor streaming. arXiv: 2211.02648. 2022.
9. Garrido-Jurado S, Munoz-Salinas R, Madrid-Cuevas FJ et al. Automatic generation and detection of highly reliable fiducial markers under occlusion. Pattern Recognit. 2014;47(6):2280–92.

Abstract: nnU-Net Revisited

Call for Rigorous Validation in 3D Medical Image Segmentation

Fabian Isensee[†1,2], Tassilo Wald[†1,2,3], Constantin Ulrich[†1,4,5], Michael Baumgartner[†1,2,3], Saikat Roy[1], Klaus Maier-Hein[‡1,2,3,4,5,6], Paul F. Jäger[‡2,7]

[1]Division of Medical Image Computing, German Cancer Research Center (DKFZ), Heidelberg, Germany

[2]Helmholtz Imaging, DKFZ, Heidelberg, Germany.

[3]Faculty of Mathematics and Computer Science, University of Heidelberg, Heidelberg, Germany

[4]National Center for Tumor Diseases (NCT), NCT Heidelberg, a partnership between DKFZ and university medical center Heidelberg, Germany

[5]Medical Faculty Heidelberg, University of Heidelberg, Heidelberg, Germany

[6]Pattern Analysis and Learning Group, Department of Radiation Oncology, Heidelberg University Hospital, Heidelberg, Germany

[7]Interactive Machine Learning Group (IML), DKFZ, Heidelberg, Germany

constantin.ulrich@dkfz-heidelberg.de

The release of nnU-Net marked a paradigm shift in 3D medical image segmentation, demonstrating that a properly configured U-Net architecture could still achieve state-of-the-art results. Despite this, the pursuit of novel architectures, and the respective claims of superior performance over the U-Net baseline, continued. In this study, we demonstrate that many of these recent claims fail to hold up when scrutinized for common validation shortcomings, such as the use of inadequate baselines, insufficient datasets, and neglected computational resources. By meticulously avoiding these pitfalls, we conduct a thorough and comprehensive benchmarking of current segmentation methods including CNN-based, Transformer-based, and Mamba-based approaches. In contrast to current beliefs, we find that the recipe for state-of-the-art performance is 1) employing CNN-based U-Net models, including ResNet and ConvNeXt variants, 2) using the nnU-Net framework, and 3) scaling models to modern hardware resources. These results indicate an ongoing innovation bias towards novel architectures in the field and underscore the need for more stringent validation standards in the quest for scientific progress [1].

References

1. Isensee F, Wald T, Ulrich C et al. nnU-Net Revisited: A Call for Rigorous Validation in 3D Medical Image Segmentation. Proc MICCAI. 2024.

[†]These authors contributed equally the most to this work.

[‡]These authors contributed equally the least to this work.

C. Palm et al. (Hrsg.), *Bildverarbeitung für die Medizin 2025*, Informatik aktuell,
https://doi.org/10.1007/978-3-658-47422-5_32

Abstract: Information Mismatch in PHH3-assisted Mitosis Annotation Leads to Interpretation Shifts in H&E Slide Analysis

Jonathan Ganz[1], Christian Marzahl[2], Jonas Ammeling[1], Emely Rosbach[1], Taryn A. Donovan[3], Samir Jabari[4], Christof A. Bertram[3], Katharina Breininger[5], Marc Aubreville[6], and the study participants

[1]Technische Hochschule Ingolstadt, Ingolstadt, Germany
[2]Gestalt Diagnostics, Spokane, USA
[3]University of Veterinary Medicine, Vienna, Austria
[4]University Hospital Erlangen, Erlangen, Germany
[3]The Schwarzman Animal Medical Center, New York, USA
[5]Universität Würzburg, Würzburg, Germany
[6]Flensburg University of Applied Sciences, Flensburg, Germany
jonathan.ganz@thi.de

The count of mitotic figures (MFs) observed in hematoxylin and eosin (H&E)-stained slides is an important prognostic marker, as it is a measure for tumor cell proliferation. However, the identification of MFs has a known low inter-rater agreement. In a computer-aided setting, deep learning algorithms can help to mitigate this, but they require large amounts of annotated data for training and validation. Furthermore, label noise introduced during the annotation process may impede the algorithms' performance. Unlike H&E, where identification of MFs is based mainly on morphological features, the mitosis-specific antibody phospho-histone H3 (PHH3) specifically highlights MFs. Counting MFs on slides stained against PHH3 leads to higher agreement among raters and has therefore recently been used as a ground truth for the annotation of MFs in H&E. However, as PHH3 facilitates the recognition of cells indistinguishable from H&E staining alone, the use of this ground truth could potentially introduce an interpretation shift and even label noise into the H&E-related dataset, impacting model performance. This study examines the effect of PHH3-assisted MF annotation on inter-rater reliability and object-level agreement through a multi-rater experiment. We also evaluated MF detectors, including a dual-stain detector, to assess the impact of PHH3-assisted labeling on model performance. While PHH3-assisted labeling significantly improved annotator agreement (F1: 0.53 to 0.74), it did not enhance H&E-based detector performance. However, the dual-stain detector benefited from the increased consistency, revealing an information mismatch between H&E and PHH3 images. Based on these findings, we propose an improved PHH3-assisted labeling procedure [1].

References

1. Ganz J, Marzahl C, Ammeling J et al. Information mismatch in PHH3-assisted mitosis annotation leads to interpretation shifts in H&E slide analysis. Sci Rep. 2024;14(1):26273.

C. Palm et al. (Hrsg.), *Bildverarbeitung für die Medizin 2025*, Informatik aktuell,
https://doi.org/10.1007/978-3-658-47422-5_33

Abstract: Multi-level Cancer Profiling through Joint Cell-graph Representations

Luis C. Rivera Monroy[1], Leonhard Rist[1], Frauke Wilm[1,2], Christian Ostalecki[3], Andreas Baur[3], Julio Vera[3], Katharina Breininger[2], Andreas Maier[1]

[1]Pattern Recognition Lab - Friedrich-Alexander-Universität Erlangen-Nürnberg, Germany [2]Department of Artificial Intelligence in Biomedical Engineering - FAU Erlangen-Nürnberg, Germany [3]Department of Dermatology - Universitätsklinikum Erlangen, Germany

luis.rivera@fau.de

Abstract

Digital pathology has enabled advanced cancer analysis, yet traditional patch-based methods struggle to capture complex, topological structures in whole-slide images (WSIs). This study introduces a graph-based framework using graph neural networks (GNNs) to model histopathology samples as multi-level cell graphs, integrating both cell- and disease-level information for improved classification. Our approach encompasses five cancer types and two staining protocols, modeling each sample as a graph to capture spatial and phenotypic relationships between cells and diseases. We implemented this framework using graph random neural networks (GRAND) [1], achieving a cell-level classification accuracy of 88% and a disease-level accuracy of 83%, significantly outperforming CNN and XGBoost baselines [2, 3]. These results emphasize the potential of GNNs to generalize across multiple cancers and staining methods, providing a valuable diagnostic tool for pathologists. Future research will extend this model to additional cancer types and explore its applicability and robustness in diverse clinical settings, with the goal of achieving interpretable and scalable computational pathology solutions [4].

References

1. Wenzheng F, Jie Z, Yuxiao D et al. Graph random neural networks for semi-supervised learning on graphs. Proc NeurIPS. 2020;33:22092–103.
2. Rivera LC, Rist L, Eberhardt M et al. Employing graph representations for cell-level characterization of melanoma MELC samples. Proc IEEE ISBI. 2023:1–5.
3. Jaume G, Pati P, Anklin V et al. HistoCartography: a toolkit for graph analytics in digital pathology. Proc MICCAI. 2021:117–28.
4. Schubert W, Bonnekoh B, Pommer AJ et al. Analyzing proteome topology and function by automated multidimensional fluorescence microscopy. Nat Biotechnol. 2006;24(10):1270–8.

C. Palm et al. (Hrsg.), *Bildverarbeitung für die Medizin 2025*, Informatik aktuell,
https://doi.org/10.1007/978-3-658-47422-5_34

Abstract: TSynD Targeted Synthetic Data Generation for Enhanced Medical Image Classification

Leveraging Epistemic Uncertainty to Improve Model Performance

Joshua Niemeijer[1], Jan Ehrhardt[2], Hristina Uzunova[3], Heinz Handels[2,3]

[1]German Aerospace Center, Braunschweig, Germany
[2]Institute of Medical Informatics, University of Lübeck, Germany
[3]German Research Center for Artificial Intelligence, Lübeck, Germany
Joshua.Niemeijer@dlr.de

Deep learning in medical applications usually faces the problem of limited training data that does not represent most of the relevant distribution. This is due to the fact that, both, the acquisition process of the data is difficult and the labeling of medical data is costly. The former is caused by the complex and expensive nature of medical sensors and strict data privacy laws. The latter is due to the high wages of medical professionals. To overcome this issue common strategies include data augmentation or the use of generative models. Both strategies however have in common that they extend the training distribution in a rather untargeted way. We presented the TSynD approach that allows for a more targeted creation of images. Targeted, in this case, means that the generated images should represent parts of the unknown distribution and, therefore, be relevant for the training of a given classifier. To generate these images we utilize an auto-encoder pre-trained on the domain of data that the classifier should be trained on. Given the frozen auto-encoder model, we aim to optimize it's latent space to create images that yield high epistemic uncertainty in the given classifier. Samples yielding a high epistemic uncertainty represent missing parts of the training distribution. During the optimization process, we maximize the Mutual Information, which is a measure of this uncertainty. In our experiments, we observe that classifiers that are trained on the resulting synthetic data yield an increased generalization and robustness. We test the generalization by applying the approach to limited training data scenarios. The robustness is measured by augmenting the test data during test time with noise and adversarial attacks. Furthermore, a qualitative evaluation shows that a classifier trained with our TSynD approach focuses on more relevant parts of an image than, e.g., the baseline classifier. This work demonstrates how to utilize generative models effectively for training data generation. Therefore, this is a first step towards alleviating the data scarcity in medical image processing [1].

References

1. Niemeijer J, Ehrhardt J, Uzunova H et al. TSynD: targeted synthetic data generation for enhanced medical image classification. Proc SASHIMI. 2025:69–78.

C. Palm et al. (Hrsg.), *Bildverarbeitung für die Medizin 2025*, Informatik aktuell,
https://doi.org/10.1007/978-3-658-47422-5_35

End-to-end Encoders Stabilize Quantum Convolutional Neural Networks for Medical Image Classification

Leyi Tang, Merlin A. Nau, Andreas K. Maier

Pattern Recognition Lab, Department of Computer Science, Friedrich-Alexander Universität Erlangen-Nürnberg, Germany
merlin.nau@fau.de

Abstract. The advent of quantum machine learning has led to the development of quantum convolutional neural networks (QCNNs) for image classification across various domains. A key limitation of current quantum hardware is the limited number of available qubits and the bandwidth required to load data, necessitating classical dimensionality reduction before inputting image data into quantum circuits. The classification performance varies significantly depending on the quantum circuit and the parameters used. We propose integrating a classical encoder for dimensionality reduction before the QCNN and training it end-to-end. Tested against principal component analysis and autoencoder methods on the Pneumonia MedMNIST dataset, our approach improves performance and stabilizes results across different quantum circuits. While our method falls short compared to the classical baseline in terms of performance, it uses significantly fewer parameters.

1 Introduction

Quantum computing is an uprising avenue in the field of high-performance computing for tasks like encryption, simulation, and optimization. Quantum computing is also actively investigated for use in machine learning (ML), a field known as quantum machine learning (QML). Whether and when QML methods will outperform classical methods remains an open question. Promising research of QML suggest quantum speedups, learning from fewer data, or recognizing computationally difficult patterns [1]. QML has also sparked interest in medical imaging where the complexity of data processing and pattern recognition pose substantial challenges [2–4]. Medical image classification is an important task in diagnostics and disease analysis. Traditional (ML) models, specifically CNNs, are widely adopted as state-of-the-art due to their ability to automatically extract features from image data and perform classification.

Among the advancements in QML, the development of quantum convolutional neural networks represents a promising frontier. QCNNs adopt the structural characteristics of classical CNNs, but leverage quantum circuits instead of classical convolutional kernels and pooling layers. By utilizing quantum effects, such as superposition and entanglement, QCNNs offer the potential to capture atypical patterns in data [5]. The pipeline of a QCNN is described in the next section. Hur et. al. [6] extended the work of Cong et al. [5] and established an open-source QCNN framework. The framework builds upon the quantum computing Python library Pennylane [7], which can be used with both classical simulators and real quantum hardware. Pennylane allows auto-differentiation capabilities when used in conjunction with classic machine learning libraries.

C. Palm et al. (Hrsg.), *Bildverarbeitung für die Medizin 2025*, Informatik aktuell,
https://doi.org/10.1007/978-3-658-47422-5_36

Hur et al. achieved promising results on MNIST and Fashion-MNIST datasets using their QCNN framework [6]. Similarly, other QML approaches were investigated for medical image classification including, quantum orthogonal neural networks [2], CNN-extraction for QCNN [4], and quantum feature extraction circuits in conjunction with classical classification networks [3].

A key hurdle in quantum computing is the bandwidth required to load classical data onto a quantum computer [8]. This process, known as data encoding, maps classical data into quantum states. Furthermore, current limitations in quantum bit (qubit) count on quantum computers and simulators necessitate dimensionality reduction before encoding image data. Techniques like PCA and AE are commonly used in QCNN for this purpose [2, 6].

In this manuscript, we want to assess the influence of the dimensionality reduction technique used in a QCNN. We evaluate the use of commonly used autoencoders (AEs) and principal component analysis (PCA) for different QCNNs on the Pneumonia MedMNIST dataset [9]. We observe large performance differences for different QCNN circuits. So, instead of training the QCNN and the AE separately [6], in this work, the dimensionality reduction technique is integrated in the QCNN and the resulting pipeline is trained end-to-end. We utilize a quantum computing simulator for all results. From the experimental results, the end-to-end QCNN pipelines not only improve the classification performance, but also provide a quantum-aware learned data encoding that stabilizes the performance across different QCNN circuits.

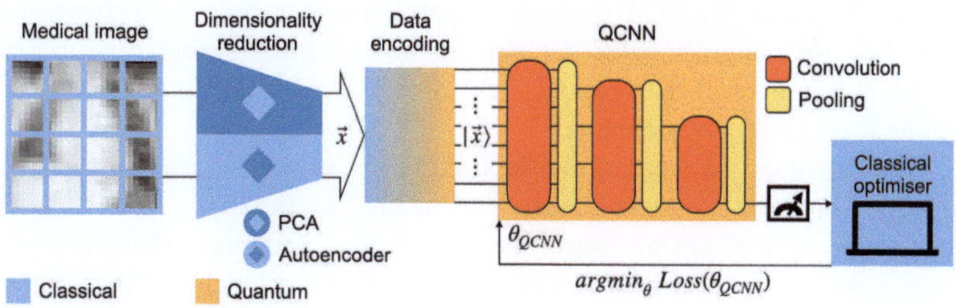

(a) The separate training pipeline of the QCNN.

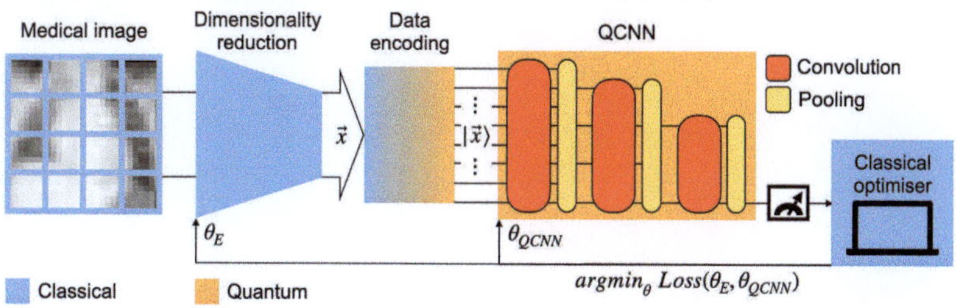

(b) The end-to-end training pipeline of the QCNN.

Fig. 1. Illustrations of the separate training pipeline and the proposed end-to-end training pipeline.

2 Materials and methods

In this study, we propose a pipeline that utilizes a QCNN model to address a light-weight binary medical image classification problem. The data for our experiments consists of the Pneumonia MedMNIST dataset [9]. The binary classification task assesses chest X-rays as pneumonia-positive or normal. Pneumonia MedMNIST provides small-scale 28×28 grayscale images, with 4,708 for training and 624 for testing. The size of the image data, however, is still too large for current quantum computers and simulators. Fig. 1a depicts the conventional QCNN pipeline. The image data undergoes a dimensionality reduction which is then encoded into a quantum state $|x\rangle$ and is then fed through a QCNN circuit with trainable parameters θ_{QCNN}. The QCNN circuit, similar to classical convolutional neural networks (CNNs), consists of a layer of feature extracting convolutional circuits applied on neighboring qubits. This is followed by a trainable pooling circuit which essentially reduces the information to half of the qubits. This procedure is applied until we arrive at one final qubit. This qubit is measured, collapsing to the $|0\rangle$ or $|1\rangle$ state indicating our binary classification result. The trainable variables θ_{QCNN} are optimized using a a classical computer. Fig. 1b shows our proposed pipeline where the CNN encoder, with paramters θ_E, is integrated into the pipeline and then trained in an end-to-end fashion.

2.1 Dimensionality reduction

The two principal dimensionality reduction techniques employed in the separate training pipeline are PCA and AE. PCA is a non-trainable linear technique for dimensionality reduction that uses singular value decomposition to extract principal components. It projects high-dimensional data onto a lower-dimensional space, aiming to maximize variance and reduce redundant features.

AE is an unsupervised neural network that compresses and decompresses input data, using an encoder to create a lower-dimensional representation and a decoder to reconstruct the original. In this work, the encoder and decoder each consist of three linear layers, with each layer followed by a ReLU activation function. Once trained, the encoder performs dimensionality reduction by extracting key features. Unlike the fixed linear PCA, AE is non-linear and learns its representation through trainable parameters.

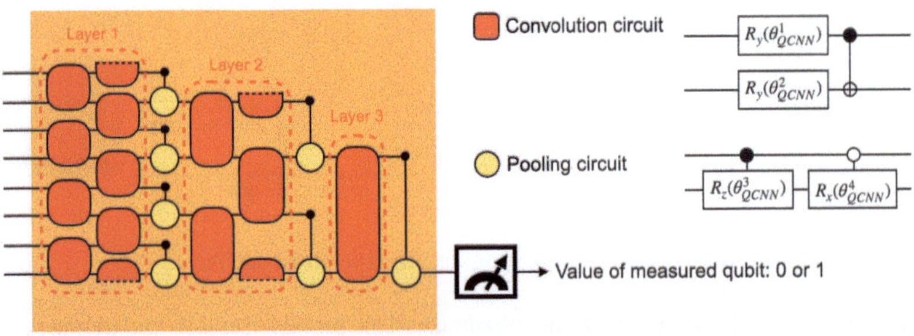

Fig. 2. Illustration of the QCNN structure with exemplary circuits.

As a third dimensionality reduction technique we utilize a simplified encoder architecture with one linear layer and integrate it before the QCNN circuit, see Fig. 1b. Pennylane allows us to perform auto-differentiation with the loss gradients from the quantum circuit to the encoder module written in PyTorch. In this way, we establish a data encoding, circuit, and classification aware dimensionality reduction technique.

2.2 Data encoding

In quantum computing, data encoding is the process of transforming classical information, stored in bits, into quantum states, which are stored in qubits. A quantum state, for a single qubit, can be expressed as a superposition of the basis states $|0\rangle$ and $|1\rangle$, with complex coefficients α and β that satisfy $|\alpha|^2 + |\beta|^2 = 1$

$$|x\rangle = \alpha|0\rangle + \beta|1\rangle \tag{1}$$

In fact, a single qubit is represented as a point on the Bloch sphere, a three-dimensional representation of the qubit's state in Hilbert space, where the top of the sphere corresponds to the $|1\rangle$ state and the bottom of the sphere corresponds to the $|0\rangle$ state. Multiple data encoding schemes exist, such as amplitude encoding, basis encoding, and angle encoding. In this work, we use angle encoding, a technique that utilizes the quantum rotation gate R_y by an angle to encode classical data x_i. Each value x_i is normalized to an angular range of $[-\pi, \pi]$. The classical data vector $\vec{x} = [x_1, x_2, ..., x_N]$ is encoded into a quantum state $|\vec{x}\rangle$, which maps N classical bits to N qubits

$$|x_i\rangle = R_y(x_i)|0\rangle + R_y(x_i)|1\rangle \tag{2}$$

2.3 Quantum gates and circuit

Quantum gates are unitary operations that act on one or more qubits, represented by matrices, commonly referred to as unitaries. The gates used in this work include the Hadamard gate H and rotation gates R_x, R_y and R_z. When multiple gates are applied in sequence, they form a quantum circuit, which processes information through transformations on qubit states. A quantum circuit is commonly referred to as a unitary, because a sequence of unitary operations remain unitary.

The overall structure of the QCNN comprises two main types of unitaries: convolutional circuits and pooling circuits (Fig. 2). We use nine different entangling convolutional circuits with different number of parameters from Hur et al. [6]. We refer to the convolutional circuits as circuits 1-9, with an example of one circuit shown in Fig. 2. Note, that a convolutional circuit is a misleading name, since it does not perform a classical convolution operation on the input data. Rather, a convolutional circuit can be thought of as a feature extracting quantum circuit similar to a convoluting kernel. Similar to classical convolutional layers, which use the same kernels across the layer, the QCNN uses identical convolutional unitary circuits in each convolutional layer. In contrast to classical CNNs, where pooling layers are not trainable, the pooling unitary circuit in the QCNN contain trainable weights. The pooling circuit reduces two qubits to one, serving a similar purpose to classical pooling layers by reducing the dimensionality of the data while preserving key features.

3 Results

We use $N = 8$ qubits on a simulator, therefore the input of the QCNN is represented by a quantum state vector $[q_1, q_2, ..., q_8]$. Consequently, in order for the QCNN to be able to classify images from our datasets, it is necessary to perform dimensionality reduction. In order to compare the proposed end-to-end pipeline, we first conduct experiments on the separate-training pipeline with PCA and AE as the reduction technique. PCA with 8 components covers 72.9% of the data variance. We train the AE on the training dataset and use the output of the encoder as input to the QCNN. Then we conduct experiment on the end-to-end pipeline with an end-to-end encoder as the reduction technique, and thus compare the experiment results. During the experiments, we alter the dimensionality reduction techniques (fixed # of parameters) and convolutional unitary circuits (varying # of parameters). We train both of our pipelines for 20 epochs and a batch size of 32. We provide the test set results in terms of accuracy of our pipelines with the different dimensionality reduction techniques and convolutional circuits in a plot in Fig. 3. Further, we show the best performing circuit pipeline for the three different dimensionality reduction techniques and compare them to the MedMNIST baseline methods [9] in terms of the accuracy and parameters in Tab. 1.

4 Discussion

for dimensionality reduction varying across different convolutional circuits, the accuracy achieved 0.71 ± 0.07 and 0.72 ± 0.05 using PCA and AE, respectively (Fig. 3). In contrast, our proposed end-to-end pipeline achieves a higher accuracy of 0.83 ± 0.01, with lower standard deviation, suggesting enhanced stability across unitary circuit configurations. Notably, this approach reaches accuracies comparable to ResNet baselines but with significantly fewer parameters. These results underscore that integrating classical and quantum components within an end-to-end framework can stabilize and enhance

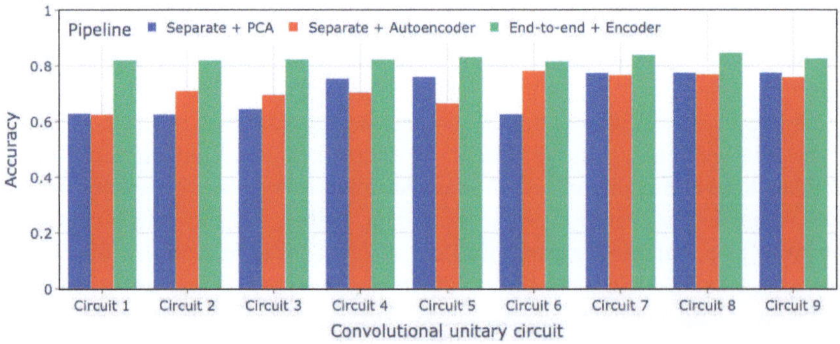

Fig. 3. Accuracy results on the PneumoniaMedMNIST dataset: nine convolutional unitary circuits are used for the separate-training pipeline with PCA and AE as well as the end-to-end pipeline.

Tab. 1. Comparison of accuracy and numbers of parameters on PneumoniaMedMNIST. The number of QCNN parameters consists of convolutional cicuit and pooling circuit parameters multiplied by the number of layers.

Pneumonia MedMNIST	Accuracy	Total Parameters	QCNN Parameters
ResNet18	0.85	11.7M	0
ResNet50	0.85	25.6M	0
Google AutoML Vision	**0.95**	–	0
AE-QCNN (Circuit 6)	0.78	218K	$(6+2)\times 3$
PCA-QCNN (Circuit 9)	0.78	0	$(15+2)\times 3$
End-to-End-QCNN (Circuit 8)	0.85	6K	$(10+2)\times 3$

QCNN performance on the Pneumonia MedMNIST dataset. Classical computation likely contributed significantly to these gains, raising important questions about the unique benefits, if any, that QCNNs offer over conventional methods. Recent research further suggests that QCNNs may even be classically simulable [10]. We encourage further research on diverse datasets to rigorously evaluate the capabilities of QCNNs in comparison with traditional approaches, larger qubit count, quantum hardware and other dimensionality reduction techniques.

References

1. Biamonte J, Wittek P, Pancotti N et al. Quantum machine learning. Nature. 2017;549:195–202.
2. Landman J, Mathur N, Li YY et al. Quantum methods for neural networks and application to medical image classification. Quantum. 2022;6:881.
3. Matic A, Monnet M, Lorenz JM et al. Quantum-classical convolutional neural networks in radiological image classification. Proc IEEE QCE. 2022:56–66.
4. Hassan E, Hossain MS, Saber A et al. A quantum convolutional network and ResNet (50)-based classification architecture for the MNIST medical dataset. Biomed Signal Process Control. 2024;87:105560.
5. Cong I, Choi S, Lukin MD. Quantum convolutional neural networks. Nat Phys. 2019;15:1273–8.
6. Hur T, Kim L, Park DK. Quantum convolutional neural network for classical data classification. Quant Mach Intell. 2022;4(1).
7. Bergholm V, Izaac J, Schuld M et al. Pennylane: automatic differentiation of hybrid quantum-classical computations. arXiv: 1811.04968. 2018.
8. Giovannetti V, Lloyd S, Maccone L. Quantum random access memory. Phys Rev Lett. 2008;100(16):160501.
9. Yang J, Shi R, Wei D et al. MedMNIST v2-A large-scale lightweight benchmark for 2D and 3D biomedical image classification. Sci Data. 2023;10(1).
10. Bermejo P, Braccia P, Rudolph MS et al. Quantum convolutional neural networks are (effectively) classically simulable. arXiv: 2408.12739. 2024.

Data Augmentation for Liver Tumor Segmentation using Structure, Texture, and Contrast

Serouj Khajarian[1,2], Oliver Amft[2,3], Stefanie Remmele[1]

[1]Research Group Medical Technolgies, University of Applied Sciences Landshut
[2]Intelligent Embedded Systems Lab (IES), University of Freiburg
[3]Hahn-Schickard
serouj.khajarian@haw-landshut.de

Abstract. We present a new data augmentation method to address the data scarcity problem in deep learning based automatic segmentation of liver tumors. A non-rigid registration algorithm was used to generate new anatomical variations of liver tumors from a publicly available benchmark dataset. Additionally, a conditional image-to-image generative adversarial network (GAN) was trained to translate the generated segmentation masks into corresponding textured CT volumes. We used a state-of the-art segmentation model to investigate the benefit of our data augmentation method. Experiments with varying amounts of synthetic data were conducted and the results show that our novel augmentation method improves tumor segmentation performance by approximately 3 %, outperforming similar data augmentation techniques.

1 Introduction

Many studies, have explored the potential of augmented reality (AR) in surgery, including markerless, non-rigid registration based on preoperative segmentation models [1, 2]. The preparation time for AR-guided liver surgery remains a significant barrier to routine clinical use. Expert surgeons often spend 3-4 hours on preparation, mainly due to the extensive time required for liver and critical tissue segmentation [3, 4].

Deep learning (DL) techniques have shown promise in automatic image segmentation, with significant advances attributed to data preprocessing methods, including HU-windowing, as well as architectural modifications, including cascading networks, attention mechanisms, and residual blocks [5, 6]. Beyond the current achievements, segmentation performance, in particular for liver tumors, remains limited due to the scarcity of labeled training data. While there is evidence that traditional data augmentation techniques can improve DL network performance [5], they often fail to capture the diversity of liver and tumor anatomies. To bridge the gap in liver segmentation, there is growing research into synthetic data generated via physical simulations or AI-based models [7]. In particular, the use of generative adverserial networks (GANs) to create synthetic data based on learned features from real data has become a popular augmentation technique, enhancing AI model performance across a range of tasks by mimicking real data variability and complexity [8]. Unlike other synthesis methods (e.g., diffusion models), GANs can achieve realistic texture synthesis based on only a limited amount of training samples [8]. Nonetheless, generating new structural information still demands substantial amounts of training data. Physical models, on the other hand, can

C. Palm et al. (Hrsg.), *Bildverarbeitung für die Medizin 2025*, Informatik aktuell,
https://doi.org/10.1007/978-3-658-47422-5_37

produce realistic deformations, provided that the biomechanical properties of the tissue are known. However, this requirement is hardly met for tumors.

This paper addresses the shortage of annotated data for liver tumor segmentation by introducing a novel data augmentation method. The contributions of this work are as follows:

1. We introduce an augmentation method that produces deformations of liver tumors (new label masks) independent of any physical priors. The method uses a GAN that enriches the synthetic label masks with realistic computer tomography (CT) textures.
2. We evaluate the benefit of the proposed method for data augmentation. In particular, we compare the performance of a state-of-the-art segmentation model across different augmentation levels. Additionally, we compare our augmentation approach against other state-of-the-art methods that use elastic deformations and GANs to generate synthetic data.

2 Materials and methods

Our proposed data augmentation method consists of two main steps: (A) Generation of new segmentation label mask with tumor deformations (B) CT volume synthesis (Fig. 1).

2.1 Generation of new segmentation masks

To generate new segmentation masks of realistic liver anatomies with varying tumor geometries and distributions, we employ a non-rigid registration algorithm commonly used for inter-patient image matching and motion tracking [9]. The algorithm follows a pyramid-based iterative approach for image matching, reducing iterations as image resolution increases. Given two liver segmentation masks from different abdominal CT scans, the algorithm generates a displacement field to deform (register) the source liver mask, aligning it with the target liver mask. The displacement field, applied with linear interpolation, deforms the source liver mask, including tumors, to conform to the target

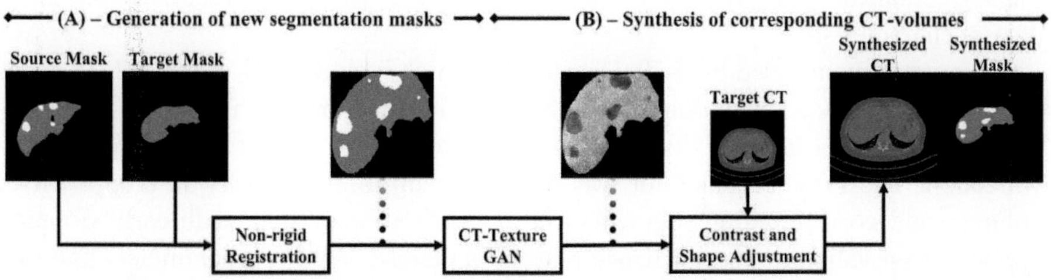

Fig. 1. Overview of our approach: (A) Generation of new segmentation masks using non-rigid image registration. (B) Synthesis of CT volumes with a GAN, adjusting texture, shape and contrast to match the target CT volume.

liver volume. We use five pyramid levels, starting with 1000 iterations at the coarsest level, reduced by 100 iterations with each level increase. The number of iterations at each level was determined experimentally to ensure complete registration from the source to the target liver mask. To smooth the displacement field, Gaussian smoothing with a standard deviation of 0.4 is iteratively applied at each level. The smoothing prevents sharp, unrealistic transitions and enhances overall registration accuracy. To avoid large-scale deformations, especially when the CT volumes vary significantly in size, both liver masks are cropped to the liver boundaries and resized to 128x128x128 before processing. Using the displacement field, we generate new segmentation masks that align with the target liver volume while deforming the source tumor volumes. This process creates new tumor geometries on an existing liver structure, allowing the data to fit seamlessly into existing patient datasets.

2.2 Synthesis of corresponding CT volumes

To translate the generated segmentation masks into textured liver CT volumes, a conditional GAN was trained to map segmentation masks to the corresponding CT textures (Fig.1B). The model is based on the Pix2Pix image-to-image translation GAN architecture [10], modified with layer adjustments to enable 3D volume translations.

The synthetic CT textures are generated for liver and tumor regions, and the synthesized liver volume is subsequently aligned within the target CT scan. Initially, the synthetic liver is resized to match the size of the liver in the target CT scan. To restore the full spatial dimensions and ensure precise alignment, padding is applied along the x, y, and z axes. Due to the limited contrast range in the synthesized liver-tumor textures, the synthetic liver intensity is adjusted to match the mean and standard deviation of the liver in the target scan. The intensity adjustment enhances visual consistency between the synthetic and original textures. Finally, the synthetic liver replaces the original liver volume in the target scan, with blurring applied around the liver edges to smooth transitions and seamlessly blend the synthesized textures with the surrounding tissues.

2.3 Experimental setup

To evaluate the benefit of our augmented data, we used the nnU-Net model [11] to segment tumors at various augmentation levels. nnU-Net provides an automated solution for segmentation tasks by configuring necessary pre- and post-processing based on dataset characteristics.

Our experiments used the LiTs Dataset [5], which includes 131 annotated CT scans with liver and tumor annotations, for both synthetic data generation and nnU-Net training. Both nnU-Net and the Pix2Pix GAN generator were trained using 5-fold cross-validation. The Pix2Pix generator was trained for up to 800 epochs on cropped liver volumes and corresponding segmentation masks from each fold, with early stopping applied when validation performance reached a plateau. All hyperparameters and loss functions followed the recommendations in the original Pix2Pix paper [10].

The baseline performance was evaluated by training the nnU-Net on the LiTs data and using the default way of data augmentation as provided by the nnU-Net implementation, using the 3D full-resolution nnU-Net variant. To evaluate the benefit of our augmentation method, we incorporated synthetic data into the training process, using augmentation levels from 100 % to 400 % in 100 % increments. Each model was trained for 1,000 epochs, with the best-performing model on the validation set chosen for testing on each one of the 5 folds. Tumor segmentation performance was measured using the Dice score, being a measure for the overlap between predicted and ground truth segmentation masks.

3 Results

Fig. 2 illustrates tumor segmentation performance across data augmentation levels ranging from 100 % to 400 %. The baseline model, achieved an average Dice score of 66 %. The highest average Dice score (69 %) was achieved at an augmentation level of 100 %, with a smaller interquartile range than the baseline, indicating improved performance and reduced variability in segmentation outcomes. At 200 % augmentation, the average Dice score (68 %) remained slightly higher than the baseline (66 %). However, increasing the augmentation levels beyond 200 % resulted in diminishing returns, with average Dice scores dropping to around 0.65, and the interquartile range expanding back to baseline levels, reflecting greater variability.

Tab. 1 presents the performance gains achieved by our approach compared to other data synthesis methods that are based on image deformation or GANs. Our method, applied to a dataset of 131 scans for liver tumor segmentation, resulted in a 3 % increase in Dice score with an augmentation factor of 100 %.

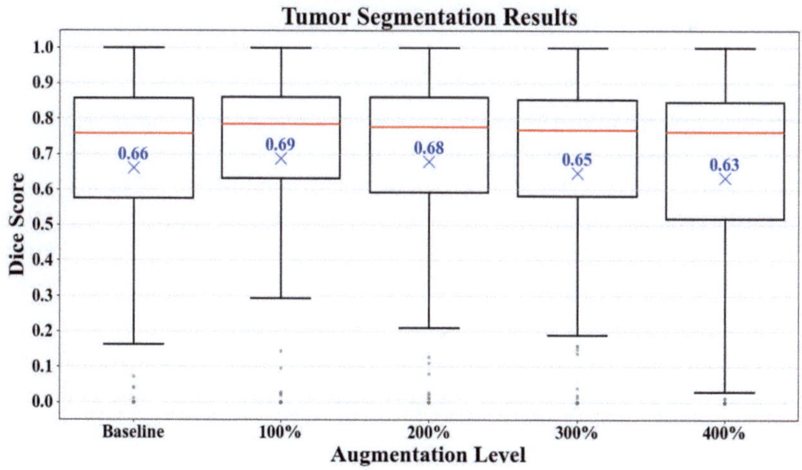

Fig. 2. Tumor segmentation performance across augmentation levels. The boxplots depict the distribution of Dice scores, with the red line representing the median and the blue 'x' indicating the mean. The best performance was achieved with 100 % augmentation, resulting in a 3 % increase in Dice score.

Tab. 1. Comparison of performance gains by related data augmentation methods to our approach.

	Segmentation task	Training data	Method	Aug. factor	Δ-Dice
Nalepa et al. [12]	Tumor from MRI brain scans	44 scans	deformation ✓ synth. texture ×	5 - 95 %	Avg. 1.5 %
Sun et al.[13]	Liver lesion from MRI/CT/PET scans	100 scans	deformation ✓ synth. texture ✓	300 %	0.5 %
Sun et al.[13]	Brain tumor from multimodal MRI scans	285 scans	deformation ✓ synth. texture ✓	500 %	1.9 %
Bowles et al.[14]	CSF from CT brain scans	500/250/50 scans	deformation × synth. texture ✓	100 %	0.4/0.9/1.5 %
Bowles et al.[14]	WMH from MRI brain scans	74/37/8 scans	deformation × synth. texture ✓	50 %	-/2.3/5 %
Ours	Liver tumor from CT scans	131 scans	deformation ✓ synth. texture ✓	100 %	3 %

4 Discussion

The proposed method for generating new tumor geometries demonstrates potential for enhancing segmentation performance of state-of-the-art models like the nnU-Net, without relying on additional real data. The achieved 3 % performance gain at 100 % augmentation level, though modest, exceeds the performance achieved of other GAN-based data augmentation methods in different segmentation tasks [8].

As shown in Tab. 1, our approach outperformed similar existing methods in improving segmentation performance. In contrast to the work by Nalepa et al. [12], which uses a non-rigid registration algorithm but generated a limited amount data, we generated up to $\frac{n(n-1)}{2}$ synthetic scans from a dataset of n scans. Additionally, the degree of deformation in each derivative can be arbitrarily manipulated.

Our findings suggest that the benefit of augmentation plateaus when synthetic data exceeds twice the size of the original training set. Excessive synthetic data may introduce biases, potentially limiting further performance gains [15]. Future work might investigate ways to leverage this unlimited range of possible data to optimize the selection of additional training data.

Bowles et al. [14] tested the effectiveness of GAN-generated synthetic data under varying conditions of real data availability and found that using synthetic training data achieved the best performance gains when the baseline amount of real data was extremely limited (5 % using only 8 real scans). In contrast to Babul et al. [15] and our work, Sun et al. [13] reported optimal gains when augmenting the real dataset with a large amount of synthetic data (300 % - 500 %). The authors used separate datasets for liver and brain lesion segmentation in MRI scans. Evidently, the segmentation results were influenced by a variety of factors including the complexity of the segmentation task, the baseline amount of real training data, and the augmentation method and level. Segmentation performance further depends on the diversity of tumor geometry, tumor-liver contrast, and intensity levels within the training data. In this study, we controlled the contrast of the synthetic tumors to match variations in the original dataset, ensuring that synthetic tumors integrate naturally within real CT scans. Although the results of this work may not yet support the practical use of automatic tumor segmentation, we anticipate the approach to greatly reduce the manual effort required to generate virtual models for AR-guided liver interventions.

References

1. Golse N, Petit A, Lewin M et al. Augmented reality during open liver surgery using a markerless non-rigid registration system. J Gastrointest Surg. 2021;25(3):662–71.
2. Khajarian S, Remmele S, Amft O. Image-based live tracking and registration for AR-guided liver surgery using Hololens2: a phantom study. Proc IEEE EMBS. 2023:1–4.
3. Okamoto T, Onda S, Yanaga K et al. Clinical application of navigation surgery using augmented reality in the abdominal field. Surg Today. 2015;45:397–406.
4. Zhao Z, Poyhonen J, Chen Cai X et al. Augmented reality technology in image-guided therapy: state-of-the-art review. Proc Inst Mech Eng H. 2021;235(12):1386–98.
5. Bilic P, Christ P, Li HB et al. The liver tumor segmentation benchmark (LiTS). Med Image Anal. 2023;84:102680.
6. Jin Q, Meng Z, Sun C et al. RA-UNet: a hybrid deep attention-aware network to extract liver and tumor in CT scans. Front Bioeng Biotechnol. 2020;8:605132.
7. Chen RJ, Lu MY, Chen TY et al. Synthetic data in machine learning for medicine and healthcare. Nat Biomed Eng. 2021;5(6):493–7.
8. Chen Y, Yang XH, Wei Z et al. Generative adversarial networks in medical image augmentation: a review. Comput Biol Med. 2022;144:105382.
9. Thirion JP. Image matching as a diffusion process: an analogy with Maxwell's demons. Med Image Anal. 1998;2(3):243–60.
10. Isola P, Zhu JY, Zhou T et al. Image-to-image translation with conditional adversarial networks. Proc IEEE CVPR. 2017:1125–34.
11. Isensee F, Jaeger PF, Kohl SA et al. nnU-Net: a self-configuring method for deep learning-based biomedical image segmentation. Nat Methods. 2021;18(2):203–11.
12. Nalepa J, Mrukwa G, Piechaczek S et al. Data augmentation via image registration. Proc IEEE ICIP. 2019:4250–4.
13. Sun Y, Yuan P, Sun Y. MM-GAN: 3D MRI data augmentation for medical image segmentation via generative adversarial networks. Proc IEEE ICKG. 2020:227–34.
14. Bowles C, Chen L, Guerrero R et al. GAN augmentation: augmenting training data using generative adversarial networks. arXiv: 1810.10863. 2018.
15. Babul KAR, Sathish R, Pattanaik M. Synthetic simplicity: unveiling bias in medical data augmentation. Proc MICCAI. 2024:64.

Abstract: IM-MoCo

Self-supervised MRI Motion Correction using Motion-guided Implicit Neural Representations

Ziad Al-Haj Hemidi, Christian Weihsbach, Mattias P. Heinrich

Institute of Medical Informatics, University of Luebeck, Luebeck, Germany
z.alhajhemidi@uni-luebeck.de

Motion artifacts in magnetic resonance imaging (MRI) arise from long acquisition times and can compromise the clinical utility of the images obtained. Traditional motion correction methods often struggle with severe motion, leading to distorted and unreliable results. Deep learning (DL) has improved upon these limitations through generalization, even though it also comes with challenges, such as vanishing structures and hallucinations. This makes its application in the medical field particularly difficult, as hallucinated structures can significantly impact diagnostic outcomes. In this work, we introduce IM-MoCo [1], an instance-based self-supervised motion correction pipeline that utilizes motion-guided implicit neural representations (INRs) to reduce motion artifacts while preserving anatomical structures. IM-MoCo operates on motion-corrupted k-spaces and consists of two stages: motion line detection and implicit motion correction. First, a U-Net pre-trained on a population predicts a motion-line sampling mask in the k-space. Next, the pipeline corrects a scan by fitting an image-INR for an artifact-free image and a motion-INR for transformations corresponding to patient movements. We then obtain a motion-corrupted k-space by applying the transformations to the image-INR output, Fourier transform the results, and sample the corresponding lines using the predicted motion sampling mask. The instance-wise optimization focuses on minimizing a data consistency loss between the predicted k-space and the acquired one while enforcing sharpness via gradient entropy regularization on the image-INR output. The final motion-corrected image is the output of the image-INR. We evaluated our method using the publicly available fastMRI dataset [2] with varying degrees of simulated motion severity. For the correction alone, we could improve over state-of-the-art motion correction methods by +5% SSIM, +5 db PSNR, and +14% HaarPSI. Clinical relevance is demonstrated by a subsequent experiment where our method improves classification outcomes by at least +1.5 accuracy percentage points over motion-corrupted images. The IM-MoCo implementation and the experiments are available[1].

References

1. Al-Haj Hemidi Z, Weihsbach C, Heinrich MP. IM-MoCo: self-supervised MRI motion correction using motion-guided implicit neural representations. Proc MICCAI. 2024:382–92.

[1] https://github.com/multimodallearning/MICCAI24_IMMoCo.git

C. Palm et al. (Hrsg.), *Bildverarbeitung für die Medizin 2025*, Informatik aktuell,
https://doi.org/10.1007/978-3-658-47422-5_38

2. Zbontar J, Knoll F, Sriram A et al. fastMRI: an open dataset and benchmarks for accelerated MRI. arXiv: 1811.08839. 2018.

Assessing Spatial Bias in Medical Imaging
An Empirical Study of PatchGAN Discriminator Effectiveness

Marc S. Seibel[1], Timo Kepp[2], Hristina Uzunova[2], Jan Ehrhardt[1,2], Heinz Handels[1,2]

[1]University of Lübeck, Institute of Medical Informatics, Lübeck, Germany
[2]German Research Center for Artificial Intelligence, Lübeck, Germany
marc.seibel@uni-luebeck.de

Abstract. Unpaired image-to-image (I2I) translation plays an important role in denoising, super-resolution and modality conversion. These methods often rely on adversarial training for matching two distributions, and they suffer from hallucinations induced by biases. In this work, we study a spatial shift bias in the case of domain translation for retinal optical coherence tomography (OCT). For one domain, the retinas are at the bottom of the image, while in the other domain, the retinas are centered. We show that the conventional PatchGAN discriminator replicates the spatial bias of the target domain. This leads to imperfectly translated images. By putting explicit limitations to the receptive field of the PatchGAN, we recover the ability of the I2I network to truthfully translate OCTs from one domain to the other. Evidence is provided by improvements of Fréchet Inception distance, increased translational equivariance, and increased Dice scores.

1 Introduction

Medical image analysis and processing applications benefit from image-to-image (I2I) translation methods which are used for denoising, super-resolution, modality conversion and image reconstruction [1]. Specifically, in the case of modality conversion, I2I methods have increased the robustness of image processing models for segmentation [2] and registration [3] by increasing the size and diversity of datasets. Examples of modality conversion are the translation of different brain MRI sequences [4], or between different Optical Coherence Tomography (OCT) devices [5].

Depending on the availability of paired images from the source and target domain, I2I methods can be categorized into paired (supervised) and unpaired (unsupervised) approaches. Since the acquisition of paired images is often technically impossible, unpaired I2I methods constitute the dominant choice in medical imaging. For example, Fig. 1 shows a case of retinal OCTs acquired from different devices with different positioning of the retina. Without pixel-wise correspondence, unpaired I2I methods are faced with the challenge of identifying corresponding structures without guidance on the pixel level. This problem is amplified, if one domain systematically contains objects (e.g., artifacts) which are not present in the other domain. Consequently, translating images from one domain to another is an ill-posed problem which can only be accurately solved if the model is appropriately designed using prior information.

Image-to-image translation methods based on the Generative Adversarial Network (GAN) approach [6] attempt to solve this problem using distribution matching. Uncontrolled adversarial distribution matching can lead to hallucinations [7]. Controlling

C. Palm et al. (Hrsg.), *Bildverarbeitung für die Medizin 2025*, Informatik aktuell,
https://doi.org/10.1007/978-3-658-47422-5_39

the training is difficult, since the discriminator will use any information in the images (e.g., pose, content, texture) to distinguish between real images in the target domain and translated images, while we are interested only in a specific set of properties (here the different texture-related characteristics of the imaging devices). Thus, to prevent the generator from following the unconstrained adversarial gradient signal, additional losses are used to guide the generator. Prominent related works to constrain (condition) the generator are, cycle-consistency [8] which makes the assumption that a bijective mapping between the source and target domain exists in the pixel space. In order to eliminate the assumption of the existence of bijective mappings entirely, contrastive unpaired image-to-image translation (CUT) [9] was proposed, which enforces semantic consistency between the source and the translated images but no cycle consistency. Unpaired neural Schrödinger bridges (UNSB) [10] combines a diffusion model with the CUT approach. All mentioned approaches use a PatchGAN discriminator [11] – a fully convolutional neural network. By keeping the receptive field of the PatchGAN small, the frequency range of the discriminator is restricted such that it can extract only particular high-frequency information from the images [11].

Our contribution in this work is an empirical analysis of the architecture of the PatchGAN discriminator for the case of a spatial bias where the retina is located at different positions in the source and target domain. Three criteria are used to quantify the impact of this spatial bias. We study the translational equivariance of the generator, the image similarity of the translated images with the original SELFF-OCT data, and lastly how good the translated images are for training a segmentation network.

2 Materials and methods

In this section, we describe the OCT data and two methods to address the spatial bias.

The dataset used in this study consists OCT images from 50 healthy subjects, which were recorded with the Spectralis OCT device (Heidelberg Engineering, Heidelberg, Germany) and a prototype of a self-examination low-cost full-field (SELFF) OCT device (Visotec GmbH, Lübeck, Germany). Images from both devices were resampled

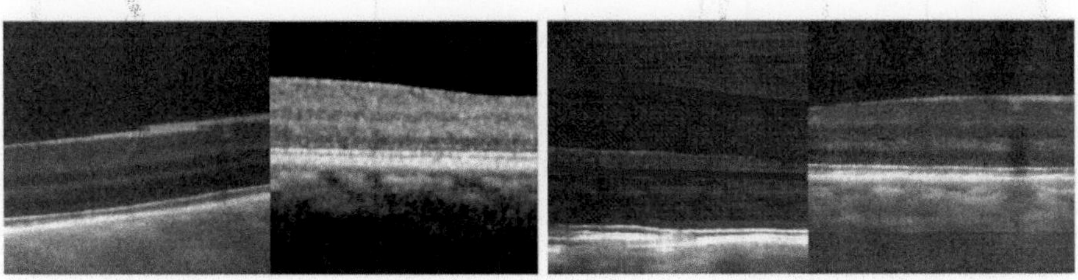

Fig. 1. Spatial bias in source and target domains. The left image compares a SELFF-OCT and a Spectralis-OCT: in SELFF-OCTs, the retina is at the bottom, while in Spectralis-OCTs, it is centered. The right image shows a Spectralis-OCT translated to the SELFF-OCT domain. The first split view, using a CycleGAN with a 70×70 PatchGAN discriminator, replicates SELFF-OCT bias and misplaces the retina (red lines indicate correct placement). The second half shows a CycleGAN with our explicit PatchGAN, which corrects the spatial bias. Image size: 192×416.

to the resolution of 11.7 × 5.6 × 11.7 (in micrometers). The resulting image sizes for the Spectralis and SELFF-OCT images were 512 × 375 × 512 and 512 × 200 × 416, respectively. For the Spectralis images, we relied on the automatically created segmentations from the Spectralis device. For ten subjects from the SELFF-OCT domain, we semi-automatically created segmentations using the Iowa Reference Algorithms [12].

The position of the retina in the Spectralis-OCTs is distributed over the entire image, while the retina in the SELFF-OCT images is located at the bottom of the image. This difference can be detected by the discriminator. During training, we randomly crop the image so that the Bruch's membrane of the retina is between 15 and 35 pixels away from the lower edge of the image. Intuitively, aligning the retina in the Spectralis images with the retina in the SELFF-OCT images, shifts the unpaired I2I problem towards a paired image-to-image problem. In Tab. 1, we refer to this method as *spatial alignment*.

The discriminator is a key component as it distinguishes real target images from translated fake images. We study how different design choices for the discriminator architecture affect the replication of the spatial bias in the translated images. As baseline, we start with a PatchGAN discriminator [11], which is a fully convolutional network. The size of the receptive field of the PatchGAN discriminator implicitly determines the patch size. By changing the depth of the network, we define three network architectures with patch sizes of 16×16, 34×34, and 70×70 pixels. Importantly, no padding is used for the discriminator, since prior work [13] provided evidence that it supports CNNs to learn the absolute position of objects in images. We design a second discriminator which explicitly divides the image into patches of size 16×16, 32×32, and 64×64. These patches are then independently fed into a PatchGAN with a receptive field of 34×34 pixels.

After training the image-to-image translation model, we evaluate the translational equivariance of the generator G. To this end, we shift the input images in the vertical direction, as denoted by $\mathcal{T}$. We then measure the difference between the fake images after shifting compared to a reference fake image. For the reference image, the retina has a distance of 20 pixels from the bottom of the image. Using the segmentations from the Spectralis images, we crop the images to the retina region. Formally, the equivariance error is defined as

$$e_{\mathcal{T}} = \frac{1}{N} \sum_{i=1}^{N} ||\mathrm{Crop}(G(x)_i) - \mathrm{Crop}(G(\mathcal{T} \circ x))_i|| \tag{1}$$

We want to evaluate the goodness of the translated Spectralis images for the purpose of segmenting SELFF-OCT images. We shifted all images such that they have a distance of 50 pixels from the bottom of the image. To this end, we train an EfficientNet B-2 [14] using only the translated Spectralis images to segment seven retinal layers with a cross-entropy loss. No further domain adaptation methods are used. The network is trained and evaluated with images from 40 subjects, while the remaining 10 subjects are used for testing the model on the SELFF-OCT images.

3 Results

We investigate three approaches to address the spatial bias in the Spectralis and SELFF-OCT images. First, we study how the size of the receptive field of an implicit PatchGAN affects the spatial bias in the translated images. Fig. 2 shows the translational equivariance error for an implicit PatchGAN with patches of size 16×16, 34×34, and 70×70 used for training a CUT network. Increasing the receptive field increases the equivariance error. The images on the right show the same Spectralis image which were translated with a CUT based I2I approach where we varied the choice of the receptive field of the PatchGAN. Only the images which were obtained from training with a PatchGAN with rf=16 are correctly located. Second, we study how a spatial alignment of the retina can reduce the spatial bias for the implicit PatchGAN. We measure how this affects the image similarity with the real SELFF-OCTs in terms of Fréchet inception distance (FID) [15], the translational equivariance error, and the segmentation performance of a downstream model which is trained on the translated images. The results of this investigation are given in Tab. 1 and Fig. 3. Debiasing through spatial alignment has a strong effect when training with an implicit PatchGAN as indicated by the reduced equivariance error and increased Dice. Third, we compare the performance of the implicit and explicit PatchGAN discriminator. The patch size of the explicit PatchGAN is 32×32 pixels and the receptive field of both PatchGANs is 34. We find that debiasing has no effect on the explicit PatchGAN. This indicates that the explicit PatchGAN naturally ignores the spatial bias.

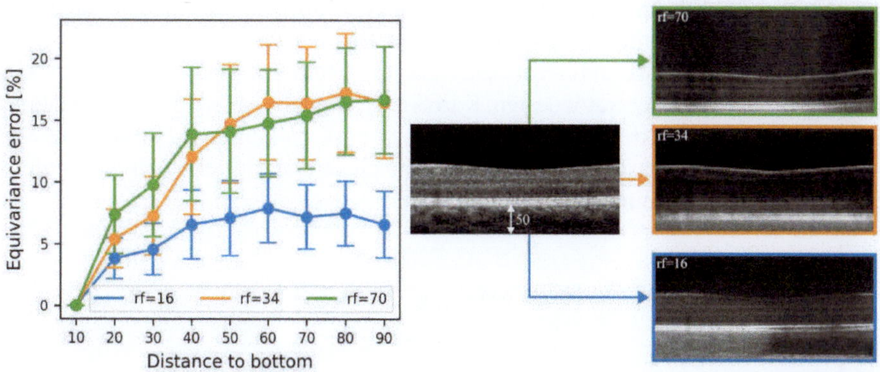

Fig. 2. Translational equivariance for three different CUT models where the discriminators had an implicit receptive field of rf=16, 34, 70. The graph on the left shows the shift equivariance error. The x-axis shows the distance of the retina from the lower edge of the image. The dots and whiskers show the mean and standard deviation of the equivariance error. The right side shows a Spectralis OCT where the retina is located 50 pixels above the bottom and which was then translated with the three models. The spatial bias of the SELFF-OCT images is only suppressed if the PatchGAN has a receptive field of 16.

Tab. 1. Evaluation of the impact of the PatchGAN design and spatial alignment on the image quality (FID), the translational equivariance error when the retina is 50 pixels above the bottom, and downstream segmentation performance (Dice). Spectralis data corresponds to the original source data.

	PatchGAN	Spat. alignment	FID ↓	Equivariance Error ↓	Dice ↑
Spectralis data	-	-	134	-	0.60
CycleGAN	implicit	×	166	0.12	0.58
CUT	implicit	×	168	0.13	0.61
CycleGAN	explicit	×	87	0.06	0.74
CUT	explicit	×	63	0.07	0.66
CycleGAN	implicit	✓	55	0.05	0.76
CUT	implicit	✓	196	0.04	0.72
CycleGAN	explicit	✓	43	0.05	0.76
CUT	explicit	✓	62	0.08	0.66

4 Discussion

Our analysis provides a new perspective on the role of the PatchGAN discriminator in the context of unpaired image-to-image translation for a case where objects are differently positioned in the source and target domain. Our results indicate that this spatial bias hurts I2I translation. Arguably, the straightforward approach to address the spatial bias is given by aligning images from both domains. Unfortunately, this is only a practical solution for simple transformations such as shifts. As an alternative, we found that the explicit PatchGAN has a similar effect on ignoring the spatial bias. One possible reason for the vulnerability of the implicit PatchGAN to spatial biases could be that CNNs lack true translation invariance and can instead exploit absolute spatial positions [16]. Despite focusing primarily on generator design, Karras et al. similarly observed that translational equivariance is hindered by padding and aliasing artifacts introduced through network nonlinearities [17]. Consistent with [18], we conclude that greater attention should be directed toward discriminator design.

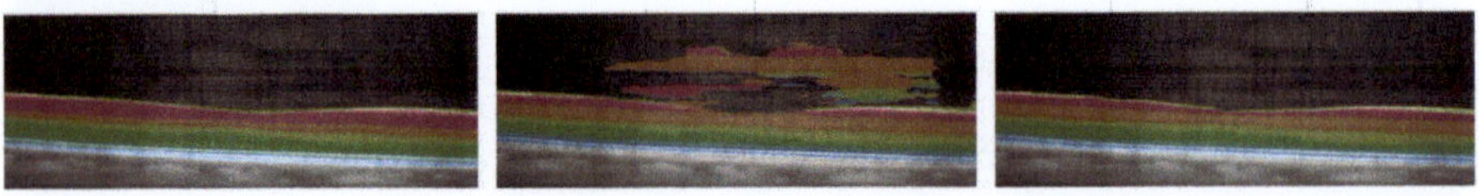

Fig. 3. B-Scan from a SELFF-OCT with segmentations overlaid. The first image shows the ground truth. The second and third images compare the segmentation quality, whereby the underlying training data was first created with a CycleGAN, with an implicit PatchGAN (receptive field=34) and secondly with an explicit PatchGAN (receptive field=32).

References

1. Kaji S, Kida S. Overview of image-to-image translation by use of deep neural networks: denoising, super-resolution, modality conversion, and reconstruction in medical imaging. Radiol Phys Technol. 2019;12(3):235–48.
2. Dorent R, Kujawa A, Ivory M et al. CrossMoDA 2021 challenge: benchmark of cross-modality domain adaptation techniques for vestibular schwannoma and cochlea segmentation. Med Image Anal. 2023;83:102628.
3. Yang Q, Li N, Zhao Z et al. MRI cross-modality image-to-image translation. Sci Rep. 2020;10(1):3753.
4. Uzunova H, Ehrhardt J, Handels H. Memory-efficient GAN-based domain translation of high resolution 3D medical images. Comput Med Imaging Graph. 2020;86:101801.
5. Seibel MS, Uzunova H, Kepp T et al. Anatomical conditioning for contrastive unpaired image-to-image translation of optical coherence tomography images. Proc IEEE ISBI. 2024:1–5.
6. Goodfellow I, Pouget-Abadie J, Mirza M et al. Generative adversarial networks. Commun ACM. 2020;63(11):139–44.
7. Cohen JP, Luck M, Honari S. Distribution matching losses can hallucinate features in medical image translation. 2018:529–36.
8. Zhu JY, Park T, Isola P et al. Unpaired image-to-image translation using cycle-consistent adversarial networks. Proc IEEE ICCV. 2017:2223–32.
9. Park T, Efros AA, Zhang R et al. Contrastive learning for unpaired image-to-image translation. Proc ECCV. 2020:319–45.
10. Kim B, Kwon G, Kim K et al. Unpaired image-to-image translation via neural Schrödinger bridge. arXiv: 2305.15086. 2024.
11. Isola P, Zhu JY, Zhou T et al. Image-to-image translation with conditional adversarial networks. Proc IEEE CVPR. 2017:1125–34.
12. Li K, Wu X, Chen DZ et al. Optimal surface segmentation in volumetric images-a graph-theoretic approach. IEEE Trans Pattern Anal Mach Intell. 2005;28(1):119–34.
13. Islam MA, Kowal M, Jia S et al. Position, padding and predictions: a deeper look at position information in CNNs. Int J Comput Vis. 2024:1–22.
14. Tan M, Le Q. EfficientNet: rethinking model scaling for convolutional neural networks. Proc ICML. 2019:6105–14.
15. Heusel M, Ramsauer H, Unterthiner T et al. GANs trained by a two time-scale update rule converge to a local nash equilibrium. Adv Neural Inf Process Sys. 2017:6629–40.
16. Kayhan OS, Gemert JCv. On translation invariance in CNNs: convolutional layers can exploit absolute spatial location. Proc IEEE CVF CVPR. 2020:14274–85.
17. Karras T, Aittala M, Laine S et al. Alias-free generative adversarial networks. Adv Neural Inf Process Syst. 2021;34:852–63.
18. Schwarz K, Liao Y, Geiger A. On the frequency bias of generative models. Adv Neural Inf Process Syst. 2021;34:18126–36.

Unsupervised Single-source Domain Generalization for Robust Quantification of Lymphatic Perfusion

Lisa K. Fischer[1], Johanna P. Müller[1], Christian Schröder[2], Anja Hanser[3], Michela Cuomo[2], Thomas Day[4], Cheng Ouyang[5,6], Oliver Dewald[2], Oliver Rompel[2], Sven Dittrich[2], Thomas Küstner[3], Bernhard Kainz[1,6]

[1]FAU Erlangen-Nürnberg, Germany
[2]University Hospital Erlangen, Germany
[3]University Hospital Tübingen, Germany
[4]King's College London, United Kingdom
[5]University of Oxford, United Kingdom
[6]Imperial College London, United Kingdom
johanna.paula.mueller@fau.de

Abstract. Infants and young children with Fontan circulation, resulting from life-saving heart surgery, experience altered hemodynamics that can lead to severe, life-threatening complications, often driven by congestion in the lymphatic system. These complications typically become more apparent as the patients grow older. Early detection and management of these complications require precise assessment of lymphatic perfusion through segmentation of lymphatic fluids. However, manual evaluation is time-intensive and subject to variability, underscoring the need for automated, reliable segmentation in clinical practice. Yet, domain shifts arising from variations in MRI acquisition protocols (e.g., BLADE versus SPACE sequences) and scanner differences present significant challenges for current segmentation models. In this work, we propose the use of causality-inspired single-source domain generalization (CISDG) to develop a robust and accurate segmentation network for lymphatic perfusion patterns across diverse imaging domains. Using a dataset of T_2-weighted MR images from 71 patients, we demonstrate that our CISDG model outperforms conventional segmentation networks, including nnU-Net, in both source and target domains. Our results indicate that the proposed method not only generalizes effectively across domain shifts but also holds promise for enhancing diagnostic efficiency and reliability in clinical settings.

1 Introduction

Congenital univentricular heart defects affect approximately 3 in 10,000 live births [1], necessitating a series of surgical interventions within the first years of life and resulting in the Fontan circulation. The significantly altered hemodynamics in patients with Fontan circulation, frequently lead to severe complications such as protein-losing enteropathy or plastic bronchitis, which are associated with congestion within the lymphatic system [2]. For early detection and effective management of these complications, regular monitoring through imaging of lymphatic perfusions is crucial. In this context a curated dataset was established by [3], it includes T_2-weighted routine MRI scans of 71 Fontan

C. Palm et al. (Hrsg.), *Bildverarbeitung für die Medizin 2025*, Informatik aktuell,
https://doi.org/10.1007/978-3-658-47422-5_40

patients, treated at the University Hospital in Erlangen between 2007 and 2020. We revised this dataset and further refined it through additional manual annotations, which were performed in collaboration with a pediatric cardiologist. Domain shifts result from variations in imaging devices, protocols, and settings often occurring even within one institution. These present a significant challenge in medical image segmentation and can lead to performance decreases in the segmentation ability when insufficient data from the target domain is available during training. How domain shifts can impede a model's performance can be seen in the variations between T_2- weighted MRI images acquired with a BLADE sequence and with a SPACE sequence. Although the nnU-Net by [4] performs well on the BLADE sequences within the dataset, it exhibits a significant performance drop when confronted with SPACE sequences. This appears due to the limited sample size of SPACE images and the intensity differences between the BLADE and SPACE images. However, domain shifts are not limited to differences between sequences, they can also occur in other contexts where imaging conditions vary. This highlights the necessity for a model that robustly and accurately segments lymphatic perfusions in images from various domains, without additional training images, which are often scarce due to privacy concerns, costs, and the labor-intensiveness of manual annotation. To find a solution that robustly segments lymphatic perfusion patterns across different domains, we explored the causality-inspired single-source domain generalization (CISDG) approach by [5]. Unlike multi-source domain generalization or conventional data augmentation, this approach does not require any target domain data during training and exclusively uses data from one domain for training. It focuses on learning domain-invariant features, that can be applied to unseen target domains. This approach has demonstrated promising results in segmenting abdominal cross-modality, cardiac cross-sequence, and prostate cross-site datasets. Nevertheless, the authors could not find an application in the context of lymphatic perfusion pattern segmentation, as proposed in this paper. The CISDG network outperformed the nnU-Net on the limited target domain data available to us and achieved slightly better results than the nnU-Net on the source domain. We propose extending the evaluation of the network across other domains, however, the results are providing a promising direction for future research.

2 Materials and methods

Since 2007, the University Hospital in Erlangen has implemented a specialized protocol for managing univentricular heart defects. This protocol incorporates a T_2-weighted MR images with fat suppression, conducted six months post-Fontan completion, to evaluate the lymphatic perfusions. By 2020 MR images had been acquired from 71 patients, forming the foundation for an underlying clinical trial, by [6]. For 67 patients, imaging was performed using the BLADE sequence, a motion-resistant, multi-shot turbo spin echo technique designed for breath-hold acquisition. BLADE incorporates intershot motion correction to effectively reduce artifacts from sources such as intestinal peristalsis, residual respiratory movement, and cardiac pulsation. In the remaining four patients, the SPACE sequence was used—a single-slab, 3D turbo spin echo sequence that employs a slab-selective, variable excitation pulse to achieve high-resolution imaging of the target region. To enhance the dataset for this study, we conducted a comprehensive

Features		Subset A	Subset B	Dataset
Domain	BLADE	58	58	73
	SPACE	0	2	4
	Abdom.	5	5	7
Region	Full	48	50	63
	Thoracic	5	5	7
	0	0	2	4
	1	12	12	13
Quality	2	27	27	36
(n)	3	16	16	19
	4	3	3	5
	1	4	4	5
Severity	2	23	24	27
(n)	3	29	30	43
	4	1	1	1
		58	60	77

Tab. 1. Number of Volumes per Dataset subset for Training and for the full Dataset. Subset A contains only BLADE sequences, Subset B contains BLADE and SPACE.

review and added detailed new annotations to improve data quality and segmentation accuracy. Within the foundational dataset from [3], annotations in the thoracic scans were confined to thoracic lymphatic perfusions, while segmentations in the abdominal scans were limited to abdominal lymphatic perfusions. However, the abdominal or thoracic lymphatic perfusions might remain visible across these scans. Throughout the dataset refinement, precise pixel-wise annotations of these lymphatic perfusions were meticulously performed in collaboration with a pediatric cardiologist, utilizing 3D Slicer, an open-source software tool. Given the similar high intensity of lymphatic perfusions and other tissues in T_2-weighted images, it was crucial to consider anatomical structures to ensure correct identification and annotation. In certain images, the thoracic scan sufficiently covered the neck, chest, and abdomen. In such cases, comprehensive annotations were made within the thoracic scans, and the corresponding abdominal scans were exempt from training. Additionally, in the underlying database ratings in diverse categories were assigned to the images. In the dataset by [3], each image received a severity rank on a scale from one to four, based on the assessments by two independent pediatric cardiologists, using the system introduced by [6, 7]. In this system, the thoracic, para-aortic, and portal-venous lymphatic perfusion patterns are individually ranked. For scans displaying multiple patterns, the mean of the individual scores was calculated. Furthermore, each scan was assigned a quality rating reaching from one, the best quality, to four, the lowest quality. Scans were also categorized by the domain and the annotated and displayed regions. Details on dataset distributions and the configuration of various data folds utilized during the training are provided in Tab. 1.

In MR images, variations in image intensity occur due to differences in acquisition protocols and sequences. These acquisition shifts are particularly visible between images acquired with BLADE and SPACE sequences. Such differences pose significant challenges to standard segmentation models such as the nnU-Net by [4]. To improve the model's performance when exposed to acquisition shifts, [5] introduced a causality-inspired data augmentation approach. The workflow is composed of two main techniques (Fig. 1), global intensity non-linear augmentation (GIN) and interventional pseudo-correlation augmentation (IPA). GIN uses randomly weighted shallow convolutional networks to generate images with different appearances, thereby preventing the model from learning acquisition-related criteria. IPA autonomously resamples the appearance of possibly confounded objects, enhancing the model's robustness against domain shifts. The efficiency of this model has been evaluated across several datasets, including an abdominal cross-modality, a cardiac cross-sequence, and a prostate cross-site dataset, demonstrating superior performance to other state-of-the-art models. Considering the differences between BLADE and SPACE sequences as examples of acquisition shifts, and the robust performance of the model on diverse test data, we selected this model for our segmentation task. By using this advanced approach adapted for our dataset, we aim to address the challenges of domain shifts and enhance the accuracy of automated segmentation. To evaluate the model's performance, we selected the 2D nnU-Net by [4] as the state-of-the-art (SOTA) method. To ensure comparability, we adopted the same 2D configuration used in the domain generalization model. Furthermore, the 3D nnU-Net did not yield improved performance in our previous work [3].

3 Results

Fig. 2 compares the label and the prediction by the CISDG model of an exemplary high-performing BLADE and SPACE scan. Tab. 2 shows the best checkpoint performance of the causality-inspired domain generalization (CISDG) network trained on Subset A compared to the performance of the 2d nnU-Net trained on Subset A and B. On the BLADE sequence, the CISDG network marginally outperformed both nnU-Net configurations by 5 % and 4 %. The nnU-Net (A) failed to deliver satisfactory results on the SPACE images, whereas the nnU-Net (B) showed 23 % better results. The CISDG model outperformed both nnU-Nets, by 13 % and 36 % on the SPACE domain. However, the CISDG network also experienced an 8 % inferior performance on the SPACE images

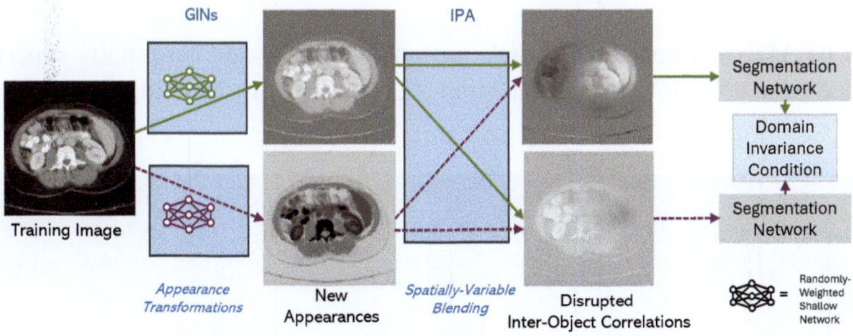

Fig. 1. Overview of the Causality-Inspired Single-Source Domain Generalization approach. During training, the input image is transformed using a generative invariant network (GIN), producing a diverse set of appearances. These transformations are then refined through invariant perturbation augmentation (IPA), which removes any residual inter-object perturbations. The resulting augmented images are used to train a segmentation network, equipping it to learn a domain-invariant representation for robust performance across diverse domains [5].

Tab. 2. Best checkpoint evaluation on the test set by T_2 sequence, best scores in bold, CISDG: causality-inspired single-source domain generalization network DSC: dice similarity coefficient, IoU: Intersection over Union, NSD: normalized surface distance.

T_2 Sequence	Measure	CISDG (A)	nnU-Net (A)	nnU-Net (B)
BLADE	DSC	**0.45 ± 0.13**	0.40 ± 0.17	0.41 ± 0.16
	IoU	**0.30 ± 0.10**	0.26 ± 0.14	0.27 ± 0.13
	NSD	0.68 ± 0.13	0.84 ± 0.06	**0.85 ± 0.05**
SPACE	DSC	**0.37 ± 0.10**	0.08 ± 0.09	0.24 ± 0.23
	IoU	**0.23 ± 0.09**	0.04 ± 0.05	0.16 ± 0.15
	NSD	0.49 ± 0.06	0.64 ± 0.06	**0.66 ± 0.10**

compared to the BLADE images. Additionally, the influence of the region, severity, and quality of the images on the model's segmentation of the BLADE images was evaluated. The performance of the CISDG network, the nnU-Net (A), and the nnU-Net (B) were compared, the results are listed in Tab. 3. The nnU-Net (A) achieved the best results on the thoracic images, followed by the abdominal images, and was the least accurate on whole-body images. Conversely, the CISDG model performed the best on whole-body images, followed by thoracic and abdominal images. In terms of quality, all networks demonstrated better performance on higher-quality images and performed the best on images with a severity rank of three. However, the CISDG model performed 15 % better than nnU-Net (A) and 3 % better than nnU-Net (B) on images with low severity, achieving similar results in this category as on images with severity rank three, and the nnU-Net (A) performed 11 % better than the CISDG model and 3 % better than nnU-Net (B) on images with quality four, even performing 16 % better than on images with quality 3. All models were least effective on images classified with a severity of two.

4 Discussion

For the BLADE sequence, the CISDG network demonstrated marginally superior performance over both nnU-Nets, indicating its robustness in handling images from the

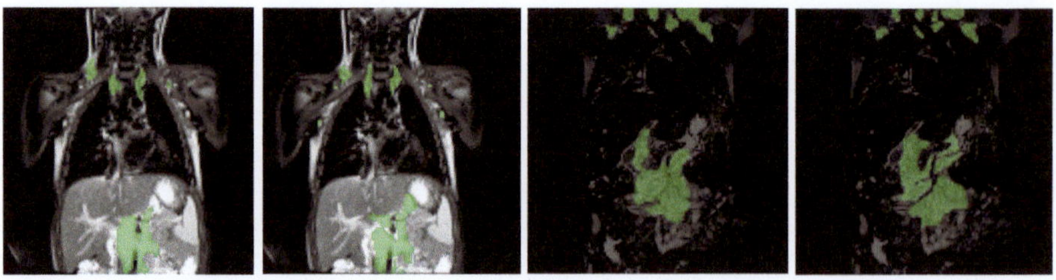

(a) BLADE Prediction. **(b)** BLADE Label. **(c)** SPACE Prediction. **(d)** SPACE Label.

Fig. 2. Comparison of high-performing BLADE (Quality 2 and Severity 3) and SPACE (Quality 0 and Severity 3) full-body prediction and label by the CISDG model.

Tab. 3. Average scores on the test set for the anatomical region, quality, and severity in the BLADE sequence, best scores in bold, CISDG: causality-inspired single-source domain generalization network DSC: dice similarity coefficient, IoU: Intersection over Union.

		CISDG (A)		nnU-Net (A)		nnU-Net (B)	
Features		DSC	IoU	DSC	IoU	DSC	IoU
Region	Abdom.	0.39 ± 0.25	0.27 ± 0.20	**0.46 ± 0.26**	**0.34 ± 0.23**	0.45 ± 0.25	0.33 ± 0.22
	Full	**0.46 ± 0.09**	**0.30 ± 0.08**	0.37 ± 0.14	0.24 ± 0.11	0.39 ± 0.14	0.25 ± 0.10
	Thoracic	0.42 ± 0.00	0.27 ± 0.00	**0.57 ± 0.00**	**0.40 ± 0.00**	0.52 ± 0.00	0.35 ± 0.00
Quality	1	0.49 ± 0.00	0.33 ± 0.00	0.51 ± 0.00	0.34 ± 0.00	**0.52 ± 0.00**	**0.35 ± 0.00**
	2	**0.49 ± 0.11**	**0.33 ± 0.09**	0.45 ± 0.15	0.30 ± 0.13	0.45 ± 0.14	0.30 ± 0.12
	3	**0.40 ± 0.05**	**0.25 ± 0.04**	0.23 ± 0.12	0.14 ± 0.07	0.28 ± 0.13	0.17 ± 0.09
	4	0.28 ± 0.15	0.17 ± 0.10	**0.39 ± 0.19**	**0.26 ± 0.14**	0.36 ±0.16	0.23 ± 0.12
Severity	1	**0.47 ± 0.00**	**0.31 ± 0.00**	0.32 ± 0.00	0.19 ± 0.00	0.44 ± 0.00	0.28 ± 0.00
	2	**0.40 ± 0.14**	**0.26 ± 0.10**	0.29 ± 0.16	0.18 ± 0.11	0.31 ± 0.15	0.19 ± 0.11
	3	0.47 ± 0.12	0.31 ± 0.10	**0.49 ± 0.14**	0.33 ± 0.12	0.48 ± 0.13	**0.33 ± 0.11**
	4	-	-	-	-	-	-

source domain. The CISDG model notably outperformed both nnU-Nets on the SPACE domain, despite being solely trained on BLADE sequences, this highlights the model's generalization abilities across unknown domains. The nnU-Net (A), which was only trained on BLADE images, failed on the SPACE domain, highlighting the limitations of the model and the necessity for a model with better generalization abilities. Incorporating a small number of SPACE samples into the training data, as in the data fold of the nnU-Net (B), significantly improved the model's performance, nevertheless, it did not reach the performance level of the CISDG network, highlighting that little data from the source domain can improve the performance but does not solve the problem of domain shifts. A closer examination of the model's performance on the BLADE images reveals that the CISDG model shows superior performance to both nnU-Nets on whole-body images, while both nnU-Nets perform better on thoracic and abdominal images and the nnU-Nets (A) achieved the best results in these categories. The overall superior performance of the CISDG model over the nnU-Nets can be attributed to its ability to segment a greater number of whole-body images with greater precision. All models demonstrated the highest performance on images with severity level three, as the majority of training images were from category three the performance increase might not be directly related to the severity of the lymphatic perfusions but rather to the increased number of training samples. On top, the performance according to severity can not be fully assessed due to the very limited data and the absence of test data in the category of severity level four. The results highlight the great potential of the CISDG approach to enhance the generalization ability of a model. However, the sample size in the SPACE domain was very small, and further testing, with a larger sample size and data from other domains, would be necessary to fully assess the capabilities of the CISDG network in the context of lymphatic perfusion segmentation.

5 Conclusion

We demonstrated the effectiveness of the CISDG approach for robust lymphatic perfusion pattern segmentation in patients with congenital univentricular heart defects. Our findings indicate that the CISDG model outperforms traditional segmentation models, such as nnU-Net, across diverse imaging protocols, including the SPACE and BLADE MRI sequences, highlighting its potential to address domain shifts. The model's ability to generalize without requiring target domain data provides a significant advantage in clinical settings where data from varied imaging protocols may be limited.

Acknowledgement. The authors gratefully acknowledge the scientific support and HPC resources provided by the Erlangen national high performance computing center (NHR@FAU) under the NHR projects b143dc and b180dc. NHR funding is provided by federal and Bavarian state authorities. NHR@FAU hardware is partially funded by the German research foundation (DFG) – 440719683. Support was also received by the DFG 513220538, 512819079, ERC - project MIA-NORMAL 101083647, DFG KA 5801/2-1, INST 90/1351-1 and by the state of Bavaria (HTA and EVUK).

References

1. Schwedler G, Lindinger A, Lange PE et al. Frequency and spectrum of congenital heart defects among live births in Germany : a study of the competence network for congenital heart defects. Clin Res Cardiol. 2011;100(12):1111–7.
2. Blum U, Meyer H, Beerbaum P et al. Kompendium angeborene Herzfehler bei Kindern: Diagnose und Behandlung. 2. Auflage. Berlin and Heidelberg: Springer, 2021.
3. Stegmaier M, Müller JP, Schröder C et al. Automatic segmentation of lymphatic perfusion in patients with congenital single ventricle defects. Bildverarbeitung für die Medizin 2024. Ed. by Maier A, Deserno TM, Handels H et al. (Informatik aktuell). Wiesbaden: Springer Fachmedien Wiesbaden, 2024:255–60.
4. Isensee F, Jaeger PF, Kohl SAA et al. nnU-Net: a self-configuring method for deep learning-based biomedical image segmentation. Nat Methods. 2021;18(2):203–11.
5. Ouyang C, Chen C, Li S et al. Causality-inspired single-source domain generalization for medical image segmentation. IEEE Trans Med Imaging. 2023;42(4):1095–106.
6. Schroeder C, Moosmann J, Cesnjevar R et al. A classification of abdominal lymphatic perfusion patterns after Fontan surgery. Eur J Cardio-Thorac Surg. 2022;62(4).
7. Biko DM, DeWitt AG, Pinto EM et al. MRI evaluation of lymphatic abnormalities in the neck and thorax after fontan surgery: relationship with outcome. Radiology. 2019;291(3):774–80.

Data-proximal Neural Networks for Limited-view CT

Simon Göppel[1], Jürgen Frikel[2], Markus Haltmeier[3]

[1]IABG, Ottobrunn, Germany
[2]Faculty of Computer Science and Mathematics , OTH Regensburg, Germany
[3]Department of Mathematics, University of Innsbruck, Austria
juergen.frikel@oth-regensburg.de

Abstract. Limited-angle computed tomography (CT) requires solving an inverse problem that is both ill-conditioned and underdetermined. In recent years, learned reconstruction methods have proven highly effective in addressing this challenge. Most of these methods follow a two-step process: first, an initial reconstruction method is applied to the data to generate an auxiliary reconstruction; second, a neural network is used to map the auxiliary reconstruction closer to the ground truth images. However, when applied to unseen data, there are no guarantees that the network's output will remain consistent with the available measurement data. To address this, we recently introduced a data-proximal network architecture. In this paper, we implement this approach for limited-angle CT and compare its performance with a standard residual network and a null space network.

1 Introduction

We consider image reconstruction in limited-data computed tomography (CT). While our concept applies to other geometries in both 2D and 3D, for the sake of clarity, we work with the limited-view Radon transform, denoted by $\mathbf{A}_I$, which maps a function $f \in L^2(\mathbb{R}^2)$ to its line integrals over a restricted set of directions I, covering an angular range of less than 180 degrees. The task is to recover the unknown function f from data

$$g = \mathbf{A}_I(f) + \eta \tag{1}$$

where η is the noise, satisfying $\|\eta\| \leq \delta$, with a noise level $\delta > 0$. The image reconstruction problem (1) is both unstable and underdetermined, requiring the use of regularization methods for its solution. One classical approach is variational regularization, which is known to be stable and convergent to the solution of the noise-free equation with the minimal value of the chosen regularizing functional as $\delta \to 0$. Moreover, it comes with error estimates under certain smoothness assumptions [1].

Recently, deep learning-based reconstruction methods have empirically demonstrated to outperform classical reconstruction methods. Specifically, the learned two-step reconstruction $f_{\alpha,\theta} = \mathbf{N}_\theta \mathbf{B}_\alpha(g)$, where a learned network $\mathbf{N}_\theta$ is applied to an initial classical reconstruction $\mathbf{B}_\alpha(g)$, is simple and works well in practice [2–4]. However, unlike classical regularization methods, these approaches lack theoretical reconstruction guarantees and may result in reconstructions for which the residual $\|\mathbf{A}_I(f_{\alpha,\theta}) - g\|$ can be arbitrarily large. This means that the data proximity $\|g - \mathbf{A}_I(f)\| \leq \delta$, which represents the actual information contained in the measurements, is destroyed.

C. Palm et al. (Hrsg.), *Bildverarbeitung für die Medizin 2025*, Informatik aktuell,
https://doi.org/10.1007/978-3-658-47422-5_41

To address this issue, so-called null-space (NS) networks have been proposed in [5, 6], ensuring that the learned component lies in the kernel of $\mathbf{A}_I$. A more general framework is given by data-proximal (DP) networks [7], which are designed to ensure data proximity and provide mathematically rigorous regularization methods. The aim of this work is to introduce DP networks as methods with theoretical guarantees and to demonstrate their strong performance in limited-view CT.

2 Material and methods

2.1 Learned two-step reconstruction

We consider the limited-view Radon transform $\mathbf{A}_I : \mathcal{D}(\mathbf{A}_I) \subseteq L^2(\mathbb{R}^2) \to L^2(I \times \mathbb{R})$ as a densely defined linear operator on $L^2(\mathbb{R}^2)$ with a nontrivial null space $\mathcal{N}(\mathbf{A}_I) \subseteq L^2(\mathbb{R}^2)$ and a dense range $\mathcal{R}(\mathbf{A}_I) \subseteq L^2(I \times \mathbb{R})$. Its Moore-Penrose inverse, $\mathbf{A}_I^+ g$, is given by the filtered back-projection (FBP) inverse applied to zero-extended data. Furthermore, the orthogonal projections onto the null space $\mathcal{N}(\mathbf{A}_I)$ and its orthogonal complement can be computed as $\mathbf{P}_{\mathcal{N}(\mathbf{A}_I)} = \mathrm{Id} - \mathbf{A}_I^+ \mathbf{A}_I$ and $\mathbf{P}_{\mathcal{N}(\mathbf{A}_I)}^{\perp} = \mathbf{A}_I^+ \mathbf{A}_I$, respectively.

Learned two-step reconstruction methods have typically the form

$$\mathbf{R}_{\alpha,\theta} : L^2(I \times \mathbb{R}) \to L^2(\mathbb{R}^2) : g \mapsto \mathbf{N}_\theta \circ \mathbf{B}_\alpha(g) \tag{2}$$

where $\mathbf{B}_\alpha : L^2(I \times \mathbb{R}) \to L^2(\mathbb{R}^2)$ is the initial reconstruction with parameter $\alpha > 0$, and $\mathbf{N}_\theta : L^2(\mathbb{R}^2) \to L^2(\mathbb{R}^2)$ is a learned neural network used to improve the initial reconstruction.

In this work, we use least squares (LS), sparse ℓ^1-minimization (SP), and total variation minimization (TV) as initial reconstruction methods, which are defined as follows

$$\mathbf{B}_0^{(1)}(g) := \operatorname*{arg\,min}_{f \in L^2([-1,1]^2)} \frac{1}{2} \|\mathbf{A}_I f - g\|_2^2 \tag{3}$$

$$\mathbf{B}_\alpha^{(2)}(g) := \operatorname*{arg\,min}_{f \in L^2([-1,1]^2)} \frac{1}{2} \|\mathbf{A}_I f - g\|_2^2 + \alpha \|\Psi f\|_{1,w} + \mathbf{1}_{\geq 0}(f) \tag{4}$$

$$\mathbf{B}_\alpha^{(3)}(g) := \operatorname*{arg\,min}_{f \in L^2([-1,1]^2)} \frac{1}{2} \|\mathbf{A}_I f - g\|_2^2 + \alpha \|f\|_{\mathrm{TV}} + \mathbf{1}_{\geq 0}(f) \tag{5}$$

where, α is the regularization parameter, Ψ the shearlet or wavelet transform, $\|\cdot\|_{\mathrm{TV}}$ the total variation, and $\mathbf{1}_{\geq 0}$ the indicator function, defined by $\mathbf{1}_{\geq 0}(f) = 0$ if $f \geq 0$ and $\mathbf{1}_{\geq 0}(f) = \infty$ otherwise.

Remark 2.1 All methods in (3), (4), (5) produce data consistent initial reconstructions, i.e., $\|\mathbf{A}_I f - g\|_2^2$ is small. Moreover, methods (4) and (5) constitute convergent regularization methods. That is, $\mathbf{B}_\alpha^{(2)}(g)$ and $\mathbf{B}_\alpha^{(3)}(g)$ converge to $\mathcal{R}$-minimizing solutions to $\mathbf{A}_I f = g$ if $\alpha = \alpha(\delta) \to 0$ and $\delta^2/\alpha \to 0$ as the noise level $\delta \to 0$ [1]. Here, $\mathcal{R}(\cdot) = \|\Psi(\cdot)\|_{1,w} + \mathbf{1}_{\geq 0}(\cdot)$ for SP, and $\mathcal{R}(\cdot) = \|\cdot\|_{\mathrm{TV}} + \mathbf{1}_{\geq 0}(\cdot)$ for TV.

It is well known that a carefully chosen prior can improve reconstructions. However, with incomplete data, such priors may still fail to produce accurate results, which is why learned post-processing networks are applied to further improve initial reconstructions.

In the second step (neural network part), we use standard residual (RS) network, null space (NS) network, and data-proximal (DP) network, defined as

$$\mathbf{N}_\theta^{\mathrm{RS}} = \mathrm{Id} + \mathbf{U}_\theta \tag{6}$$

$$\mathbf{N}_\theta^{\mathrm{NS}} = \mathrm{Id} + (\mathrm{Id} - \mathbf{A}_I^+\mathbf{A}_I)\mathbf{U}_\theta \tag{7}$$

$$\mathbf{N}_\theta^{\mathrm{DP}} = \mathrm{Id} + (\mathrm{Id} - \mathbf{A}_I^+\mathbf{A}_I)\mathbf{U}_\theta + \mathbf{A}_I^+\Phi_\beta\mathbf{A}_I\mathbf{U}_\theta \tag{8}$$

where $(\mathbf{U}_\theta)_{\theta\in\Theta}$ is the standard UNet, and $\Phi_\beta\colon \mathcal{R}(\mathbf{A}_I) \to \mathcal{R}(\mathbf{A}_I)$ is a function satisfying $\|\Phi_\beta(f)\| \le \beta$ for some $\beta > 0$. In our numerical experiments, we use the data-proximity function defined by $\Phi_\beta(f) := f$ if $\|f\|_2 \le \beta$, and $\Phi_\beta(f) := \beta \cdot f/\|f\|_2$ otherwise.

Note that all networks (6)–(8) are of residual type, as they add a learned component to the identity. While the RS network adds an arbitrary residual, the NS network is designed to add a residual $\mathbf{P}_{\mathcal{N}(\mathbf{A}_I)}\mathbf{U}_\theta = (\mathrm{Id} - \mathbf{A}_I^+\mathbf{A}_I)\mathbf{U}_\theta$ that lies in the null space of $\mathbf{A}_I$. The DP network allows for updating both the null space component and its complement. Importantly, the bound $\|\Phi_\beta(f)\| \le \beta$ ensures that $\|\mathbf{A}_I[f - \mathbf{N}_\theta^{\mathrm{DP}}(f)]\| \le \beta$. Consequently, unlike the RS network, the DP network provably preserves the data proximity of the initial reconstruction. In particular, letting $\beta \to \infty$ yields the RS network, and choosing $\beta = 0$ we obtain the NS network.

2.2 Numerical aspects

All computations are performed in a discrete setting, with $f \in \mathbb{R}^{N\times N}$ and $g \in \mathbb{R}^{P\times M}$, where $N, P, M \in \mathbb{N}$ are the discretization values for the image space $[-1, 1]^2$, angles are given in $I := [0, 3\pi/4]$, and the distance variable in $[-1.5, 1.5]$. The Radon transform $\mathbf{A}_I\colon \mathbb{R}^{N\times N} \to \mathbb{R}^{P\times M}$ and the FBP $\mathbf{A}_I\colon \mathbb{R}^{P\times M} \to \mathbb{R}^{N\times N}$ on I are computed using the Torch Radon package [8]. The full-view Radon transform is given as $\mathbf{A} := [\mathbf{A}_I, \mathbf{A}_I^c]$, with truncated projections for the forward map and zero extension for the inverse. The LS reconstruction (3) is computed using 1000 iterations of the Landweber algorithm, while regularized reconstructions are computed with the ADMM algorithm for SP (4) and the Chambolle-Pock algorithm for TV (5).

In our experiments, we use two different datasets. The first dataset consists of synthetic self-generated Shepp-Logan type phantoms and corresponding parallel-beam CT data with $N = 128$, $M = 200$ and $P = 121$. We generate 1000 training and 200 test pairs (f_n, g_n), where $g_n = \mathbf{A}_I f_n + 0.03\eta_n$, with $\eta_n \sim \|\mathbf{A}_I f_n\|_\infty \cdot \mathcal{N}(0, 1)$. The second dataset is the LoDoPaB-CT dataset, consisting of clinical low-dose CT measurements and corresponding ground truth images with $f_n \in \mathbb{R}^{362\times 362}$ [9]. CT measurement data are provided in parallel beam geometry with a total of $M = 513$ spatial sensors and 1000 projections of the full angular range. For $\mathbf{A}_I$, we restricted the directions to the angular range $[0, 3\pi/4]$, resulting in $P = 751$ projection angles. We use 1500 data pairs for training and 300 data pairs for testing. Following the learning paradigm, the network parameters are chosen to minimize the empirical risk $\mathcal{L}_N(\theta) := \sum_n \|\mathbf{N}_\theta(\mathbf{B}_\alpha(g_n)) - f_n\|^2$. By precomputing $\mathbf{B}_\alpha(g_n)$, the application of $\mathbf{B}_\alpha$ is not required during training, which makes it computationally efficient. We use $\beta := \sum_n \|\mathbf{A}_I f_n - g_n\|_2/N$, with N training samples, for both data sets.

Tab. 1. Average PSNR (peak signal-to-noise ratio) and SSIM (structural similarity index measure) computed over reconstructions from the test set of the Shepp-Logan type phantoms (Fig. 1).

	PSNR				SSIM			
Init.	Initial	RS	NS	DP	Initial	RS	NS	DP
LS	22.6356	32.5292	23.6555	26.6165	0.2510	0.8731	0.3092	0.4622
TV	29.6028	34.2014	32.9212	33.9671	0.8423	0.9600	0.8991	0.9504
SP	28.2054	34.3616	32.4811	34.1929	0.7901	0.9610	0.8621	0.9490

3 Results

In the following, $f_{(i)}$ $(i = 1, 2, 3)$ represents the initial reconstructions of the ground truth image $f_\star$ obtained via (3)–(5). The networks (6)–(8) are then applied to these reconstructions, resulting in $f_{(i)}^{\mathrm{RS}}$, $f_{(i)}^{\mathrm{NS}}$, and $f_{(i)}^{\mathrm{DP}}$. Fig. 1 and 2 show reconstructions for randomly selected examples from the synthetic and LoDoPaB datasets, where all examples were chosen outside the training data. In Fig. 1, LS fails to remove noise, while the NS network struggles due to its limitation to modifying the null space $\mathcal{N}(\mathbf{A}_I)$, leaving noise in the orthogonal complement $\mathcal{N}(\mathbf{A}_I)^\perp$. SP and TV reduce noise and limited-view artifacts but introduce new characteristic Gibbs-type artifacts, which remain present even after applying the NS network. In contrast, RS and DP architectures effectively

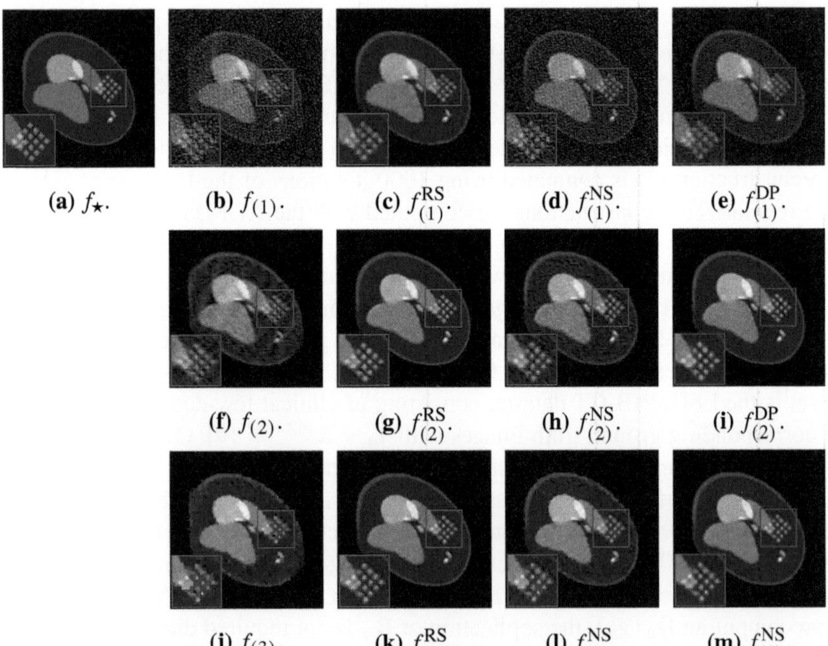

(a) $f_\star$. **(b)** $f_{(1)}$. **(c)** $f_{(1)}^{\mathrm{RS}}$. **(d)** $f_{(1)}^{\mathrm{NS}}$. **(e)** $f_{(1)}^{\mathrm{DP}}$.

(f) $f_{(2)}$. **(g)** $f_{(2)}^{\mathrm{RS}}$. **(h)** $f_{(2)}^{\mathrm{NS}}$. **(i)** $f_{(2)}^{\mathrm{DP}}$.

(j) $f_{(3)}$. **(k)** $f_{(3)}^{\mathrm{RS}}$. **(l)** $f_{(3)}^{\mathrm{NS}}$. **(m)** $f_{(3)}^{\mathrm{NS}}$.

Fig. 1. Reconstruction results for a random example from the Shepp-Logan phantom class.

Tab. 2. Average ℓ^2 reconstruction errors in the Radon domain for the Shepp-Logan like phantom class (as in Fig. 1), indicating data proximity for each reconstruction method.

	$\|\mathbf{A}_I f - g\|$	$\|\mathbf{A}_I (f - f_\star)\|$	$\|\mathbf{A}_I^c (f - f_\star)\|$
$f_{(1)}$	1.0283	0.2723	0.4889
$f_{(2)}$	0.6934	0.0377	0.2453
$f_{(3)}$	0.7278	0.0385	0.1259
$f_{(1)}^{\mathrm{NS}}$	1.0110	0.2549	0.0277
$f_{(2)}^{\mathrm{NS}}$	0.6937	0.0362	0.0142
$f_{(3)}^{\mathrm{NS}}$	0.7257	0.0350	0.0148

	$\|\mathbf{A}_I f - g\|$	$\|\mathbf{A}_I (f - f_\star)\|$	$\|\mathbf{A}_I^c (f - f_\star)\|$
$f_{(1)}^{\mathrm{RS}}$	0.7933	0.0371	0.0396
$f_{(2)}^{\mathrm{RS}}$	0.7547	0.0220	0.0179
$f_{(3)}^{\mathrm{RS}}$	0.7566	0.0223	0.0192
$f_{(1)}^{\mathrm{DP}}$	0.8256	0.0694	0.0577
$f_{(2)}^{\mathrm{DP}}$	0.7543	0.0204	0.0160
$f_{(3)}^{\mathrm{DP}}$	0.7520	0.0197	0.0154

remove these artifacts, delivering visually superior reconstructions. Notably, $f_{(2)}^{\mathrm{RS}}$, $f_{(2)}^{\mathrm{DP}}$, $f_{(3)}^{\mathrm{RS}}$, and $f_{(3)}^{\mathrm{DP}}$ show no significant visual differences. Similar observations can be made for the LoDoPaB example.

Our visual findings match the quantitative results in Tab. 1, which shows average reconstruction errors. To assess data consistency, Tab. 2 compares the differences between the Radon transforms of the reconstructions and the ground truth $f_\star$. By the Fourier slice theorem, this is in one-to-one correspondence with the parts in the null space of $\mathbf{A}_I$ and its orthogonal complement. These results confirm our previous findings.

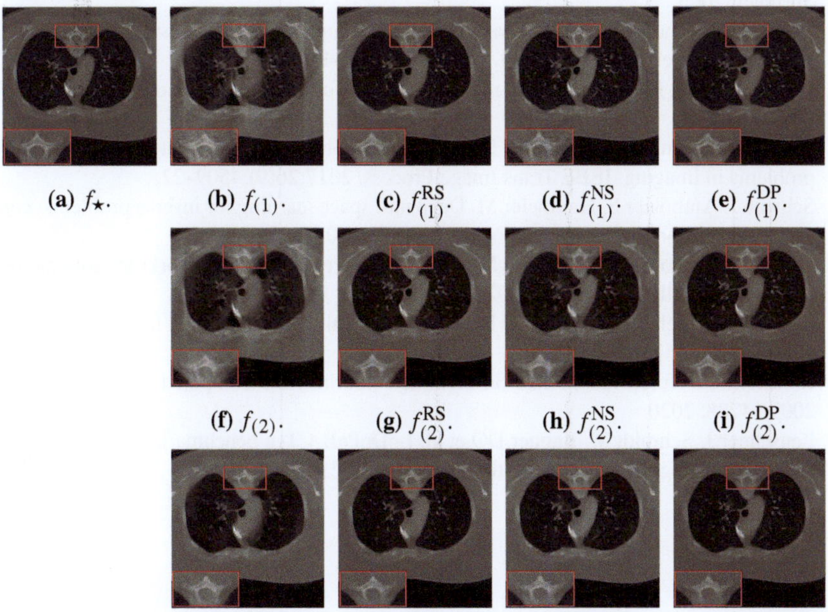

(a) $f_\star$. (b) $f_{(1)}$. (c) $f_{(1)}^{\mathrm{RS}}$. (d) $f_{(1)}^{\mathrm{NS}}$. (e) $f_{(1)}^{\mathrm{DP}}$.

(f) $f_{(2)}$. (g) $f_{(2)}^{\mathrm{RS}}$. (h) $f_{(2)}^{\mathrm{NS}}$. (i) $f_{(2)}^{\mathrm{DP}}$.

(j) $f_{(3)}$. (k) $f_{(3)}^{\mathrm{RS}}$. (l) $f_{(3)}^{\mathrm{NS}}$. (m) $f_{(3)}^{\mathrm{DP}}$.

Fig. 2. Results for a random example from the LoDoPaB-CT data set.

4 Discussion

In this paper, we introduced data-proximal (DP) networks for limited-view CT. Standard residual (RS) networks update both the range and null space components but lack data consistency. Null space (NS) networks, introduced in [5], effectively handle the null space but cannot correct the range component, resulting in insufficient denoising performance. DP networks combine the strengths of both approaches, ensuring data consistency while providing accurate reconstructions. They match the performance of RS networks and offer theoretical guarantees, making them a promising and reliable method for use in medical imaging. Future work includes investigating scenarios where RS networks hallucinate range components, examining how parameters (e.g., β) affect DP performance, exploring alternative architectures, and assessing robustness under varying noise levels or sparse data.

Both DP and NS networks are designed to avoid hallucinations and they come with mathematical guarantees, ensuring reliability in practice. However, they require data-proximal initial reconstruction. Since FBP reconstructions from limited-view data have unbounded support, truncation to the region of interest (ROI) is required, which compromises data consistency – an aspect not widely discussed in the literature.

References

1. Scherzer O, Grasmair M, Grossauer H et al. Variational methods in imaging. New York: Springer, 2009.
2. Antholzer S, Haltmeier M, Schwab J. Deep learning for photoacoustic tomography from sparse data. Inverse Probl Sci Eng. 2019;27(7):987–1005.
3. He K, Zhang X, Ren S et al. Deep residual learning for image recognition. Proc IEEE CVPR. 2016:770–8.
4. Jin KH, McCann MT, Froustey E et al. Deep convolutional neural network for inverse problems in imaging. IEEE Trans Image Process. 2017;26(9):4509–22.
5. Schwab J, Antholzer S, Haltmeier M. Deep null space learning for inverse problems: convergence analysis and rates. Inverse Probl. 2019;35(2):025008.
6. Schwab J, Antholzer S, Haltmeier M. Big in Japan: regularizing networks for solving inverse problems. J Math Imaging Vis. 2020;62(3):445–55.
7. Göppel S, Frikel J, Haltmeier M. Data-proximal null-space networks for inverse problems. arXiv: 2309.06573. 2023.
8. Ronchetti M. TorchRadon: fast differentiable routines for computed tomography. arXiv: 2009.14788. 2020.
9. Leuschner J, Schmidt M, Baguer DO et al. LoDoPaB-CT, a benchmark dataset for low-dose computed tomography reconstruction. Sci Data. 2021;8(1):109.

Towards Robust Zero-shot Chest X-ray Classification
Exploring Data Distribution Bias in Chest X-ray Datasets

Sheethal Bhat[1,2], Adarsh Bhandary Panambur[1], Awais Mansoor[3], Bogdan Georgescu[3], Sasa Grbic[3], Andreas Maier[1],

[1]Fakultät für Pattern Recognition, FAU Erlangen-Nürnberg
[2]Digital Technology and Innovation, Siemens Healthineers, Erlangen
[3]Digital Technology and Innovation, Siemens Healthineers, USA
sheethal.bhat@fau.de

Abstract. In recent years, unsupervised classification models have become increasingly significant, primarily due to the difficulties associated with data labeling and its costs. This trend is also notable in the field of medical imaging, particularly with chest X-rays (CXRs). Among the various unsupervised pretraining methodologies, image-text models like CLIP are highlighted for their considerable enhancements in zero-shot classification. In this study, we perform a detailed analysis of CLIP's performance using multiple large CXR datasets, investigating how the batch size, dataset size, and distribution biases differentially influence outcomes across various findings. In two distinct experiments, we show an average of 3% enhancement in the macro average zero-shot AUC scores when the batch size is increased, and a corresponding 8% improvement for pneumothorax by the addition of a second dataset. For pleural effusion, where performance is nearly saturated and previous changes had little effect, we examine adding weak supervisory meta-labels and image-to-image contrastive loss, achieving an average 1% improvement in zero-shot AUC. Consequently, our work shows incorporating dataset insights, meta-information and contrastive learning strategies enhances the robustness and accuracy of CLIP-CXR for specific findings.

1 Introduction

The high cost and expertise required for annotating medical images, particularly chest X-Rays (CXRs), make unsupervised pretraining methods like DINO [1] and MoCo [2] invaluable. Among these, a contrastive image-text pretraining method called CLIP [3], offers the additional advantage of zero-shot capabilities, as model exposure to class names during pretraining can reduce the need for additional finetuning. However, the most commonly used large-scale CXR image-text dataset, MIMIC-CXR [4], faces challenges, including significant class imbalance and a high negative-to-positive label ratio, especially for critical findings such as pneumothorax (ptx). Furthermore, large interobserver variability and non-standardized terminology lead to inconsistent reporting. For instance, terms like "lesions" and "nodules" are used interchangeably in reports, compounding the uncertainty in model predictions.

Several studies [5–9] have applied CLIP [3] to CXR datasets [4]. In Ekin et al. [5], only frontal views were considered, and a text encoder with knowledge distillation was included to demonstrate high zero-shot classification in multiple categories of the

C. Palm et al. (Hrsg.), *Bildverarbeitung für die Medizin 2025*, Informatik aktuell,
https://doi.org/10.1007/978-3-658-47422-5_42

CheXPert dataset [10]. On the other hand, Wu et al. [6], used RadGraphs [11] for weak supervision of class labels and locations, thereby improving the zero-shot AUC score by 1.5-2% across various findings in multiple datasets. The RadGraphs provided additional meta information as weak supervision to the pretraining models. Similarly, various image-text pretraining methods [7–9] focus on enhancing the textual context, such as through additional medical literature such as medical Twitter [9] or specific anatomy and disease notebooks [6].

Most CLIP [3] evaluations in CXR focus on a few key findings or aggregate dataset-level metrics [6–9]. This may not lead to a complete understanding of the model's limitations across diverse findings. Another key limitation of CLIP [3] in CXRs is its reliance solely on image-text correlations, without an image-to-image contrastive loss. In the medical context, humans naturally learn by contrasting images alongside correlating images with external cues, enabling a more robust understanding of visual distinctions. Integrating these mechanisms could enhance the model's ability to distinguish subtle differences in medical images, leading to improved diagnostic performance.

The main contributions of our research are as follows, 1) We assess how batch sizes and CXR views impact CLIP-CXR's zero-shot classification across multiple findings, showcasing its scalability; 2) We explore the effects of data distribution biases with respect to varying dataset sizes, revealing 1-8% improvement in classification results in two specific scenarios with different class representations; 3) We conduct preliminary experiments incorporating meta-label information and SimCLR-based image-to-image contrastive loss (SLIP) [12], resulting in a 1% improvement in zero-shot classification accuracy for specific finding.

2 Materials and methods

The MIMIC-CXR [4] pretraining dataset is a large and publicly available collection of 350,000 de-identified chest radiographs, of 65,000 plus patients along with their corresponding radiograph text reports. Each image is associated with rich clinical metadata, including patient demographics, radiographic findings, and relevant clinical notes. The Zwanger-Pesiri dataset from Zwanger-Pesiri Radiology, LLP. [13], an outpatient imaging center with multiple locations in United States, is additionally used for pretraining. The dataset includes 250,000 frontal and lateral images from multiple vendors along with clinical report, and comprises patients 18 years or older. CheXpert [10] includes 224,316 chest radiographs of 65,240 patients with both frontal and lateral views. A random subset of non-overlapping 2000 images is taken as the validation dataset.

ChestX-ray14[1] (CXR14) consists of 112,120 frontal-view X-ray images from 30,805 individual patients. It features fourteen common disease labels extracted through natural language processing (NLP) techniques from clinical text reports. Two distinct random and non-overlapping subsets of 2000 images are taken as test and validation datasets. Additionally, an internal dataset of 16,000 images are acquired from multiple sites in the United States and Europe. The overall study includes frontal and lateral chest exams from adult cohorts. Two general radiologists independently reviewed all CXRs for 16 findings, with a third radiologist resolving any discrepancies. A test dataset with binary

[1]https://www.kaggle.com/datasets/nih-chest-xrays/data

Text prompt	MIMIC-CXR (Pos labels)	Zwanger-Pesiri
Pleural effusion	207,139 (53,188)	13,476
Pneumothorax	220,778 (9,317)	10,676
Cardiomegaly	45,147 (39,094)	7,258
Aorta enlargement	5	0
Aorta	27,781	31,442
Pleural thickening	5,169	3,201

Tab. 1. The case insensitive word count of some findings in MIMIC-CXR and Zwanger-Pesiri datasets with the number of positive findings in brackets (where available).

labels is created for ptx $\mathcal{A}$ (412 images, 154 positive samples) and pleural effusion $\mathcal{B}$ (331 images, 74 positive samples).

The associated CXR-reports from both pretraining datasets are minimally processed to extract mainly the impressions and findings sections. Redundant sentences and filler words are removed to shorten the text length, and the remaining section of the report is ignored at the moment. Tab. 1 shows the word count of the key findings in the processed text report for each dataset. As CLIP [3] requires significant prompt engineering, the Tab. 1 indicates how the diversity of clinical reports could negatively impact correlation results. For example, the word count of "aorta" v.s. "aorta enlargement" illustrates the potential impact in correlation results. We find the model assigns higher probability scores to phrases that appear frequently and consistently in reports, compared to those with more variation. Secondly, the number of positive findings included in brackets demonstrates the small negative to positive sample ratio for certain findings like ptx. Following the methodology in CLIP [3], the model is pretrained both with and without the lateral images, utilizing different batch sizes, and is assessed on the evaluation datasets without additional finetuning. The corresponding class name of interest is provided as a *text prompt* to evaluate the classification score [14]. The best checkpoint of each independent run is selected based on the step resulting in the highest validation AUC score. To improve the generalizability of the model, the validation dataset includes a subset of images in all categories in CXR-14 and ChexPert [10].

To further boost the model performance, two additional experiments are conducted. First, a meta label file is created for pleural effusion which is extracted from the CXR clinical reports in MIMIC-CXR [4]. This is used as a weak supervision label in addition to the contrastive image-text loss. Secondly, we include an additional image-to-image contrastive loss SLIP [12] during pre-training and verify the performance for a single finding "pleural effusion".

3 Results and discussion

The experiments were performed on a single node with eight V100-SXM2-16GB GPUs, employing a batch size of 32 or 64 in conjunction with a ViT-B/32 architecture. Pretraining used an initial learning rate of 0.0001, with evaluations performed without finetuning. Data pre-processing included only image normalization; no augmentations were used. Average results of multiple runs are reported.

Fig. 1 indicates the mean and standard deviation of the zero-shot AUC classification score of the top 5 checkpoints for the categories in the CXR-14 dataset. Blue values are from study [5], orange values show model performance with frontal and lateral

MIMIC-CXR [4] images. Green bars (batch size 32) and red bars (batch size 64) are scores using only frontal views from MIMIC-CXR [4].

From the plot, it is observed that in some findings such as ptx, consolidation and pleural thickening there is a performance gain achieved by including both the frontal and lateral views. This is attributed to the data distribution; for example, ptx has only 9,300 positive samples in MIMIC with more than 220,000 mentions in the reports. The inclusion of both views provides a greater number of images for learning. However, in many cases, the increased standard deviation when using both frontal and lateral views suggests greater performance instability. This is especially noticeable in findings such as Edema, Hernia and Pleural thickening. The observed increase in performance variance can be attributed to the challenges associated with accurately identifying the finding in the lateral views, leading to a loss of accuracy.

Moreover, when using only frontal views, the macro average performance improves by 3% as the batch size is increased from 32 to 64. This is anticipated, given that CLIP [3] employs a contrastive learning loss that relies on the choice of contrasting samples contained in a batch. Finally, findings such as pleural thickening show baseline AUC scores below 50%, indicating very poor model performance and the failure to learn this phrase from the clinical reports.

The classification performance across various findings correlate to the number of positive samples in the pretraining dataset. To further understand the impact of the data distribution, we investigate the zero-shot AUC score as a function of dataset size for ptx and pleural effusion as illustrated in Fig. 2. These two findings are selected based on the class distribution involving negative to positive sample ratio of MIMIC-CXR as seen in Tab. 1. In this experiment we pretrain using both the MIMIC-CXR [4] and Zwanger-Pesiri dataset.

The imbalance of positive samples within MIMIC-CXR [4] results in performance instability when using a smaller subset of MIMIC-CXR [4] dataset for pretraining as seen in Fig. 2. In the case of ptx in Fig. 2a, incorporating the second dataset leads to a significant 8% rise in the AUC score. In contrast, as seen in Fig. 2b conducting the same experiment with pleural effusion yields only a 1% enhancement, indicating the model is already near saturation for this finding.

As the performance for pleural effusion does not benefit much from increasing batch size or dataset size, we explore additional loss functions to boost classification. Tab. 2

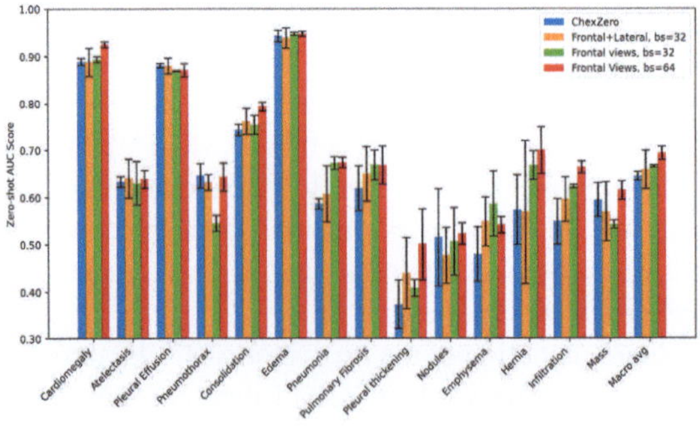

Fig. 1. Comparison of mean zero-shot AUC classification scores across various findings in the CXR-14 dataset. Baseline in blue is from ChexZero [5]. bs is the batch size.

Method	*Zero-shot AUC Score*
Baseline	95.16 ± 0.003
Baseline + Meta Label info	96.48 ± 0.004
Baseline + SLIP [12] Loss	96.70 ± 0.003

Tab. 2. Comparison of average pleural effusion AUC scores with std dev for different methods on dataset $\mathcal{B}$ when pretraining only with MIMIC-CXR [4].

denotes the performance improvement for pleural effusion when adding the image-to-image contrastive loss SLIP [12] to the baseline CLIP [3] implementation using MIMIC-CXR. In addition, a separate experiment adding the weak supervision from the meta labels shows a similar performance gain, showcasing the potential for improvement for all the findings in the dataset.

4 Conclusion

Recent studies suggest that DINOv2 [15] outperforms CLIP [5] in chest X-rays (CXRs), yet CLIP-CXR remains a strong option for zero-shot classification, benefiting from the easy availability of clinical text reports paired with images. Performance analyses conducted in our work indicate that improvements can be achieved by increasing batch size, standardizing clinical reports, extracting weakly supervised meta-class labels, and expanding dataset size. Moreover, current experiments use the ViT-B/32 model, which may limit the learning of small findings due to downsampling to CLIP's standard 224x224 resolution. These improvements can optimize a computer-aided diagnostic system for high classification accuracy without label-specific finetuning, enabling scalable models using large CXR datasets. Future work will explore higher model capacities, with increased image resolution and a more capable text encoder, to enable such a system.

Acknowledgement. This study is funded by Siemens-Healthineers.

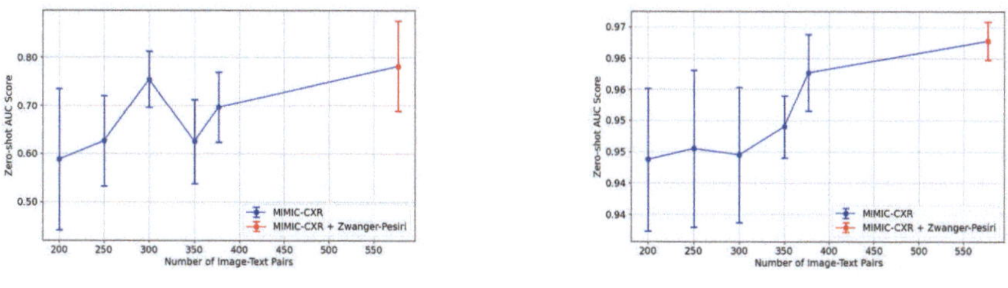

(**a**) Pneumothorax test set $\mathcal{A}$

(**b**) Pleural effusion test set $\mathcal{B}$

Fig. 2. Mean zero-shot AUC classification performance vs. size of dataset. Impact of additional dataset shown in red. Scores for subset of MIMIC-CXR [4] indicate higher standard deviation denoting unstable results.

References

1. Oquab M, Darcet T, Moutakanni T et al. DINOv2: learning robust visual features without supervision. arXiv: 2304.07193. 2023.
2. Sowrirajan H, Yang J, Ng AY et al. MoCo pretraining improves representation and transferability of chest X-ray models. Proc MIDL. 2021:728–44.
3. Radford A, Kim JW, Hallacy C et al. Learning transferable visual models from natural language supervision. Proc ICML. 2021:8748–63.
4. Johnson AE, Pollard TJ, Berkowitz SJ et al. MIMIC-CXR: a de-identified publicly available database of chest radiographs with free-text reports. Sci Data. 2019;6(1):317.
5. Tiu E, Talius E, Patel P et al. Expert-level detection of pathologies from unannotated chest X-ray images via self-supervised learning. Nat Biomed Eng. 2022;6(12):1399–406.
6. Wu C, Zhang X, Zhang Y et al. MedKLIP: medical knowledge enhanced language-image pre-training. Proc IEEE CVF ICCV. 2023.
7. Kim C, Gadgil SU, DeGrave AJ et al. Fostering transparent medical image AI via an image-text foundation model grounded in medical literature. Nat Med. 2024;30(4):1154–65.
8. Zhang Y, Jiang H, Miura Y et al. Contrastive learning of medical visual representations from paired images and text. Proc MLHC. 2022;182:2–25.
9. Huang Z, Bianchi F, Yuksekgonul M et al. A visual-language foundation model for pathology image analysis using medical Twitter. Nat Med. 2023;29:2307–16.
10. Irvin J, Rajpurkar P, Ko M et al. CheXpert: a large chest radiograph dataset with uncertainty labels and expert comparison. Proc AAAI. 2019;33(1):590–7.
11. Jain S, Agrawal A, Saporta A et al. RadGraph: extracting clinical entities and relations from radiology reports. arXiv: 2106.14463. 2021.
12. Mu N, Kirillov A, Wagner D et al. SLIP: self-supervision meets language-image pre-training. Proc ECCV. 2022:529–44.
13. Mansoor A, Schmuecking I, Ghesu FC et al. Large-scale study on AI's impact on identifying chest radiographs with no actionable disease in outpatient imaging. Acad Radiol. 2024;31(12):5300–13.
14. Rajpurkar Lab. CheXzero: zero-shot chest X-ray classification. `https://github.com/rajpurkarlab/CheXzero`. Accessed: 2024-10-28. 2023.
15. Bensaid R, Gripon V, Leduc-Primeau F et al. A novel benchmark for few-shot semantic segmentation in the era of foundation models. arXiv: 2401.11311. 2024.

Precision ICU Resource Planning
A Multimodal Model for Brain Surgery Outcomes

Maximilian Fischer[†1,2,3], Florian M. Hauptmann[†1], Robin Peretzke[†1,2], Paul Naser[4,5], Peter Neher[1,6,7], Jan-Oliver Neumann[‡4], Klaus Maier-Hein[‡1,2,6,7]

[1]Medical Image Computing Group, Deutsches Krebsforschungszentrum (DKFZ), Heidelberg
[2]Medical Faculty Heidelberg, Heidelberg University, Heidelberg
[3]Research Campus M^{2}OLIE, Mannheim, Germany
[4]Department of Neurosurgery, Medical Faculty Heidelberg, Heidelberg University, Germany
[5]AI Health Innovation Cluster, German Cancer Research Center (DKFZ), Heidelberg, Germany
[6]German Cancer Consortium (DKTK), partner site Heidelberg
[7]Pattern Analysis and Learning Group, Heidelberg University, Heidelberg
robin.peretzke@dkfz-heidelberg.de

Abstract. Although advances in brain surgery techniques have led to fewer post-operative complications requiring intensive care unit (ICU) monitoring, the routine transfer of patients to the ICU remains the clinical standard, despite its high cost. Predictive Gradient Boosted Trees based on clinical data have attempted to optimize ICU admission by identifying key risk factors pre-operatively; however, these approaches overlook valuable imaging data that could enhance prediction accuracy. In this work, we show that multimodal approaches that combine clinical data with imaging data outperform the current clinical data only baseline from 0.29 [F1] to 0.30 [F1], when only pre-operative clinical data is used and from 0.37 [F1] to 0.41 [F1], for pre- and post-operative data. This study demonstrates that effective ICU admission prediction benefits from multimodal data fusion, especially in contexts of severe class imbalance.

1 Introduction

Advanced neurosurgical techniques have significantly reduced the incidence of post-operative complications that require intensive care unit (ICU) admission, even among elderly patients [1]. Despite these advancements, many medical institutions still routinely transfer patients to the ICU following brain surgeries for the highest medical attention, even though ICU care is much more expensive [2]. Recent studies have challenged this practice in postoperative care, prompting a reevaluation of its necessity [3, 4].

A challenge in the field is the small number of patients who truly require ICU transfer, leading to few true positive cases in cohorts. Consequently, the class that demands the highest predictive accuracy is most impacted by the limited data available. The approach presented in [4] addresses this issue with a gradient-boosted tree (GBT) trained on clinical data and demonstrates better prognostic pattern recognition than traditional uni- or multivariate logistic regression. However, a limitation of previous approaches is its reliance solely on clinical data, overlooking valuable imaging information.

[†]These authors contributed equally the most to this work.
[‡]These authors contributed equally the least to this work.

C. Palm et al. (Hrsg.), *Bildverarbeitung für die Medizin 2025*, Informatik aktuell,
https://doi.org/10.1007/978-3-658-47422-5_43

In this work, we enhance this predictive model by incorporating T1 MRI imaging data alongside clinical data, aiming to improve accuracy in ICU admission predictions, which has already been proven effective in other applications, such as Alzheimer's disease prediction [5]. Furthermore, we especially focus on the evaluation of the model performances for true positive ICU subjects, which is of utmost importance.

Our study involves different architectures and approaches to fuse tabular information with imaging data. As baseline, we consider the same GBT approach as [4] and we use autoencoders (AE) to incorporate imaging data to generate latents from the input images.

In our work, we show that plane fusion of tabular and imaging data does not automatically lead to improved classification performances, even for deeper ResNet models than GBTs. For improved fusion of multimodal data for ICU admission prediction, dynamic fusion strategies, such as [5] are required. Combined with a brain foundation model as an image feature extractor, we observe promising results compared to existing GBT approaches and outperformed ResNet-based approaches.

To the best of our knowledge, this is the first approach to integrate multimodal data for predicting ICU admission in postoperative neurosurgical care.

2 Dataset

For our experiments, we used the same cohort presented in [4]. All subjects underwent brain surgery at the University Hospital Heidelberg, with various clinical parameters available, including demographic information and pre- and post-operative clinical data. Subject labels were assigned based on post-operative information, depending on whether one or more of nine events requiring ICU admission occurred post-surgery: CPR, re-intubation, return to the operation room, mechanical ventilation, vasopressor use, impaired consciousness, intracranial hypertension, swallowing disorders, or death. An overview of the available clinical information is provided in [4].

In contrast to [4], we additionally incorporated imaging data, aiming to improve predictive accuracy. Since T1 scans were not available for all subjects that were used in [4], our cohort was reduced to 611 subjects. For the remaining subjects, we created a segmentation mask of the tumor by using a pretrained nnU-Net [6]. Within the dataset, a significant class imbalance was observed, with 552 ICU-negative and 59 ICU-positive labels, offering insights into the extent of potentially unnecessary ICU resource allocation. Fig. 1 displays a random subject with a tumor, alongside example distributions from the tabular data of the cohort both before and after surgery.

3 Materials and methods

In this work, we employed multiple architectures to improve prediction accuracy. The used models can be distinguished into feature extraction and classification models.

Feature extraction is a key method for aligning or reducing data dimensionality across domains. Here, we use AEs to derive compact representations from the image domain. These encoder-decoder models are pretrained on an image reconstruction task, compressing high-dimensional data into a lower-dimensional latent space that retains essential features while reducing overall dimensionality.

Extreme gradient boosting is a decision-tree-based machine learning technique that efficiently processes 2D structured or tabular data. In [4], this approach was applied to predict ICU admissions using clinical data. In our work, we extend this method by incorporating imaging based latents alongside the clinical data.

In contrast to XGBoost models, Residual Neural Networks are deep learning (dl) architectures with residual connections to facilitate the training of very deep networks. These connections enable efficient capturing of complex patterns. For our experiments, we use this model architecture as a more advanced approach than XGBoost.

Along with introducing more advanced dl architectures, we hypothesize, that plane combinations of clinical and imaging data might not be sufficient for improved ICU-admission prediction. Thus we considered the dynamic affine feature map transform (DAFT) [5], which enables the dynamic scaling and shifting of feature maps in a dl model, depending on the clinical data of a subject. This improved fusion of 3D imaging data with tabular clinical data has shown great results in predicting the outcome of Alzheimer's disease.

4 Experiments

This section provides an overview of the conducted experiments, divided into two parts: (i) feature extraction from T1-scans and (ii) the ultimate classification task. Each feature extractor was trained using five-fold cross-validation, generating latents only for the data in its respective validation fold. For the classification experiments, data splits were further stratified by label and tumor volume, and for the classification training suitable sampling strategies, such as undersampling, were applied to address the severe class imbalance in the data. A threshold of 0.5 was used to assign labels based on predicted probabilities. Evaluation metrics included F1-score and ROC-AUC, both of which are well-suited for capturing the effects of class imbalance.

For feature extraction, we implemented two approaches. First, we generated latent representations using our own pretrained 2D AE. Second, we leveraged a publicly available large-scale pretrained 3D model (SSL) [7]. Both models were trained on image reconstruction tasks. The 2D AE was trained on our dataset using the ADAM optimizer with a learning rate of $1e^{-2}$, a batch size of 16, over 50 epochs. For the

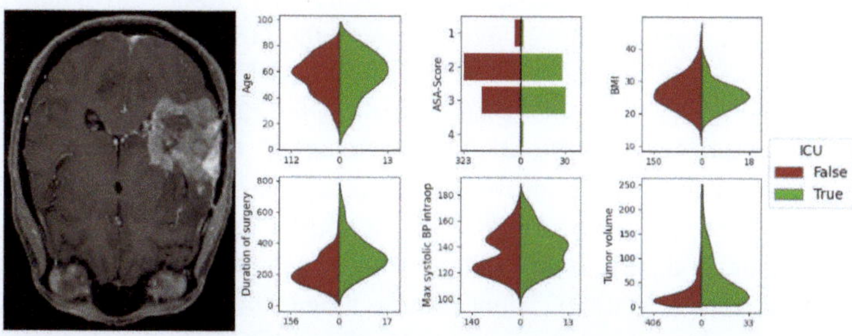

Fig. 1. Left: Brain slice of a random subject of the cohort. Right: Overview of six tabular feature distributions.

downstream task, we extracted latent representations from one axial slice of the T1 scan per subject showing the largest tumor diameter based on the segmentation mask, resulting in dimensions of $(128 \times 16 \times 16)$.

For the 3D approach, we used the pretrained model from [7], where the authors trained a masked AE on 44,000 multicenter images on different MRI modalities. This 3D model was fine-tuned during five fold CV on our data with a learning rate of $1e^{-5}$ over 15 epochs. For the classification task, we extracted latents from a 3D region of interest (ROI) centered on the tumor, defined by each subject's tumor segmentation mask. This ROI, sized at 160 mm^3 with dimensions ($320 \times 5 \times 5 \times 5$), was used to capture relevant latent features based on the T1 scan around the tumor. For clarity, we refer to the latents from the 2D AE as 2D latents and from the 3D AE as 3D latents.

For the GBT model, we conducted experiments using three different input scenarios: (i) solely on tabular data, (ii) solely on latents from the 2D images, and (iii) the concatenated tabular and flattened latent data from the 2D image. For all three scenarios, we used the same hyperparameters as [5].

The ResNet18-Classifier[1] experiments followed a similar structure, utilizing the same three input scenarios: tabular data alone, latent data alone, and a combination of both. For all scenarios, the data was shaped into a 2D array, using zero-padding. For all ResNet experiments, we trained 500 epochs using the ADAM optimizer with a learning rate of $1e^{-2}$ and a batch size of 32.

Since the DAFT model is specifically designed for multimodal purposes, we limited these experiments to combining clinical and imaging data. In our DAFT experiments, we integrated clinical tabular data with three types of latents: the 2D latents, where we stacked the same latent 16 times to meet DAFT's dimensionality requirements; the latents generated by DAFT's integrated 3D encoder; and 3D SSL latents. For all DAFT experiments, we used the ADAM optimizer with a learning rate of $1e^{-3}$ and a batch size of 16, training each DAFT model until convergence. The 2D model converged after 100 epochs, while the 3D model converged after 25 epochs, as the batchgenerators [8]framework was applied in the 3D scenario.

5 Results

The models incorporate both pre- and postoperative data demonstrated a consistent trend towards better performance compared to those using only pre-operative data across all pure tabular data scenarios (Fig. 2). For instance, the GBT model, when using only tabular data, achieved an F1-score of 0.37 and a ROC-AUC of 0.77. However, when the GBT model relied exclusively on 2D latent features for classification, its performance dropped, with an F1-score of 0.08 and a ROC-AUC of 0.5. Combining tabular data with 2D latent features also did not improve the model's performance over the tabular-only setup, yielding a lower F1-score of 0.28 and a ROC-AUC of 0.71.

With only tabular data it was similar for the ResNet: a F1-score of 0.37 and a lower ROC-AUC of 0.75. With 2D latent features alone, however, the ResNet classifier's performance declined, reaching an F1-score of 0.18 and a ROC-AUC of 0.53. Combining

[1] https://pytorch.org/vision/main/models

tabular data with 2D latents led to further reductions, with an F1-score of 0.18 and a ROC-AUC of 0.66, performing even worse than the GBT under the same conditions.

In contrast, the DAFT model demonstrated the most potential for integrating tabular and imaging data. Using only 2D latents, DAFT achieved an F1-score of 0.35 and a ROC-AUC of 0.74, outperforming prior attempts at combining data types, though still slightly trailing the GBT trained solely on tabular data. When using a complete 3D ROI as input, the DAFT model maintained an F1-score of 0.35 but improved its ROC-AUC to 0.77. Finally, employing 3D latents from the pretrained SSL model yielded the best performance, achieving an F1-score of 0.41 and a ROC-AUC of 0.76.

6 Discussion

In our experiments, we progressively applied increasingly complex dl approaches to the problem of ICU admission prediction. Initially, we applied a GBT model trained on clinical data which, despite its outdated architecture, remains the most performant method currently published for this problem. In addition to clinical data, we have gradually integrated imaging data into the cohort, starting with 2D slices and extending to 3D volumes. To push the boundaries further, we applied a more contemporary architecture, ResNet, to leverage a deeper model with more parameters to extract richer correlations between the imaging and tabular data. However, without specific fusion techniques designed to effectively combine imaging and tabular data, this approach was limited due to the dimensionality differences between the two data domains.

The most promising approach, as revealed by our experiments, is the DAFT architecture. DAFT, with its specialized DAFT block, is specifically designed to fuse high-dimensional image data with low-dimensional tabular data (in our case, clinical data). Like other studies, our work was limited by the sparse availability of true positive ICU subjects. This is the main reason for generally low F1 scores across all methods. However, we were able to further enhance the performance by using a brain foundation model as feature extractor (see DAFT 3D ROI vs. 3D SSL latent).

Another challenge for our work and other multimodal approaches, was the fusion of different domains. In our case, the tabular clinical data was tremendously smaller

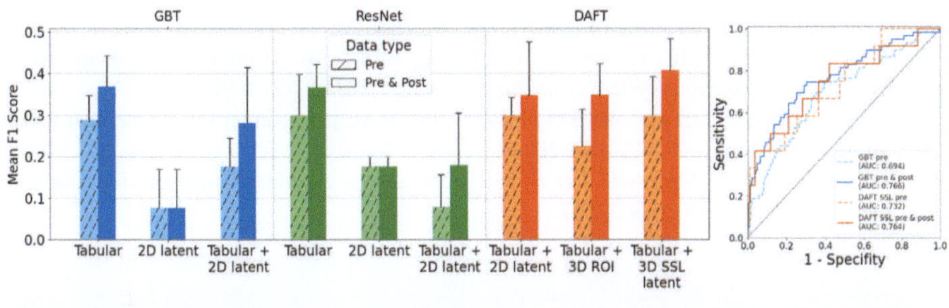

Fig. 2. Left: F1-scores of different scenarios. The bar in the lighter color and dashed lines present the performance when only pre-operative data is used. Right: ROC-AUC curve of the GBT-baseline and our best performing method for only pre- and for pre- and post-operative data.

than the imaging data, even after feature extraction. For problems where prognostic markers for classification are present in smaller tabular data (see GBT on tabular data), it is important that these features are not lost in noise after being combined with image information. To solve this problem, we have combined two approaches: (i) the DAFT model which is capable of maintaining attention on low dimensional tabular data (ii) reducing noise in the image latents by using a foundation model as feature extractor.

Our work was task-driven, aiming towards an improved ICU-admission scheme, especially for those patients that require ICU treatment. We have thus decided against exhaustive ablations, such as general 2D vs. 3D scenarios in our model development. In the future, we are planning to consider further experiments with 3D latents and ResNet models, other fusion strategies, and introducing more modalities such as different acquisition sequences to further improve the performance. Additionally, it is crucial to consider weighting strategies that prioritize accurately identifying true ICU patients. While misclassifying non-ICU patients as needing ICU admission may result in unnecessary resource allocation, the reverse—failing to identify patients who truly require ICU care—poses a serious risk to patient safety and could lead to fatal outcomes.

In conclusion, our experiments show that ICU-admission prediction is not a task that can be solved solely based on a single modality. However, combining different modalities can help to improve the classification performance. Moreover, large pretrained models as feature extractors are beneficial especially for heavy class imbalanced cohorts. Insights from this work can streamline future experiments to achieve clinical relevant results.

References

1. Schär RT, Tashi S, Branca M et al. How safe are elective craniotomies in elderly patients in neurosurgery today? A prospective cohort study of 1452 consecutive cases. J Neurosurg. 2021;134(4):1113–21.
2. Costa DK, Moss M. The cost of caring: emotion, burnout, and psychological distress in critical care clinicians. Ann Am Thorac Soc. 2018;15(7):787–90.
3. Beauregard CL, Friedman WA. Routine use of postoperative ICU care for elective craniotomy: a cost-benefit analysis. Surg Neurol. 2003;60(6):483–9.
4. Neumann JO, Schmidt S, Nohman A et al. Routine ICU surveillance after brain tumor surgery: patient selection using machine learning. J Clin Med. 2024;13(19).
5. Pölsterl S, Wolf TN, Wachinger C. Combining 3D image and tabular data via the dynamic affine feature map transform. Proc MICCAI. 2021:688–98.
6. Naser PV, Maurer MC, Fischer M et al. Deep learning aided preoperative diagnosis of primary central nervous system lymphoma. iScience. 2024;27(2):109023.
7. Wald T, Ulrich C, Lukyanenko S et al. Revisiting MAE pre-training for 3D medical image segmentation. arXiv: 2410.23132. 2024.
8. Isensee F, Jäger P, Wasserthal J et al. batchgenerators – a python framework for data augmentation. Zenodo. 2020;3632567.

Systematic Analysis of Input Modalities for Fracture Classification of the Paediatric Wrist

Ron Keuth[1], Maren Balks[2], Sebastian Tschauner[3], Ludger Tüshaus[4], Mattias Heinrich[1]

[1]Institute of Medical Informatics, University of Lübeck
[2]Institut of Radiology and Nuclear Medicine, University Hospital Schleswig-Holstein
[3]Paediatric Radiology, Medical University of Graz
[4]Paediatric Surgery, University Hospital Schleswig-Holstein
r.keuth@uni-luebeck.de

Abstract. Fractures, particularly in the distal forearm, are among the most common injuries in children and adolescents, with approximately 800 000 cases treated annually in Germany. The AO/OTA system provides a structured fracture type classification, which serves as the foundation for treatment decisions. Although accurately classifying fractures can be challenging, current deep learning models have demonstrated performance comparable to that of experienced radiologists. While most existing approaches rely solely on radiographs, the potential impact of incorporating other additional modalities, such as automatic bone segmentation, fracture location, and radiology reports, remains underexplored. In this work, we systematically analyse the contribution of these three additional information types, finding that combining them with radiographs increases the AUROC from 91.71 to 93.25. Our code is available on `https://github.com/multimodallearning/AO_Classification`.

1 Introduction

Fractures, particularly in the distal forearm, are among the most common injuries in children and adolescents, with approximately 800 000 cases treated annually in Germany. The risk of suffering a fracture by the end of the growing years is estimated to be between 15 % and 45 % [1]. However, due to child-specific factors like skeletal growth, fracture treatment decisions can differ fundamentally from those in adults. To determine the appropriate treatment, factors beyond the patient's age and growth stage must be considered, including fracture location, degree of displacement, fracture pattern, and any accompanying injuries. These considerations are incorporated in the AO/OTA Paediatric Comprehensive Classification of Long Bone Fractures system, developed and validated specifically for paediatric fractures [2]. Since 2006, it is now the most widely adopted framework worldwide, serving as the standard for documentation, communication, and treatment planning for paediatric fractures.

In recent years, deep learning has supported clinicians in radiograph interpretation, matching the performance of human experts in fracture detection [3]. For fracture classification, evidence shows similar results for distal forearm fractures (AUC of 0.89)[4]. While further work focuses on tweaking the feature extraction by comparing different CNN-based encoders (AUC of 0.94) [5], others employ a classical and deep learning-based feature fusion (F1 of 0.81) [6]. Hierarchical classification approaches, including

C. Palm et al. (Hrsg.), *Bildverarbeitung für die Medizin 2025*, Informatik aktuell,
https://doi.org/10.1007/978-3-658-47422-5_44

multilabel subgrouping for ankle fractures (AUC of 0.9) [7] and multistage models for radius fractures (AUC of 0.82) [8], offer further refinement. However, while some multistage methods use fracture location for classification [8], the impact of additional modalities remains underexplored. Further motivation is provided by other classification settings, demonstrating the positive impact of intermediate representations, e.g., depth, and flow field in autonomous driving [9], landmarks for facial emotion classification [10], as well as segmentation facial expression classification [11]. In this work, we systematically analyse the contribution of three modalities, namely automatic bone segmentation, fracture location, and radiology reports as additional input to the radiograph for fracture classification of the paediatric wrist within the AO/OTA system. We found providing all modalities improves the performance, with the impact of fracture location being significant.

2 Materials and methods

2.1 Dataset

The GRAZPEDWRI-DX dataset [12] is a publicly available dataset containing over 20k radiographs of 5900 children and adolescents. For fractures, it provides bounding box annotations, their AO/OTA codes, and the corresponding radiology report for each radiograph. Since we only have segmentations for the 10k AP perspectives, we exclude the lateral views. For our classification task, we use the seven most common AO/OTA classes (adding "no fracture") to ensure that each class includes at least 100 examples and split the dataset into 7809/1978 radiographs for training/testing.

2.2 Setup

Fig. 1 shows a schematic overview, how we incorporate the additional modalities into our classification pipeline. For the spatial input (radiograph, bone segmentation, and

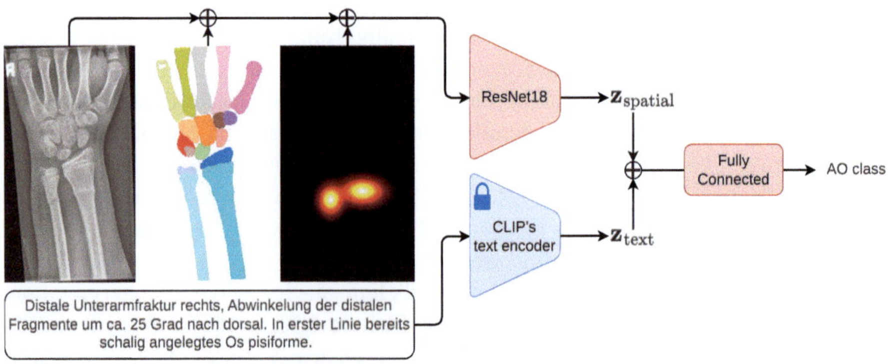

Fig. 1. Usage of the four modalities for fracture classification. The radiograph, the bone segmentation, and the heatmap encoding the fractures' location are feed to the ResNet18. The report embedding of the frozen CLIP text encoder $\mathbf{z}_{\text{text}} \in \mathbb{R}^{512}$ is fused to the ResNet's latent vector $\mathbf{z}_{\text{spatial}} \in \mathbb{R}^{512}$. $\bigoplus$ describes channel-wise concatenation.

fracture location), we concatenate them channelwise $\bigoplus$ and feed them into a ResNet18 embedding them into $\mathbf{z}_{\text{spatial}} \in \mathbb{R}^{512}$. The non-learnable radiology report embedding $\mathbf{z}_{\text{text}} \in \mathbb{R}^{512}$ is then concatenated to $\mathbf{z}_{\text{spatial}}$, constructing the latent space for the classifier, which linear projects its 1024 dimensions onto the eight fracture classes likelihoods.

2.2.1 Different modalities. In this section, we will briefly introduce the four different modalities used by our classifier. 1) The *radiograph* itself, which we z normalize and resize to 384 × 224, where small details like fractures are still visible. 2) The multilabel *segmentations* of 17 bones. Those were created in a semi-supervised setting, starting with 40 annotated images and using label propagation with a SAM-based mask refinement to enable training on all unlabelled data (reaching a Dice of 84.2 % on nine annotated test images)[13]. 3) We encode the *fracture's locations* (h_f, w_f) using a heatmap $\mathbf{H} \in \mathbb{R}^{H \times W}$. For this, we extract the parameters of the multivariate Gaussian kernel from the fracture's bounding box, where its centre (h_f, w_f) represents the means and its axis lengths (l_h, l_w) the standard derivations

$$\mathbf{H}(h, w) = \frac{1}{2\pi l_h l_w} \exp\left[-\frac{1}{2}\left(\frac{(h_f - h)^2}{l_h^2} + \frac{(w_f - w)^2}{l_w^2}\right)\right] \tag{1}$$

As a last step, we normalize $\mathbf{H}$ to [0,1]. While we use the ground truth bounding boxes during training, we use a YOLOv10x to estimate the fracture locations during inference. We train the model on the same train/test split and achieve an accuracy of 90 % and an area under the precision-recall curve of 93.4 % on the test data. 4) As a last modality, we include the *radiology report*, which we encode with a distilled variant of a pretrained multilingual BERT model (`distilbert-base-cased` on Hugging Face). Since an end-to-end approach, trying to classify solely based on the text embedding, did not converge (15 % precision, 100 % recall), we follow a more complex CLIP approach, where the text embedding gets aligned with the corresponding radiograph embedding in a self-supervised fashion. The radiograph embedding is thereby learned by a ResNet18 encoder. We employ a two-layer MLP on top of the BERT model, projecting the text embedding to 512 dimensions. During training (same routine as in Sec. 2.2.2, batch size of 256), we minimize the InfoNCE loss, forcing CLIP to lean semantically cluster and only adapt the ResNet18 and projection MLP, leaving the text model frozen. Since the usability of the learned clusters for our fracture classification is not guaranteed, we provide a proof of concept, where we fit a single fully-connected layer on CLIP's frozen latent space. As a comparison, we choose ImageNet features (provided by a ResNet18) and the latent representation of an Autoencoder, which we train with an L1-norm to reconstruct the radiographs (same routine as in Sec. 2.2.2 with no data augmentation).

2.2.2 Training routine. Since a wrist can suffer from multiple fractures, we formulate our problem as a multilabel classification. Hence, we use the binary cross entropy, which is weighted to balance recall and precision. The loss is minimized by the ADAM optimiser with a learning rate of $1e-3$ over 100 epochs and a batch size of 64. To prevent overfitting, we introduce dropout with a rate of 60 % on $[\mathbf{z}\_\text{spatial}, \mathbf{z}\_\text{text}]^\top$ and use spatial data augmentation by applying for each training example a random affine

Tab. 1. Quantitative results on the test split. ✓ describes the use of the modality radiograph (Img), bone segmentation (BoneSeg), heatmap encoding fracture's location (FracLoc), and CLIP's text embedding of the radiology report (Report). All metrics are computed over the eight fracture types independently and macro averaged.

Img	BoneSeg	FracLoc	Report	Accuracy	F1	Precision	Recall	AUROC
✓				85.16	60.69	49.25	82.12	91.71
✓	✓			84.16	59.26	47.21	85.09	91.60
✓		✓		84.90	61.66	48.75	87.40	93.08
✓	✓	✓		**86.89**	**63.51**	**53.67**	84.04	93.15
✓	✓	✓	✓	84.80	61.70	49.51	**88.83**	93.16
✓		✓	✓	86.60	63.47	51.73	84.48	**93.26**

transformation on the fly, with its parameters sampled from $\mathcal{U}(-30°, 30°)$ for rotation, from $\mathcal{U}(-10\,\%, 10\,\%)$ for translation, and $\mathcal{U}(85\,\%, 115\,\%)$ for scaling (percentage of spatial image dimensions).

3 Results

We train a model for each of the eight possible modality combinations of radiograph, multilabel bone segmentation, fracture's location (as heatmap), and CLIP's text embedding of the radiology report. Tab. 1 shows a selection of the quantitative results obtained from a single training run of each model. These results include accuracy, F1, precision, recall, and area under the receiver operating characteristic curve (AUROC), which are calculated independently for each class and averaged in a macro-fashion. The standard approach, only considering the radiograph, already yields a competitive baseline with an AUROC of 91.71 % and F1 of 60.69 %. While providing the segmentation as additional input, the balance of precision and recall shifted towards the latter by remaining a comparable AUROC but decreasing F1. However, using the fracture's heatmap instead of segmentation, we obtain an increase of recall by over 5 % compared to the baseline, resulting in a rise of 1.3 % in AUROC. When both are used, we obtain the best trade-off between precision and recall, yielding the overall best F1 of 63.51 %. CLIP's report embedding further increases recall and AUROC to 88.83 % and 93.26 %, respectively.

To create further insights into the individual improvement each modality provides, we compare all experiments with the equivalent experiments without this modality. We test for significance with the Wilcoxon paired signed-rank test on the AUROCs of the eight classes with a significance level $\alpha = 0.05$. Since the test includes four comparisons for each modality, we reduce $\alpha' = \frac{\alpha}{4} = 0.0125$ for multiple comparisons with the Bonferroni correction. In our setting with α', we could not find any significant improvement in providing the bone segmentation ($0.5 < p_{\max}$), fracture heatmap ($0.019 < p_{\max}$), or CLIP's report embedding ($0.07 < p_{\max}$) independently of the availability of the other modalities. However, when just the addition to the radiograph is considered, the fracture heatmap provides a significant improvement ($p < 0.007 < \frac{\alpha}{1}$).

Regarding the linear evaluation of CLIP's latent space as proof of concept concerning its usability for fracture classification, Tab. 2 shows, that both CLIP image and text

Encoder	Accuracy	F1	AUROC
CLIP's img encoder	73.97	48.10	85.40
CLIP's txt encoder	72.35	46.90	83.77
ResNet18 ImageNet	67.80	40.68	77.49
AE on GRAZPEDWRI	64.65	39.23	76.33

Tab. 2. Linear evaluation of CLIP's latent space demonstrates its potential for fracture classification, compared to ImageNet features and an autoencoder's latent vector. All encoders are frozen.

encoder provide suitable features, yielding an AUROC of 85.4 and 83.77 respectively. With this, CLIP outperforms the features provided by an ImageNet pretrained ResNet18 and an autoencoder trained in reconstructing the radiographs. Since we are interested in using the reports as an additional modality, we only considered CLIP's text embeddings.

Fig. 2 shows the ROC of two fracture types, where the benefit of using multiple modalities as input is especially visible. Both AO/OTA classes correspond to torus fracture (incomplete fracture with intact periost) of the radius and ulna. Due to their subtle and incomplete fracture lines, torus fractures can be especially hard to notice in radiographs. In such cases, the fracture heatmap can provide guidance.

4 Discussion

Our analysis reveals that providing bone segmentation, fracture location, and radiology reports in addition to the radiographs increases the performance for fracture classification regarding accuracy, precision, recall, and AUROC. However, by adding each modality alone to the radiograph, we could only prove the significance of the fracture location. The added value by the fracture's location becomes visible by considering the ROCs of two AO/OTA codes (Fig. 2) describing a torus fracture with fine fracture lines, which can be easily missed in the radiograph alone or is not represented in the bone segmentation. However, regarding the results, including bone segmentations, it should be noted, that since the GRAZPEDWRI dataset natively lacks segmentation, the use of our predicted ones (Dice of 84.2 % on nine test samples) still has some potential for improvement. Hence, those results could be underestimated due to their quality. While we demonstrated that CLIP's self-supervised training enables the use of radiology

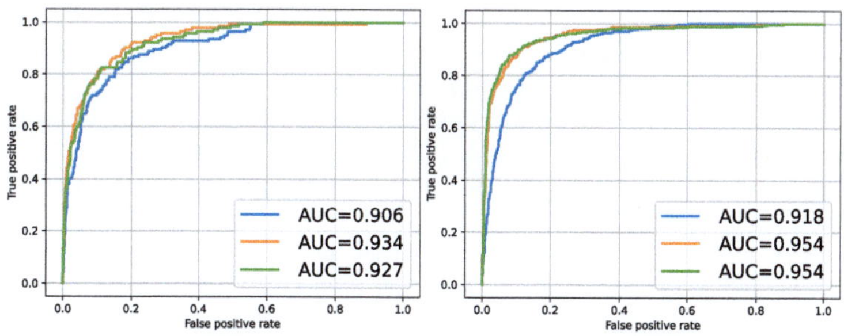

(a) 23-M/2.1. **(b)** 23u-E/7.

Fig. 2. AUROC comparison for fracture types (AO/OTA codes in captions) shows the benefit of including fracture location as input. Blue: Img, orange: Img + FracLoc, green: all modalities.

reports as an input modality for our fracture classification (Tab. 2), it alone does not provide a significant improvement. This could be due to the relatively short and not necessary detailed description of the fractures in the radiology report, lacking direct information on the AO/OTA class (Fig. 1). In future work, we will investigate the different modalities' potential for reducing the amount of training data while remaining the same performance, as it has been already demonstrated for segmentation in other settings [11]. Moreover, considering a hierarchical [7] or multistage [8] approach instead of a multilabel one could be beneficial, as both are better suited to the hierarchy of the AO/OTA system.

Acknowledgement. This research has been funded by the state of Schleswig-Holstein, Grant Number 22023005.

References

1. Kraus R, Schneidmüller D, Röder C. Häufigkeit von Frakturen der langen Röhrenknochen im Wachstumsalter. Dtsch Arztebl International. 2005;102(12):A–838-.
2. Slongo T, Audigé L, Schlickewei W et al. Development and validation of the AO pediatric comprehensive classification of long bone fractures. J Pediatr Orthop. 2006;26(1):43–9.
3. Kuo RYL, Harrison CJ, Curran TA et al. Artificial intelligence in fracture detection: a systematic review and meta-analysis. Radiol. 2022:211785.
4. Binh LN, Nhu NT, Vy VPT et al. Multi-class deep learning model for detecting pediatric distal forearm fractures based on the AO/OTA classification. J Imaging Inform Med. 2024;37(2):725–33.
5. Gan K, Liu Y, Zhang T et al. Deep learning model for automatic identification and classification of distal radius fracture. J Imaging Inform Med. 2024.
6. Yang F, Cong R, Xing M et al. Study on AO classification of distal radius fractures based on multi-feature fusion. J Phys: Conference Series. 2021;1800(1):012006.
7. Olczak J, Emilson F, Razavian A et al. Ankle fracture classification using deep learning. Acta Orthop. 2020;92:101–7.
8. Min H, Rabi Y, Wadhawan A et al. Automatic classification of distal radius fracture using a two-stage ensemble deep learning framework. Phys Eng Sci Med. 2023;46(2):877–86.
9. Zhou B, Krähenbühl P, Koltun V. Does computer vision matter for action? Sci Robot. 2019;4(30):eaaw6661.
10. Hasani B, Mahoor MH. Facial expression recognition using enhanced deep 3D convolutional neural networks. Proc IEEE CVPR. 2017:2278–88.
11. Keuth R, Hansen L, Heinrich MP. Der Einfluss von Segmentierung auf die Genauigkeit eines CNN-Klassifikators zur Mimik-Steuerung. Proc BVM. 2020:294–300.
12. Nagy E, Janisch M, Hržić F et al. A pediatric wrist trauma X-ray dataset for machine learning. Sci Data. 2022;9(1):222.
13. Keuth R, Hansen L, Balks M et al. SAM carries the burden: a semi-supervised approach refining pseudo labels for medical segmentation. arXiv: 2411.12602. 2024.

Intrinsic Correspondence of Classification Ground Truth and Image Content on the Example of Endoscopic Images

Johannes Schuiki, Andreas Uhl

Dept. of Artificial Intelligence and Human Interfaces, University of Salzburg, Austria
jschuiki@cs.sbg.ac.at

Abstract. On what basis class labels ("ground truth") get assigned to images heavily depends on the application scenario, sometimes even without visual inspection of the data. Therefore, it can be of interest to evaluate whether distinguishing intrinsic structures exist within the image data. In this study, it is investigated if images from five small-scale endoscopic datasets where class labels were assigned based on domain-specific criteria can be algorithmically clustered into the desired classes. The image classification task is treated as a clustering comparison problem by comparing ground truth labels with clustering results derived from a variety of image representations.

1 Introduction

Image classification is one of the fundamental tasks in the domain of computer vision. It involves assigning a label or category to a given image based on its visual content. With rapid advances in deep learning techniques, image classification has become more accurate and efficient, enabling machines to perceive and interpret visual information with human-like accuracy. However, having properly labeled data points for learning and evaluation is paramount to satisfying results. Such labels are a subset of metadata widely known in the machine learning and computer science community as "ground truth" and used to train a model via supervised learning. This labeled data provide the "correct answers" that the model should learn to predict. Throughout various domains of science employing computer vision tools, the understanding of ground truth and also the process of obtaining slightly differs. In the domain of medicine (and therefore heavily influenced is the discipline of medical imaging), the term "gold standard" is used for the benchmark that is available under reasonable conditions [1]. For data annotations, experts often rely on the results from gold standard methods.

Because the process of assigning a class label to images does not necessarily rely on visual inspection, it can be unclear whether relevant structures for distinguishing actually exist within the image data. Also, some domains require experts for data labeling while it is known [2] that, especially in the medical fields, an inter-observer discrepancy exists. Furthermore, there is also the possibility that learning based approaches learn something unintended but rather forced by labeling. Thus, it is of interest to explore if a collection of images can be grouped according to the defined class labels, i.e. to assess the extent of correspondence between class label and visual content.

In this work, we investigate the correspondence between label and image content experimentally for five small-scale datasets. To evaluate this correspondence, a variety

C. Palm et al. (Hrsg.), *Bildverarbeitung für die Medizin 2025*, Informatik aktuell,
https://doi.org/10.1007/978-3-658-47422-5_45

of image representations are first grouped into clusters using a number of clustering algorithms and obtained cluster labels are afterwards compared to the ground truth labels using a clustering comparison metric.

2 Materials and methods

2.1 Data

For the experiments in this work, five small-scale endoscopic image datasets are employed where data labeling happened under supervision of domain experts. Two image sets deal with celiac disease while the other three focus on colonic polyps. Although the datasets provide annotations for various stages of the respective conditions, the labels are always collapsed to a two-class scenario (healthy vs. pathologic or benign vs. malignant). In the following, every dataset is briefly introduced. A property shared across all the employed datasets is their imbalance in terms of class distribution and that classes can be further subdivided according to patient-ids. Thus, dataset statistics can be visualized using nested pie charts as depicted in Fig. 1. Example patches for every dataset are shown in Fig. 2.

2.1.1 Celiac disease. Celiac disease (CD) is a chronic autoimmune condition that affects approximately 1% of the global population. Currently, the gold standard for diagnosing CD is endoscopy with biopsy. Specimen are then classified in a histological analysis according to the modified Marsh classification proposed in [3] which distinguishes between classes Marsh-0 to Marsh-3, with subclasses 3A, 3B, and 3C. The used dataset includes classes Marsh-0, Marsh-3A, Marsh-3B and Marsh-3C. For this dataset, patient-level biopsy results were available rather than area-specific data. Consequently, final patch labeling incorporated both histological and visual criteria. Within this work, class 0 is used as the healthy class and classes 3A, 3B & 3C are collapsed to form the disease class. Imaging techniques within the scope of this work include the modified immersion technique (MIT) under traditional white-light (WL) illumination, as well as MIT under narrow band imaging (NBI). The green (the two left-most) pie charts in Fig. 1 visualize the distribution for the celiac samples. Further information about the dataset can be found in [4].

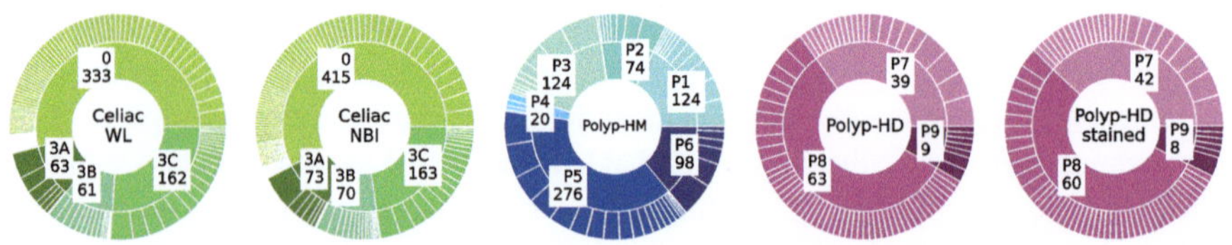

Fig. 1. Distribution of the data for all datasets used in this work. The inner ring depicts the proportion of the data for each class; segments in the outer ring indicate images from the same patient. The accompanying integer value indicates the number of samples per class.

2.1.2 Colonic polyps. Colonic polyps are growths that develop on the inner lining of the colon or rectum. For colon examination, the current gold standard is colonoscopy. Colonoscopy allows to investigate the inside of the colon using an endoscope. This work employs three such datasets, acquired using different imaging techniques:

- Polyp-HM: This dataset was acquired using a high magnification (HM) colonoscope together with a contrast staining. Images within this image set are classified based on six classes, known as pit patterns [5]. These class labels are assigned solely based on the visual content. The data distribution of the six classes, denoted as P1 - P6, are visualized by the blue (center) pie chart in Fig. 1. They can be summarized as P1 and P2 including benign polyps and P4 - P6 including malignant polyps. Additional information about the data can be found in [6].
- Polyp-HD: Two further image datasets were acquired using a high definition (HD) endoscope with and without additional staining. For these datasets, however, images are only divided into three classes, "normal", "non-invasive" and "invasive" based on their histological diagnosis (abbreviated as P7 - P9, where P7 is treated as the healthy class and P8 & P9 together are viewed as the pathologic class). The data distribution is depicted in the magenta (the two right-most) pie charts in Fig. 1. For further information the interested reader is referred to [7].

2.2 Image representation

In our experiments, we employ a variety of image representations to evaluate the intrinsic correspondence between ground truth labels and image content. This approach is necessitated by the absence of a universally optimal image representation. By evaluating multiple representations, we aim to comprehensively assess the intrinsic relationship between image content and ground truth labels across different levels of abstraction.

- Raw pixel values: We begin with flattened raw pixel values, which provide the closest approximation to a "natural description" of the image. While this representation preserves all original information, it lacks desirable properties such as spatial invariance.

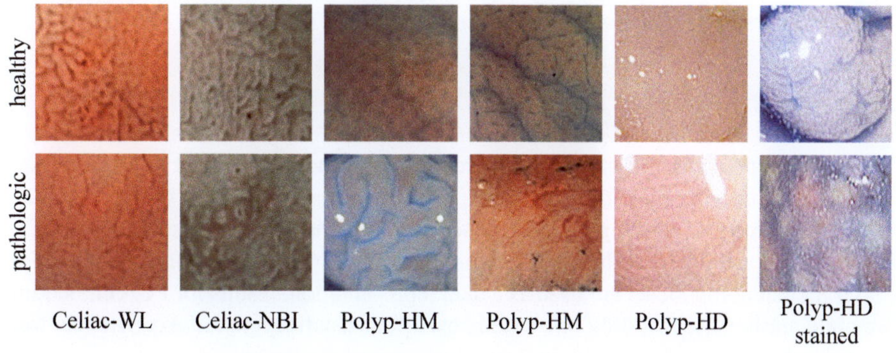

Fig. 2. Example patches from all datasets included in this work.

- Dimensionality reduction: We apply principal component analysis (PCA) to reduce the dimensionality of the raw pixel data. This step helps to mitigate the curse of dimensionality and potentially reveals latent structures in the data.
- Neural Networks: We utilize feature embeddings extracted from pre-trained deep learning models. These representations excel at identifying relevant structures in images due to their ability to capture complex relations within the data. However, it is important to note that these networks, trained on ImageNet, introduce biases inherent to their training data. Yet, in pursuit of finding a "natural representation" of the images and also to avoid learning something unintended by force, we explicitly refrain from fitting a model to our data. Network model architectures are taken from the PyTorch Image Models collection[1] which encompasses a large variety of state-of-the-art model architectures. In particular, seven different architectures are employed in this work: ResNet-18 & ResNet-50, MobileNetv3, TinyNet, EfficientNet, Vision Transformer (ViT) & Mobile-ViT. Within this work, models are utilized such that images are embedded into a feature representation using a pre-trained network where the final classification layer is removed.

2.3 Consensus of ground truth and image content

To quantify the alignment between the assigned ground truth and the image descriptors outlined in Section 2.2, these descriptors are grouped using a variety of algorithmic approaches for data clustering. Three clustering algorithms are employed for the experiments in this work: k-means clustering, hierachical (or agglomerative) clustering and spectral clustering. Implementations from the *scikit-learn* python library are used. After clustering, images have both a ground truth class label and a newly generated cluster label. For comparing both label assignments, the ground truth assignment can be treated as a different clustering result and thus the comparison be treated as a case of clustering comparison. One such comparison method is the adjusted mutual information (AMI) [8] metric, which is a version of mutual information that introduces a correction for chance by considering the expected similarity of all pairwise comparisons. For calculation of an expected similarity value, a random model must be chosen based on how the data points can be clustered. According to [8], the right random model to choose for experiments within this work is the *one-sided* (always comparing against the same basis, i.e. ground truth) comparison with a *fixed number of clusters*.

3 Results

This section presents the experimental results. Bar charts in Fig. 3 depict the AMI values for comparing the clustering labels with the ground truth labels for every image representation and clustering algorithm used in this work. As mentioned in Section 2.1, image classes are always collapsed to a two-class scenario. Regardless of how many of the first principal components are used as a data representation, results for PCA embedding are quite similar. Hence, only one case is used for visualization. All experiments were carried out ten times. Error bars indicate the standard deviation.

[1] `https://github.com/rwightman/pytorch-image-models`

4 Discussion

The overview presented in Fig. 3 indicates that raw and PCA representations result in an overall low AMI value, suggesting their unsuitability for our analysis. Except for Polyp-HM, every dataset has a configuration achieving a metric value of 0.4 of higher. One particular combination even yields a metric value exceeding 0.5 AMI. Here, 0.5 AMI can be interpreted as roughly 90% of agreement between class label and clustering, as discussed in Section 4.1. It is interesting to observe that the Polyp-HM dataset (labels assigned solely based on visual appearance) appears to yield the lowest agreement of labels and algorithmic clustering, whereas the AMI values for other datasets (labels assigned also/solely based on histological analysis) are relatively high. We can further observe that the choice of clustering algorithm and feature embedding has a high impact on the results. Hence, we can conclude that the employed methodology appears to only provide insight into coarse trends, but seems insufficient to give a definitive answer to the correspondence between image labels and visual content.

4.1 Relationship between AMI and classification accuracy

In an attempt to establish a relationship between the AMI and an estimation of the classification accuracy, two artificial clusterings were gradually alienated and the corresponding metrics calculated. Fig. 4 depicts the simulated relationship between AMI and accuracy for a two-class setup. Two cases for label randomization are considered: (i) permutation, where the starting point is an equal amount of elements per cluster and on every step of scrambling the labels, every cluster receives exactly one element from the other cluster. Doing so, the number of elements per cluster does not change, merely

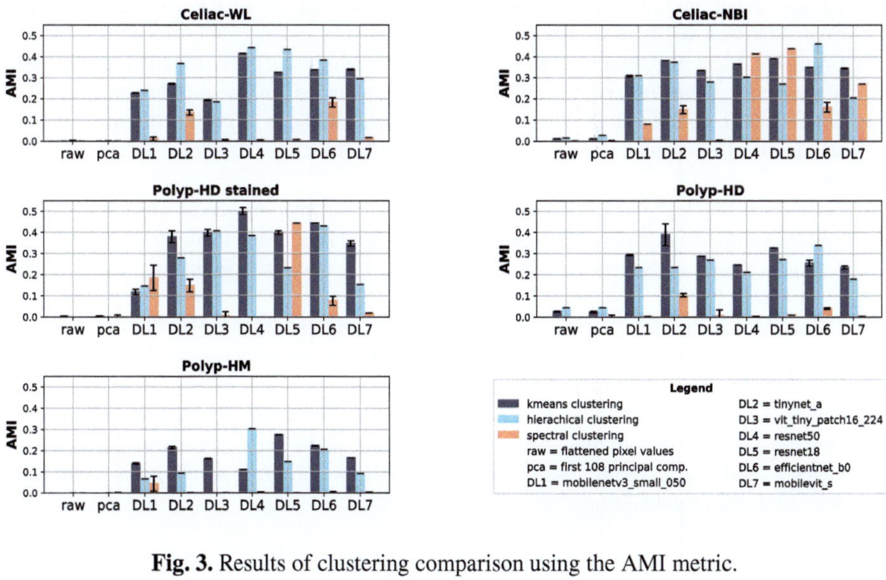

Fig. 3. Results of clustering comparison using the AMI metric.

the labels get permuted. (ii) randomized, which also considers imbalanced clusters. Depending on the step, a number of elements are picked and assigned to the other cluster in a random fashion. The second case is more realistic but doing so, however, does not result in an unambiguous relationship between AMI and accuracy. The relationship can be understood as: *The clustering algorithm was able to separate the feature embeddings as if a classifier model would score x% accuracy.* Note that 0.5 accuracy corresponds to random guessing in a two-class scenario.

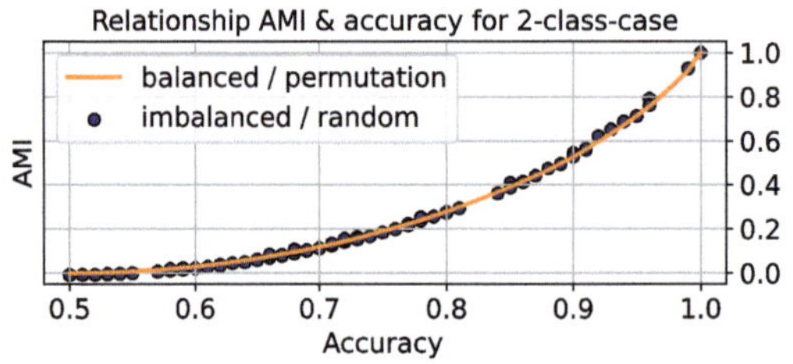

Fig. 4. Simulated relation between AMI and accuracy for a two-class-scenario.

Acknowledgement. This work has been partially supported by the Salzburg State Government WISS2025 Research and Transfer Lab on “Artificial Intelligence in BioMedical Image Analysis (AIBIA)”.

References

1. Cardoso J, Pereira L, Iversen M et al. What is gold standard and what is ground truth? Dental Press J Orthod. 2014;19:27–30.
2. Corona R, Mele A, Amini M et al. Interobserver variability on the histopathologic diagnosis of cutaneous melanoma and other pigmented skin lesions. J Clin Oncol. 1996;14(4):1218–23.
3. Oberhuber G, Granditsch G, Vogelsang H. The histopathology of coeliac disease: time for a standardized report scheme for pathologists. Eur J Gastroenterol Hepatol. 1999;11(10):1185–94.
4. Gadermayr M, Hegenbart S, Kwitt R et al. Narrow band imaging versus white-light: what is best for computer-assisted diagnosis of celiac disease? Proc IEEE ISBI. 2016:355–9.
5. Kudo S, Hirota S, Nakajima T et al. Colorectal tumours and pit pattern. J Clin Pathol. 1994;47(10):880–5.
6. Häfner M, Liedlgruber M, Uhl A et al. Delaunay triangulation-based pit density estimation for the classification of polyps in high-magnification chromo-colonoscopy. Comput Methods Programs Biomed. 2012;107(3):565–81.
7. Ribeiro E, Häfner M, Wimmer G et al. Exploring texture transfer learning for colonic polyp classification via convolutional neural networks. Proc IEEE ISBI. 2017:1044–8.
8. Gates AJ, Ahn YY. The impact of random models on clustering similarity. J Mach Learn Res. 2017;18(1):3049–76.

Abstract: Real-world Federated Learning in Radiology

Hurdles to Overcome and Benefits to Gain

Markus Bujotzek[1,2], Ünal Akünal[1], Stefan Denner[1,3], Peter Neher[1], Maximilian Zenk[1,2], Klaus Maier-Hein[1], Andreas Bucher[4], Rickmer Braren[5]

[1]Division of Medical Image Computing, German Cancer Research Center Heidelberg, Germany
[2]Medical Faculty Heidelberg, University of Heidelberg, Germany
[3]Faculty of Mathematics and Computer Science, Heidelberg University, Germany
[4]Institute for Diagnostic and Interventional Radiology, University Hospital Frankfurt, Germany
[5]Institute for Diagnostic and Interventional Radiology, Klinikum rechts der Isar, Technical University of Munich, Germany
markus.bujotzek@dkfz-heidelberg.de

Federated learning (FL) enables collaborative model training while keeping data locally. Currently, most FL studies in radiology are conducted in simulated environments due to numerous hurdles impeding its translation into practice. The few existing real-world FL initiatives rarely communicate specific measures taken to overcome these hurdles. To bridge this significant knowledge gap, we propose a comprehensive guide for real-world FL in radiology. Minding efforts to implement real-world FL, there is a lack of comprehensive assessments comparing FL to less complex alternatives in challenging real-world settings, which we address through extensive benchmarking. We developed our own FL infrastructure within the German Radiological Cooperative Network (RACOON)[1] and demonstrated its functionality by training FL models on lung pathology segmentation tasks across six university hospitals. Insights gained while establishing our FL initiative and running the extensive benchmark experiments were compiled and categorized into the guide. The proposed guide outlines essential steps, identified hurdles, and implemented solutions for establishing successful FL initiatives conducting real-world experiments. Our experimental results prove the practical relevance of our guide and show that FL outperforms less complex alternatives in all evaluation scenarios. Our findings justify the efforts required to translate FL into real-world applications by demonstrating advantageous performance over alternative approaches. Additionally, they emphasize the importance of strategic organization, robust management of distributed data and infrastructure in real-world settings. With the proposed guide, we are aiming to aid future FL researchers in circumventing pitfalls and accelerating translation of FL into radiological applications. This work was originally published in the Journal of American Medical Informatics Association [1].

References

1. Bujotzek MR, Akünal Ü, Denner S et al. Real-world federated learning in radiology: hurdles to overcome and benefits to gain. J Am Med Inform Assoc. 2024;32(1):193–205.

[1]https://racoon.network/

C. Palm et al. (Hrsg.), *Bildverarbeitung für die Medizin 2025*, Informatik aktuell,
https://doi.org/10.1007/978-3-658-47422-5_46

Abstract: Contrastive Learning Approach for Assessment of Speech in Patients with Tongue Cancer using MRI Data

Tomás Arias-Vergara[1,2], Paula A. Pérez-Toro[1,2], Xiaofeng Liu[3], Fangxu Xing[2], Maureen Stone[4], Jiachen Zhuo[4], Jerry L. Prince[5], Maria Schuster[6], Elmar Nöth[1], Jonghye Woo[2], Andreas Maier[2]

[1]Pattern Recognition Lab. Friedrich-Alexander University, Erlangen, Germany
[2]Massachusetts General Hospital - Harvard Medical School, Boston, MA, USA
[3]Department of Radiology and Biomedical Imaging, Yale University, New Haven, CT, USA
[4]University of Maryland, Baltimore, MD, USA
[5]Johns Hopkins University, Baltimore, MD, USA
[6]Department of Otorhinolaryngology, Ludwig-Maximilians University, Munich, Germany
tomas.arias@fau.de

The analysis of human speech with magnetic resonance imaging (MRI) provides essential information on the dynamic processes involved in speech production, allowing unobtrusive monitoring of the complete vocal tract during speech production. In clinical applications, personalized monitoring and increased speed of speech rehabilitation can be achieved through targeted phonological therapy i.e., by breaking down spoken words into their linguistic units. While MRI provides detailed visualization of the anatomical structures involved in speech production, the acoustic information provided by synchronized audio signals allows higher temporal resolution to process speech sounds. However, having access to reliable acoustic information is not always possible; thus, in this work, we proposed the use of contrastive learning for the automatic detection of vowels and consonants grouped into nine phonological classes from MRI data, aiming to analyze speech disorders in tongue cancer patients. The aim is to train a multi-modal system (image and acoustic signals) that only uses one modality during inference (e.g. the MRI frames) while keeping a high performance for the selected task i.e., phoneme-based speech recognition. During training, a single video frame and its corresponding acoustic signal are processed by two different transformer-based encoders. For this, we ensure that the image and acoustic encoders are projected to have the same dimensions using linear layers and maximize the similarity between these embeddings. Then, a linear multilayer perceptron with a softmax activation function is used for phonological classification. We demonstrated that frame-wise recognition improves from an average F1-score of 0.74 to 0.85 when the contrastive loss approach is implemented. Furthermore, we show the utility of our approach in the clinical application of using such phonological classes to assess speech disorders in patients with tongue cancer [1].

References

1. Arias-Vergara T, Pérez-Toro PA, Liu X et al. Contrastive learning approach for assessment of phonological precision in patients with tongue cancer using MRI data. Proc Interspeech. 2024:927–31.

C. Palm et al. (Hrsg.), *Bildverarbeitung für die Medizin 2025*, Informatik aktuell,
https://doi.org/10.1007/978-3-658-47422-5_47

Active Learning Pipeline for Biomedical Image Instance Segmentation with Minimal Human Intervention

Shuo Zhao[1], Yu Zhou[1,2], Jianxu Chen[1],

[1]Leibniz-Institut für Analytische Wissenschaften - ISAS - e.V.
[2]Faculty of Computer Science, Ruhr University Bochum
jianxu.chen@isas.de

Abstract. Biomedical image segmentation is critical for precise structure delineation and downstream analysis. Traditional methods often struggle with noisy data, while deep learning models such as U-Net have set new benchmarks in segmentation performance. nnU-Net further automates model configuration, making it adaptable across datasets without extensive tuning. However, it requires a substantial amount of annotated data for cross-validation, posing a challenge when only raw images but no labels are available. Large foundation models offer zero-shot generalizability, but may underperform on specific datasets with unique characteristics, limiting their direct use for analysis. This work addresses these bottlenecks by proposing a data-centric AI workflow that leverages active learning and pseudo-labeling to combine the strengths of traditional neural networks and large foundation models while minimizing human intervention. The pipeline starts by generating pseudo-labels from a foundation model, which are then used for nnU-Net's self-configuration. Subsequently, a representative core-set is selected for minimal manual annotation, enabling effective fine-tuning of the nnU-Net model. This approach significantly reduces the need for manual annotations while maintaining competitive performance, providing an accessible solution for biomedical researchers to apply state-of-the-art AI techniques in their segmentation tasks. The code is available at `https://github.com/MMV-Lab/AL_BioMed_img_seg`.

1 Introduction

Image segmentation is crucial in biomedical image analysis, as it allows precise delineation of structures, which could be used for downstream quantification and modeling. The field of biomedical image segmentation has evolved significantly with deep learning techniques. Although traditional methods such as thresholding or graph-based methods were foundational, they often yield much worse performance on challenging tasks (e.g., noisy data) compared to deep learning-based approaches such as U-Net [1].

Traditional neural networks such as nnU-Net further improved this by automating model configuration for different segmentation tasks [2], which has become a strong baseline method in segmentation benchmarks. nnU-Net can adapt to various biomedical imaging datasets without extensive manual tuning, effectively overcoming the challenges associated with manual network design and configuration. Empirical selection requires a complete training set or sufficient data for five-fold cross-validation. However, obtaining labeled data for nnU-Net, especially in 3D image analysis, is time-consuming and requires knowledge and expertise. In practice, data often has no labels.

C. Palm et al. (Hrsg.), *Bildverarbeitung für die Medizin 2025*, Informatik aktuell,
https://doi.org/10.1007/978-3-658-47422-5_48

Unsupervised active learning advances core-set selection for efficient training and lower annotation costs but faces challenges in feature selection and initialization. [3].

Meanwhile, different network architectures, such as transformer-based models and hybrid models combining convolutional neural networks (CNNs) with transformers, have also been proposed to improve segmentation by capturing long-range dependencies in images [7]. Recent developments in large foundation models, such as SAM [8], SAM2 [9], cellSAM [4], microSAM [10], medSAM [11], have further advanced the field toward generalist models for biomedical image segmentation. However, large foundation models often struggle with specific datasets, such as unique tissue environments or drug-treated cells, limiting their effectiveness in direct downstream analysis.

We address the two bottlenecks with an active learning pipeline based on the idea of data-centric AI to solve these two bottlenecks, which focuses on data quality and diversity rather than model complexity [12]. This pipeline combines traditional neural networks and large foundation models with minimal human input. A 3D mitochondrial segmentation [13] was used as an example. Pseudo-labels generated from a foundation model for raw images can be used to create a training set for self-configuration and pre-training. This approach enables nnU-Net to work with unlabeled images. A core-set is a small, representative subset that approximates the properties of the full dataset. Then a core-set was selected for manual annotation and fine-tuning the pre-rained nnU-Net, leading to a robust model with minimal manual effort. It is worth mentioning that this paper focuses on an active learning pipeline to address key bottlenecks in traditional neural networks and large foundation models. So we focus on demonstrating and validating the effectiveness of this pipeline rather than competing on leaderboards.

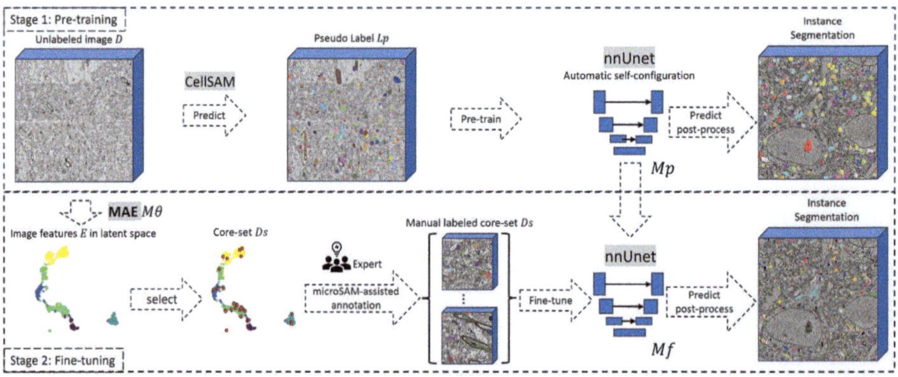

Fig. 1. An active learning pipeline for 3D unlabeled biomedical image instance segmentation. This pipeline consists of two main stages: Pre-training and Fine-tuning. Stage 1: Pre-training. Pseudo-labels were generated from CellSAM [4] for unlabeled raw images, forming a training set for nnU-Net to run self-configuration and pre-training. Stage 2: Fine-tuning. Unlabeled images were mapped into a latent space to select a representative core-set [5], using features from a pre-trained foundation model MAE [6] via self-supervised learning. The pre-trained nnU-Net model was fine-tuned by using minimal microSAM-assisted annotations.

2 Materials and methods

2.1 Methods

The proposed pipeline (Fig. 1) consists of two main stages: pre-training and fine-tuning.

1. *Pre-training*: To enable nnU-Net M_p to run self-configuration and pre-training, avoiding manual design, pseudo-labels L_p were generated from CellSAM [4] for unlabeled raw images D. Then D and L_p formed a train set for nnU-Net M_p.
2. *Fine-tuning*: The selected core-set D_s and its manual label were used to fine-tune the pre-trained nnU-Net M_p. We selected raw images based on their latent space features. An MAE model M_θ using U-net architecture was trained with unlabeled images D via self-supervised learning. According to $E = M_\theta(D)$, D were mapped into a latent space as the features E. Pre-trained MAE models excel in scalability, speed, and feature extraction, outperforming supervised models [14]. According to $d = 1 - E \cdot E^T$, a cosine distance matrix d was computed between features E.

Unlabeled images D consists of a selected core-set D_s [5] and unselected set D_u. The core-set selection algorithm, initialization, k ($k = 3$) samples were selected randomly from D_u. Then, each sample S in D_u was traversed, find the minimum distance $d_{\min}(S, D_s)$ for each S to D_s. Then the sample S in D_u with the maximum $d_{\min}$ was selected to D_s. We repeated this process, and finally get a core-set D_s of size N.

The unlable selected core-set D_s was checked and annotated by experts with minimal manual effort, assisted by microSAM [10]. Then D_s and manual labels were used to fine-tune the nnU-Net M_p, resulting in M_f. Connected components were applied to make instance segmentation as in MitoEM Challenge [13].

2.2 Validation on the 3D unlabeled dataset MitoEM

The MitoEM Grand Challenge [13] is an international competition focused on segmenting mitochondria in electron microscopy images. The 3D MitoEM dataset [15] contains two high-resolution volumes, each measuring $30 \times 30 \times 30$ μm with voxel dimensions of $1000 \times 4096 \times 4096$ at $30 \times 8 \times 8$ nm resolution. Each volume is divided into training (400 slices), validation (100 slices), and test (500 slices) sets. Although it has ground truth (GT), we assume no GT is available for training, as in real-world tasks.

3 Experiment

All experiments were run on 8 NVIDIA A100 GPUs (40GB). For fair experiments, we simply adopt the hyperparameters in the original nnU-Net codebase for training.

For dataset preprocessing, train and test sets were padded and cropped into 1024 patches ($32 \times 512 \times 512$). 2D pseudo-labels were generated by CellSAM and combined into 3D patch labels. nnU-Net was pre-trained and fine-tuned automatically. MAE models were trained on 1000 raw 2D images with a 0.75 mask ratio for 400 epochs. Then the pre-trained encoders were used to extract image features. Patches were selected by the core-set selection algorithm ($k = 3$). Core-sets were annotated by microSAM

Tab. 1. Evaluation metrics for fine-tuning with different core-set sizes. Where the 1024 core-set represents the full manually labeled set. Each double row displays the score and percentage of the full set score. Bold text highlights when the score first surpasses 90% of the full set performance.

Core-set Size Percentage (%)	0 (0.00)	8 (0.78)	16 (1.56)	32 (3.13)	64 (6.25)	128 (12.50)	256 (25.00)	512 (50.00)	1024 (100.00)
F1 Score	0.4025	0.4462	0.5297	0.5630	**0.5884**	0.6003	0.6011	0.6294	0.6350
Percentage (%)	63.38	70.26	83.41	88.66	**92.65**	94.53	94.65	99.12	100.00
Accuracy	0.2521	0.2882	0.3603	0.3918	0.4170	**0.4291**	0.4298	0.4593	0.4652
Percentage (%)	54.19	61.95	77.45	84.22	89.63	**92.23**	92.39	98.72	100.00
Panoptic	0.3628	0.3962	0.4723	0.5038	**0.5284**	0.5405	0.5421	0.5689	0.5750
Percentage (%)	63.09	68.90	82.13	87.61	**91.89**	93.99	94.26	98.93	100.00
Precision	0.2824	0.3300	0.4181	0.4599	0.4926	**0.5045**	0.5058	0.5411	0.5554
Percentage (%)	50.85	59.42	75.29	82.81	88.70	**90.85**	91.08	97.43	100.00

with the `vit_b` model. Fine-tuned models segmented the test set, with post-processing and evaluation following the MitoEM Challenge [13]. For ablation experiments, we compared nnU-Net models trained on the core-set with those pre-trained on pseudo-labels. We also assessed the impact of various core-set sizes, from 8 to 1024 samples.

4 Results

We observed that simply relying on pseudo-labels from large foundation models may be insufficient. As shown in Fig. 2, pseudo-labels (Fig. 2a) closely resemble the manual labels in (Fig. 2b). However, yellow arrows highlight labeling errors, e.g., imprecise boundaries and false negatives. The white arrows indicate that, compared to GT (Fig. 2f), the segmentation after pre-training (Fig. 2c) detects mitochondria but has inaccuracies. The selected core-sets are reasonable and effective. Fig. 3 shows the latent space distribution of image features, with red points marking diverse, representative patches that enhance information density. Fine-tuning with the selected core-set is effective. As shown in Fig. 2, fine-tuning with 12.5% and 100% manual labels (Fig. 2d, Fig. 2e) improves segmentations closer to the GT (Fig. 2f). Fig. 4 and Tab. 1 show fine-tuning

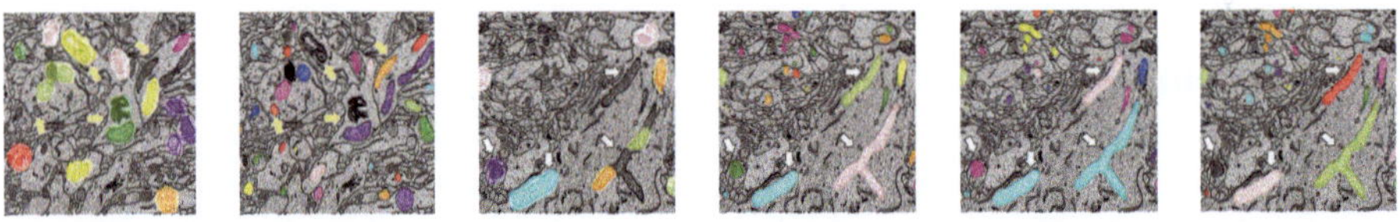

(a) (b) (c) (d) (e) (f)

Fig. 2. Labels for the train set: (a) pseudo-labels from cellSAM and (b) manual labels. Segmentations for the test set: (c) pre-trained with pseudo-labels, (d) fine-tuned with 12.5% manual labels, (e) fine-tuned with 100% manual labels, and (f) GT. Yellow arrows in (a) and (b) show differences between pseudo and manual labels, while white arrows in (c)–(f) highlight discrepancies between segmentations and the GT.

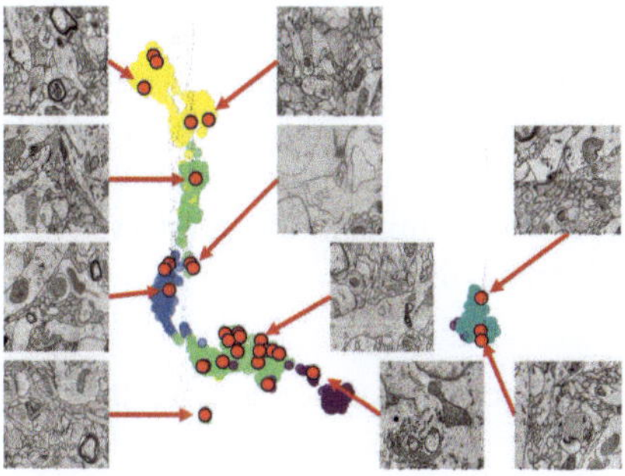

Fig. 3. Examples of patches in the selected core-set. The plot visualizes the latent features of all patches in latent space after UMAP dimensionality reduction. Red dots represent the selected image patches. The selected patches cover a wide range but have different features. Compared with random selection, the selected core-set is both representative and diverse, with high information density.

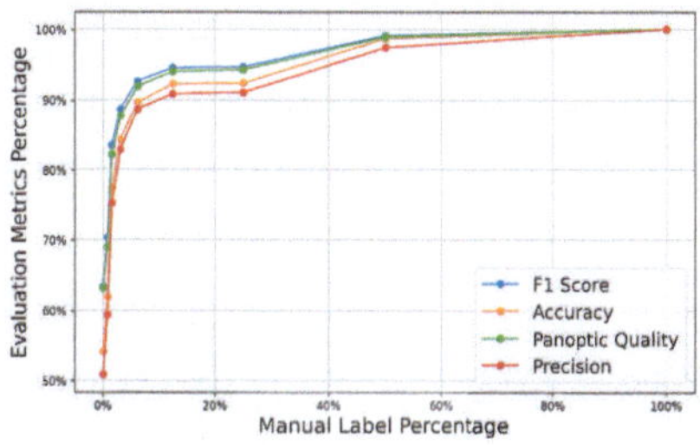

Fig. 4. Instance segmentation metrics: The X-axis shows manual annotation percentage, and the Y-axis shows performance relative to full labels. As manual annotations increase, the model's performance improves. At about 12.5% annotations, the model achieves 90% of the full annotation performance.

Tab. 2. Evaluation metrics for Core-set and Random selection. A train set of 128 (12.5%) samples was selected to compare the performance of the core-set selection and randomly selection. W/ indicates nnU-Net was pre-trained on pseudo-labels before fine-tuning, while w/o means it was trained directly on the selected set without pre-training.

	Pre-trained	F1 score	Accuracy	Panoptic	Precision
Core-set	w/	0.6003	0.4291	0.5405	0.5045
Core-set	w/o	0.5939	0.4225	0.5342	0.4953
Random	w/	0.5773	0.4058	0.5173	0.4697
Random	w/o	0.5793	0.4076	0.5183	0.4732

results with different core-set sizes. Tab. 1 highlights that F1 score and Panoptic metrics surpassed 90% at 6.25% (64 samples), and Accuracy and Precision at 12.5% (128 samples). Fine-tuning surpasses pseudo-label-only pre-training (core-set = 0). nnU-Net leverages pseudo-label pre-training for auto-configuration.. As shown in Tab.1, core-set fine-tuned models consistently outperformed pseudo-label-only pre-trained models. Core-set selection outperforms random selection. Tab.2 shows that with 128 (12.5%) samples, the core-set improved F1 score, accuracy, panoptic, and precision, making core-set selection with pre-training the most effective for fine-tuning nnU-Net.

5 Discussion and conclusion

Pseudo-labels from CellSAM enable nnU-Net training without manual annotations. MicroSAM refines these labels semi-automatically, reducing effort. This pipeline integrates foundation models with traditional networks for efficient raw data use. Core-set fine-tuning surpasses pseudo-label pre-training and random selection.

In summary, this work presents an active learning workflow addressing two major pain-points in existing methods: (1) nnU-Net requires considerable ground truth, but usually not available in real applications, for auto-configuration, (2) foundation models cannot always provide completely satisfactory results off-the-shelf. The proposed framework seamlessly streamlines two powerful methods with minimal human intervention. Future work will enable continuous learning for dynamic datasets.

Disclaimer. The authors declare that there is no conflict of interest regarding the publication of this paper.

Acknowledgement. This work is supported by the by the Federal Ministry of Education and Research (BMBF) in Germany under the funding reference 161L0272, and also supported by the Ministry of Culture and Science (MKW) of the State of North Rhine-Westphalia.

References

1. Ronneberger O, Fischer P, Brox T. U-Net: convolutional networks for biomedical image segmentation. Proc MICCAI. 2015:234–41.
2. Isensee F, Jaeger PF, Kohl SA et al. nnU-Net: a self-configuring method for deep learning-based biomedical image segmentation. Nat Methods. 2021;18(2):203–11.
3. Ash JT, Zhang C, Krishnamurthy A et al. Deep batch active learning by diverse, uncertain gradient lower bounds. arXiv: 1906.03671. 2019.
4. Israel U, Marks M, Dilip R et al. A foundation model for cell segmentation. bioRxiv. 2024:2023–11.
5. Yang L, Zhang Y, Chen J et al. Suggestive annotation: a deep active learning framework for biomedical image segmentation. Proc MICCAI. 2017:399–407.
6. He K, Chen X, Xie S et al. Masked autoencoders are scalable vision learners. Proc IEEE CVF CVPR. 2022:16000–9.
7. Alexey D. An image is worth 16x16 words: transformers for image recognition at scale. arXiv: 2010.11929. 2020.
8. Kirillov A, Mintun E, Ravi N et al. Segment anything. Proc IEEE CVF ICCV. 2023:4015–26.
9. Ravi N, Gabeur V, Hu YT et al. Sam 2: segment anything in images and videos. arXiv: 2408.00714. 2024.
10. Archit A, Nair S, Khalid N et al. Segment anything for microscopy. bioRxiv. 2023:2023–8.
11. Ma J, He Y, Li F et al. Segment anything in medical images. Nat Commun. 2024;15(1):654.
12. Zha D, Bhat ZP, Lai KH et al. Data-centric artificial intelligence: a survey. arXiv: 2303.10158. 2023.
13. Franco-Barranco D, Lin Z, Jang WD et al. Current progress and challenges in large-scale 3d mitochondria instance segmentation. IEEE Trans Med Imaging. 2023.
14. Zhou L, Liu H, Bae J et al. Self pre-training with masked autoencoders for medical image classification and segmentation. IEEE ISBI. 2023:1–6.
15. Wei D, Lin Z, Franco-Barranco D et al. Mitoem dataset: large-scale 3d mitochondria instance segmentation from em images. Proc MICCAI. 2020:66–76.

Improving Segmentation by Combining Preoperative CT and Intraoperative CBCT using Synthetic Data

Maximilian E. Tschuchnig[1,2], Philipp Steininger[3], Michael Gadermayr[1]

[1]Salzburg University of Applied Sciences, Applied Data Science Lab
[2]University of Salzburg, Department of Artificial Intelligence and Human Interfaces
[3]MedPhoton GmbH
maximilian.tschuchnig@fh-salzburg.ac.at

Abstract. Computer-assisted interventions enable clinicians to perform precise, minimally invasive procedures, often relying on advanced imaging methods. Cone-beam computed tomography (CBCT) can be used to facilitate computer-assisted interventions, despite often suffering from artifacts that pose challenges for accurate interpretation. While the degraded image quality can affect image analysis, the availability of high quality, preoperative scans offers potential for improvements. Here we consider a setting where preoperative CT and intraoperative CBCT scans are available, however, the alignment (registration) between the scans is imperfect to simulate a real world scenario. We propose a multimodal learning method that fuses roughly aligned CBCT and CT scans and investigate the effect on segmentation performance. For this experiment we use synthetically generated data containing real CT and synthetic CBCT volumes with corresponding voxel annotations. We show that this fusion setup improves segmentation performance in 18 out of 20 setups investigated.

1 Introduction

To establish computer-assisted interventions, precise and reliable imaging, especially intraoperative imaging, is crucial. Mobile robotic medical imaging systems, like cone-beam computed tomography (CBCT) [1], enable intraoperative medical imaging with real time capabilities. CBCT is an imaging method that utilizes a cone-shaped X-ray beam and a flat-panel detector to capture detailed, three-dimensional images of a patient's anatomy using a potentially mobile system [2]. However, using CBCT as an intraoperative imaging system often comes with the disadvantage of suffering from more artifacts than preoperative CT imaging, affecting the performance of downstream tasks like segmentation [3].

While this degraded image quality can affect medical imaging tasks, the availability of high quality preoperative scans represents potential to integrate highly detailed information based on the idea of multimodal learning [4–6]. Multimodal learning is an approach that involves fusing information from multiple domains to improve machine learning models for a downstream task like segmentation. In 3D medical imaging, a common approach is to enrich computed tomography (CT) scans, focusing on dense structures, with magnetic resonance imaging data for soft tissue analysis [4, 5]. Multimodal learning is typically separated into three fusion strategies [4, 6]: early, late and hybrid.

C. Palm et al. (Hrsg.), *Bildverarbeitung für die Medizin 2025*, Informatik aktuell,
https://doi.org/10.1007/978-3-658-47422-5_49

Early-fusion combines images of different modalities before being processed by an image processing model. Typically, the two domains are fused along a dimension additional to the spatial volume dimensions and processed jointly [4, 7]. Late-fusion merges different streams before the final layer of the downstream task and hybrid fusion combines ideas of both early and late-fusion.

We propose a method that combines CBCT with misaligned, preoperative CT scans using early-fusion to improve semantic segmentation performance. Additionally, we examine how varying CBCT quality impacts segmentation performance in both baseline and multimodal configurations.

2 Methodology

We investigate multimodal learning of intraoperative CBCT volumes and misaligned, high quality, preoperative CT volumes using early-fusion, similar to Ren et al. [7] with both scans showing approximately the same section of the body. Evaluation is performed on the CBCT liver tumor segmentation (CBCTLiTS) [8] dataset with the two different semantic segmentation targets, liver and liver tumor segmentation.

To perform segmentation we used a holistic 3D U-Net introduced by Çiçek et al. [9] as the basis of our segmentation model and our baseline for all investigated settings. The 3D U-Net was adapted to process multimodal data by adding a paired and misaligned, preoperative CT as a second channel, resulting in a 4D data structure (early fusion). The 3D U-Net used for segmentation is shown in Fig. 1 and consists of an encoder with 3 double convolution layers and $3 \times 3 \times 3$ convolutional kernels, connected by 3D max pooling. The latent space consists of one double convolution block followed by the U-Net decoder, mirroring the encoder. As is typical for U-Net, each double convolutional output in the encoder is also connected to the decoder double convolutional block of the

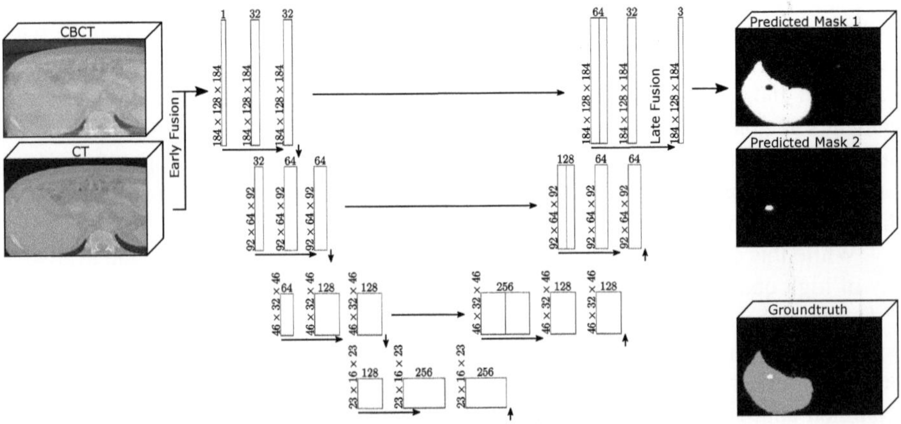

Fig. 1. Multimodal model configuration. After fusing the intraoperative CBCT and preoperative CT (early fusion), the data was processed by the shown 3D U-Net (displayed are the number of filters and filter dimensions), segmenting liver and liver tumors. The figure further shows where late fusion would be applied.

same order. Additionally, one 3D convolutional layer is added to the decoder with a filter size of $1 \times 1 \times 1$ and the number of filters set to the number of segmentation classes. The number of feature maps were set to $\{32, 64, 128, 256\}$. Batch norm was applied after each layer in the double convolutional blocks. The model was trained utilizing a sum of binary cross-entropy and Dice similarity. For our baseline, the same U-Net was used [9], with only the CBCT as input.

2.1 Data

CBCTLiTS is an addition to the well studied liver tumor segmentation (LiTS) [10] dataset. LiTS is an abdominal CT dataset with liver and liver tumor segmentations. CBCTLiTS [8] expands on that by adding perfectly aligned, synthetic CBCT volumes. Fig 2 shows exemplar CT and corresponding CBCT volumes (with the varying parameter α_{np}) of subject 28, and the provided segmentation mask.

The factor α_{np} corresponds to the undersampling of digitally reconstructed radiographs (DRRs) in the CBCT reconstruction process of CBCTLiTS. In detail, Tschuchnig et al. [8] synthetically generated CBCTLiTS by simulating digitally reconstructed radiographs (DRRs) from the LiTS CT volumes, followed by filtered backprojection to generate the CBCT scans in CBCT geometry. By adjusting undersampling based on the parameter $\alpha_{np} \in \{32, 64, 128, 256, 490\}$, the quality of the synthetic CBCT can be adapted.

Since we aim to generate a realistic evaluation scenario, we synthetically generate misalignment between the perfectly aligned CT and CBCT pairs. We further aim to reduce the number of parameters controlling misalignment to one. Misalignment is established by the factor α_a. Misalignment augmentation was performed using TorchIO RandomAffine and RandomElasticDeformation. In detail, affine misaligned was performed using random (non-isotropic) scaling, with the scaling parameter sampled from $\mathcal{U}(1-0.5\cdot\alpha_a, 1+0.5\cdot\alpha_a)$, rotation, parameters sampled from $\mathcal{U}(-22.5\cdot\alpha_a, 22.5\cdot\alpha_a)$, and translation, with the parameter sampled from $\mathcal{U}(0, 0.5\cdot\alpha_a)$ with tri-linear interpolation. Elastic misalignment was applied with a maximum displacement sampled from $\mathcal{U}(0, 20\cdot\alpha_a)$ with 7 control points and no locked borders. Fig. 3 shows 3 unprocessed volumes and examples of affine and elastic misalignment with $\alpha_a = 0.25$. Fig. 3 displays the elastic transformation in isolation from affine transformations for improved readability.

During training and validation, only affine transformations were used to streamline data loading. In testing, both affine and elastic transformations were applied for a

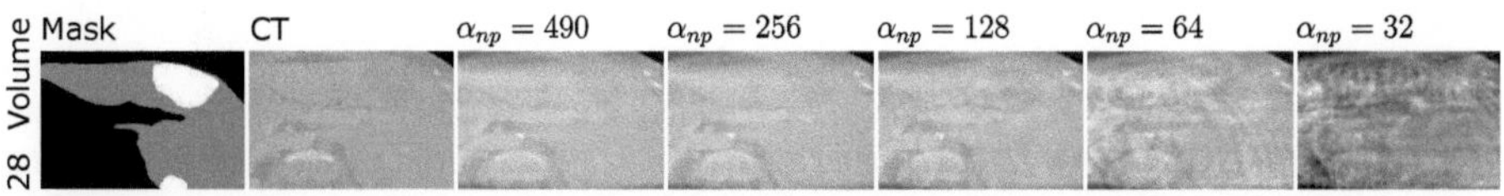

Fig. 2. Sample CBCTLiTS data (subject 28): From left to right, the segmentation mask, CT scan, and various CBCT scans are shown, with CBCT quality degraded according to the undersampling factor α_{np}.

single evaluation per sample for a more realistic evaluation. The CBCTLiTS training set contains 131 paired samples. Since the CBCTLiTS testing data lacks segmentation masks, it was excluded from this study.

2.2 Experimental details

The models were trained on a Ubuntu server using NVIDIA RTX A6000 graphics cards. Due to the large data size and 48 GB VRAM memory limit, volumes were downscaled (isotropic) by the factor of two [11]. To binarize the masks, a threshold of 0.5 was applied to each channel of the U-Net output. The data was separated into training-validation-testing data. The separation was performed using the ratios 0.7 (training), 0.2 (validation), 0.1 (testing). All experiments were trained and evaluated 4 times to facilitate stable results with the same random splits as well as the same random CT misaligned for comparable result. Adam was used as an optimizer with a learning rate of 0.005 for liver and liver tumor segmentation

3 Results

Experimental results are shown as boxplots in Fig. 4. The top row shows the results of liver and the bottom row of liver tumor segmentation. The left column shows results evaluated on affine misalignment, while the right columns show combined affine and elastic misalignment. The undersampling factor α_{np} is shown on the x axis and Dice similarity coefficients on the y axis. Blue boxes show Baseline results and green boxes the multimodal learning approach results. Additionally the mean values are plotted in the corresponding box, for easy comparison.

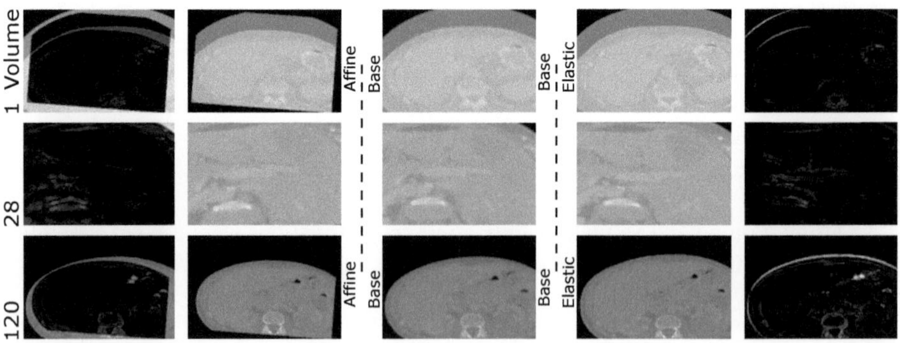

Fig. 3. Here, samples of affine and elastic misalignment are shown. Left, results of random affine augmentation (α_a = 0.25) and the corresponding absolute difference image of 3 different CBCTLiTS volumes are shown. The centered column shows the original data. Right, resulting volumes of random elastic misalignment (α_a = 0.25) of the same volumes and corresponding difference images are shown. Elastic misalignment is shown separate from affine misalignment for easier readability.

4 Discussion

The results show that enriching intraoperative CBCT with roughly aligned, preoperative CT improves medical imaging tasks like semantic segmentation. Most multimodal setups improved segmentation performance with the only exception in liver tumor segmentation with $\alpha_{np} = 490$ in the combined affine and elastic misaligned case.

Several trends are notable. First, the worse the CBCT quality, the more can be gained by adding high quality CT, leading to a maximum increase of Dice from 0.78 to 0.88 for liver and from 0.03 to 0.17 for liver tumor segmentation. This shows that adding the preoperative CT partly mitigates the decreasing image quality of the intraoperative CBCT. This also shows that there might be some implicit registration taking place, however, further experimentation with different degrees of misalignment are needed to investigate this effect further. Overall, tumor segmentation performed poorly, especially compared to liver segmentation. Qualitative evaluation shows that poor performance in these cases is mainly dependent on the visual quality of the provided CT/CBCT pairs.

Since we generate a dynamic dataset for both training and testing through the misalignment process, the misalignment itself can be seen as data augmentation. We assume that this effect can further improve the positive effect of the proposed multimodal setup however, this has to be evaluated on real, imperfectly aligned volume pairs. Furthermore,

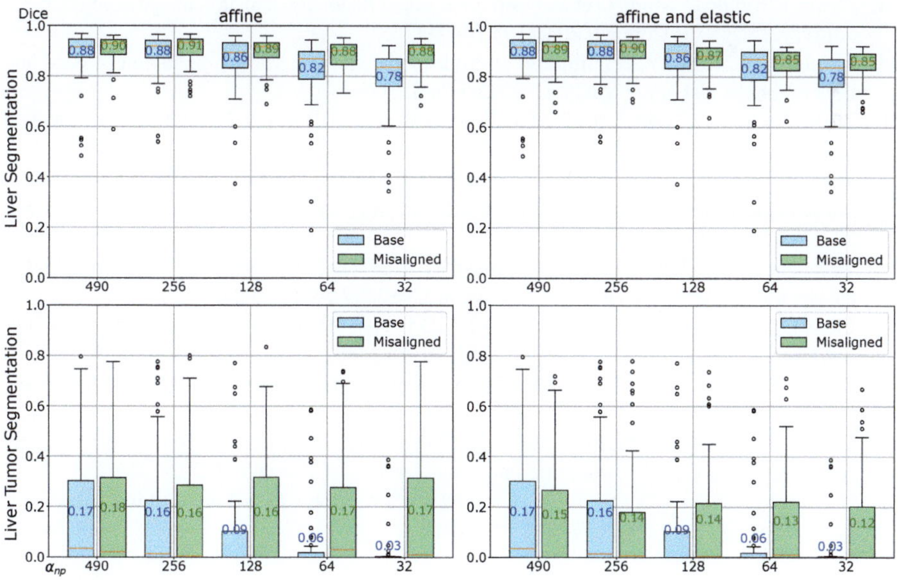

Fig. 4. Experimental results shown as boxplots. In the top row, results for liver segmentation are shown with Dice score on the y axis and the volume quality (α_{np}) on the x axis. The median is shown as an orange bar and the mean value is printed in the corresponding box. Baseline results are displayed in blue and our proposed, multimodal method in green. The bottom row shows liver tumor segmentation. In the first column, experiments were performed on affine and the second column on combined affine and elastic transformed volumes.

this form of multimodal learning is theoretically applicable to other medical imaging applications and architectures like architectures including attention [12] or to facilitate tasks like image reconstruction.

Acknowledgement. This project was partly funded by the Austrian research promotion agency (FFG) under the bridge project "CIRCUIT: Towards Comprehensive CBCT Imaging Pipelines for Real-time Acquisition, Analysis, Interaction and Visualization" (CIRCUIT), no. 41545455 and by the county of Salzburg under the project AIBIA and the Salzburg University of Applied Sciences under the project FHS-trampoline-8 (Applied Data Science Lab).

References

1. Rafferty MA, Siewerdsen JH, Chan Y et al. Intraoperative cone-beam CT for guidance of temporal bone surgery. Otolaryn Head Neck Surg. 2006;134(5):801–8.
2. Jaffray DA, Siewerdsen JH, Wong JW et al. Flat-panel cone-beam computed tomography for image-guided radiation therapy. Int J Rad Onc Biol Phys. 2002;53(5):1337–49.
3. Wei C, Albrecht J, Rit S et al. Reduction of cone-beam CT artifacts in a robotic CBCT device using saddle trajectories with integrated infrared tracking. Med Phys. 2024.
4. Zhang Y, Sidibé D, Morel O et al. Deep multimodal fusion for semantic image segmentation: a survey. Image Vis Comput. 2021;105:104042.
5. Podobnik G, Strojan P, Peterlin P et al. Multimodal CT and MR segmentation of head and neck organs-at-risk. Proc MICCAI. 2023:745–55.
6. Zhang Y, Yang J, Tian J et al. Modality-aware mutual learning for multi-modal medical image segmentation. Proc MICCAI. 2021:589–99.
7. Ren J, Eriksen JG, Nijkamp J et al. Comparing different CT, PET and MRI multi-modality image combinations for deep learning-based head and neck tumor segmentation. Acta Oncol. 2021;60(11):1399–406.
8. Tschuchnig ME, Steininger P, Gadermayr M. CBCTLiTS: a synthetic, paired CBCT/CT dataset for segmentation and style transfer. arXiv: 2407.14853. 2024.
9. Çiçek Ö, Abdulkadir A, Lienkamp SS et al. 3D U-Net: learning dense volumetric segmentation from sparse annotation. Proc MICCAI. 2016:424–32.
10. Bilic P, Christ P, Li H et al. The liver tumor segmentation benchmark (LiTS). Med Image Anal. 2023;84.
11. Tschuchnig ME, Coste-Marin J, Steininger P et al. Multi-task learning to improve semantic segmentation of CBCT scans using image reconstruction. Proc BVM. 2024:243–8.
12. Hatamizadeh A, Tang Y, Nath V et al. UNETR: transformers for 3D medical image segmentation. Proc IEEE CVF WACV. 2022:574–84.

Automatic Thyroid Scintigram Segmentation using U-Net

Moritz A. Mau, Marius Krusen, Floris Ernst

Institut für Robotik und Kognitive Systeme, Universität zu Lübeck
ma.krusen@uni-luebeck.de

Abstract. Thyroid scintigraphy is an important tool to determine thyroid function and pathologies. The manual segmentation of these images is a time-intensive and error-prone task required to evaluate the scintigram. In this paper, a 5-layer U-Net is presented that automatically detects and evaluates thyroids in scintigrams by segmenting the left and right lobe and calculating the uptake used for diagnosis. The dataset used to train the network contains 2 734 different thyroid scintigrams collected over the course of four years from a medical office. The network reaches a median Dice score of 0.921 for the thyroid lobes and 0.937 for the complete thyroid, while maintaining a median difference of $3.520\,\text{cm}^2$ for the size of the thyroid and 0.029 percentage points for the uptake. Overall, the trained network has the potential to speed up the diagnostic process, while improving the consistency and accuracy of medical diagnoses of thyroid scintigrams.

1 Introduction

The thyroid is an endocrine gland in the anterior neck, which produces and stores hormones in a greater quantity [1]. It is composed of two lobes that have an elliptical appearance (Fig. 1, top left). Thyroid disorders are one of the most common types of endocrine diseases. While typically easily treatable, they can substantially impact well-being and lead to significant complications if undiagnosed [2]. Widespread testing and accurate diagnosis therefore play a critical role in decreasing the economical and health impact of thyroid diseases.

Various imaging modalities are used to examine and evaluate thyroid diseases. Ultrasonography is the cost-effective first choice modality for diagnosis, while cross-sectional imaging modalities, like computed tomography (CT) and magnetic resonance imaging (MRI), can be used for additional evaluation, in particular for tumor staging. Radionuclide scintigraphy plays a critical role in analyzing functional information about the thyroid gland by recording the radiation emitted by a previously injected tracer, typically ^{99m}Technetium (^{99m}Tc) pertechnetate. A common use-case for this is the classification of thyroid nodules as hot, warm or cold based on the relative uptake of the nodule [3].

Evaluation of these images is a time-intensive task and prone to errors due to subtle details and the subjectivity of the medical assistant. Thyroid scintigrams in particular are typically segmented by manually placing regions of interest (ROIs) around both thyroid lobes. Using these ROIs, the ^{99m}Tc thyroid uptake (TcTU) can be calculated, which describes the percentage of ^{99m}Tc that the thyroid absorbs and is an important indicator for thyroid function. The high inter- and intraobserver variability of manually segmenting these scintigrams can affect the resulting uptake calculation and therefore the diagnosis of the physician.

C. Palm et al. (Hrsg.), *Bildverarbeitung für die Medizin 2025*, Informatik aktuell,
https://doi.org/10.1007/978-3-658-47422-5_50

In recent years, deep learning-based approaches have shown great potential in automating this evaluation across all imaging modalities to reduce the workload of the physician and increase the accuracy of pathology detection and classification [4, 5]. Compared to traditional image analysis methods, these approaches are more robust to noise and adapt better to problematic data, like one-sided or low uptake thyroids. For thyroid scintigraphy specifically, there have been a number of deep learning approaches to automate the diagnosis of different pathologies based on scintigraphy images [5–7].

In this work, a deep learning approach is presented, which automatically segments the thyroid lobes in a thyroid scintigram using a U-Net architecture and allows subsequent uptake calculation without intervention by a medical assistant. For this purpose, the segmentations and resulting uptake values are compared to the ground truth data labeled by medical assistants. The resulting approach has the potential to speed up the evaluation process significantly and makes it more consistent while avoiding the ethical and social challenges of fully automatic diagnoses.

2 Materials and methods

The dataset consists of 2 734 ^{99m}Tc pertechnetate scans from 2 388 different patients taken in a single medical office over the course of four years (August 2019 until August 2023). Around 79 % of the patients were female and around 21 % male. The mean age is 58.89 ± 14.40 years, ranging from 18 to 95 years. Each scan consists of an unprocessed and a processed thyroid scintigram stored in the DICOM format. The unprocessed scintigrams are images of 128 × 128 pixels and represent the input for the U-Net. The processed scintigrams were created by different medical assistants and were used for diagnosis and treatment planning. They contain an outline of the right and left lobe of the thyroid, as well as additional diagnostic information, like the calculated TcTU. The differentiation between left and right lobe is not crucial but can assist the physician in recognizing asymmetries in thyroid function. From this data, one-hot encoded ground truth segmentation maps of the same size as the input were created with three channels for the three labels right lobe, left lobe and background. Additionally, the ground truth TcTU was extracted from the processed scintigram to compare with the TcTU calculation based on the U-Net segmentation. The average TcTU across the whole dataset is 1.02 % ± 1.18 % and the average ROI size is 21.40 cm^2 ± 8.12 cm^2, with the ROIs of female patients being an average of 4.65 cm^2 smaller than that of male patients.

The final dataset was divided into 3 subsets for training, validation and evaluation. 100 samples were held back for validation and the remaining data was split into 75 % for training and 25 % for evaluation. Segmentation is done using a U-Net [8]. With its U-shaped structure and skip-connections between the contracting and expansive path to preserve spatial information, it is specifically designed for biomedical segmentation tasks. The used architecture is 5 layers deep, with padding after each convolution layer, leading to a 8 × 8 resolution with 1 024 channels after the contracting path (Fig. 1). The activation function used throughout the network is ReLU. To mitigate the class imbalance caused by the large backgrounds, weighted cross entropy loss was chosen as the loss function, with the weights being the inverse of the total number of samples per class in the training subset. Training was done with the PyTorch framework using the

Adam optimizer [9] with an initial learning rate of 0.001 in combination with a step learning rate scheduler decaying the learning rate with a factor of 0.9 every 25 epochs. The batch size was set to 128. The model with the lowest loss on the validation subset over 1 000 epochs was chosen as the best model.

The resulting model was evaluated on the evaluation subset using different metrics. First, the Dice scores for the segmentation of the left and right lobe were calculated individually. The average of both scores gives the total Dice score. In addition, the Dice score of the full thyroid segmentation, without distinguishing left and right lobe, was determined by combining both segmentations and treating them as a single class.

Apart from the Dice score, the TcTU was calculated based on the ROI provided by the segmentation of the model and the equation

$$\mathrm{TcTU} = \frac{n}{A \cdot t \cdot \eta} \tag{1}$$

where A is the applied activity, t is the acquisition frame duration and η is the efficiency, all of which were extracted from the corresponding DICOM file. n is the number of impulses from the thyroid in the scintigram, which can be calculated by subtracting the average background radiation across the ROI from the total activity inside the ROI. This uptake was compared to the same calculation done on the ground truth segmentation and the mean absolute error is reported.

Finally, the size differences between the predicted and actual thyroid lobes were evaluated.

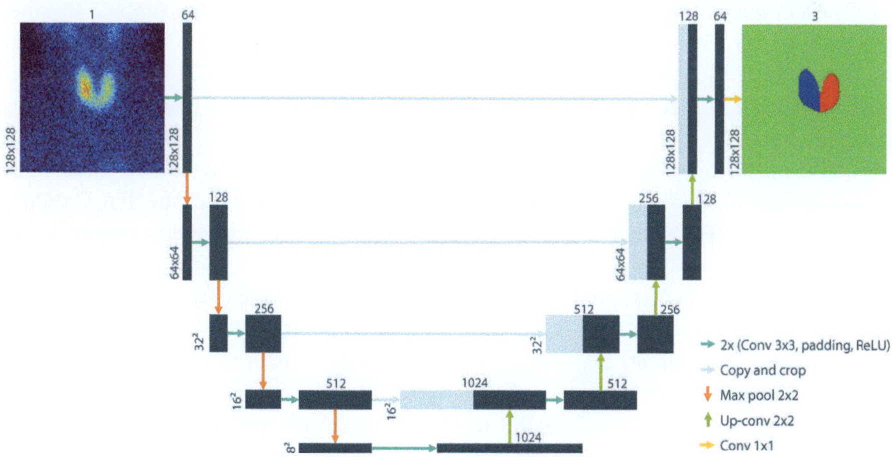

Fig. 1. Diagram of the used U-Net architecture with example input and output. The input image in the top left is a thyroid scintigram as produced by the gamma camera, with the horseshoe shaped thyroid in the center. Each blue box in the following U-Net represents a multi-channel feature map, with the number of channels indicated on top. The x-y-size of the image is provided on the lower-left edge. The light blue boxes signify copied feature maps and the arrows indicate various operations as denoted in the bottom right. In the top right is the output mask generated by the U-Net.

3 Results

The mean Dice scores for the segmentation of the left and right lobe are 0.882 ± 0.135 and 0.877 ± 0.151, respectively, for an overall Dice score of 0.879 ± 0.129. The full distribution (Fig. 2a) shows the majority of Dice scores above 0.85 and a few outliers with some scores as low as 0. The median of 0.921 is therefore even higher than the mean. Combining both classes and looking at it as a single-class segmentation results in a Dice score of 0.907 ± 0.097 with a median of 0.937 instead.

The mean error of the TcTU resulting from the segmentation is 0.051 percentage points (pp) $\pm$ 0.076 pp, the left lobe contributing an average of 0.029 pp and the right lobe 0.033 pp. The median error is 0.029 pp (Fig. 2b). For the size, the mean error of the left lobe of $1.762\,cm^2$ is also marginally smaller than the right one of $1.945\,cm^2$. The mean error of the total size is $3.520\,cm^2 \pm 3.692\,cm^2$ and the median is $2.475\,cm^2$ (Fig. 2c).

4 Discussion

The segmentations of the U-Net achieve a high median Dice score of 0.921. The average is a bit lower due to some outliers with Dice scores as low as 0. These particular cases happen when there is only one of the two lobes visible in the scintigram and the network and ground truth disagree which of the two it is (Fig. 2g). Most commonly the ground truth is incorrect due to human mistakes. Evaluating the segmentation as a single class reduces the impact of these outliers, increasing the median Dice score to 0.937.

The comparatively larger ROI size errors are mainly due to low-uptake thyroids (Fig. 2e and 2f). These thyroids show barely any discernible structures in the scintigram because less ^{99m}Tc gathers in the thyroid or has already decayed. This makes it more difficult for the U-Net but also for the medical assistant labeling the ground truth to segment correctly. The result can be large discrepancies between network output and ground truth for these scintigrams. However, the TcTU error is much less affected by this since the TcTU is very low in these cases either way. The error of the diagnostically more relevant TcTU is very low in general and highlights the promising results of this approach.

As seen in previous examples, the ground truth labels of the dataset are not without mistakes. While samples with incomplete or incorrect labels were filtered out ahead of time, there remains an uncertainty for some samples caused by human error and interobserver variability. This can affect the final U-Net during training, but especially during evaluation this can cause the results to seem less accurate than they are in reality. Human errors in this process can be caused by stress, fatigue, inexperience or other factors and are unavoidable. These errors also highlight the need for an automatic segmentation of thyroid scintigrams that is not affected by these factors.

The network gives consistent results and eliminates the inter- and intraobserver variability of manual segmentation. Another advantage of this approach is the speed. While a medical assistant could take up to several minutes to place the ROIs on a scintigram, the U-Net takes less than a second to create a segmentation, allowing for a much higher throughput.

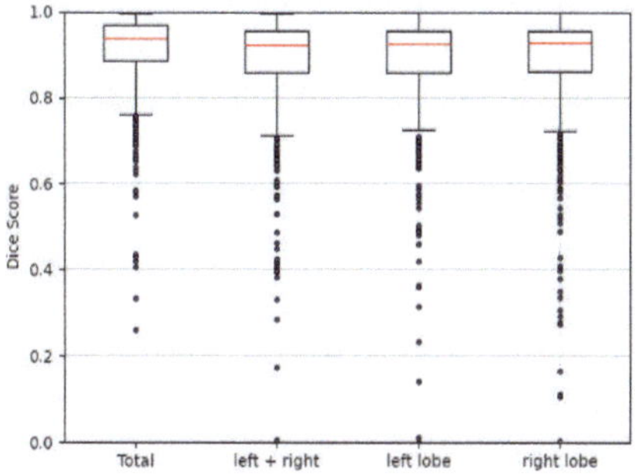

(a) Dice scores.

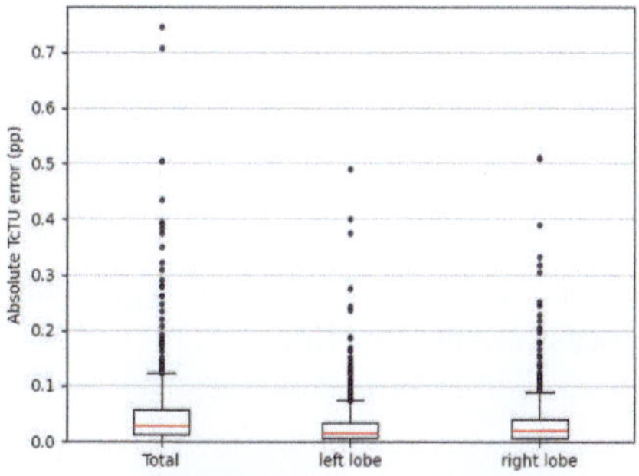

(b) Absolute TcTU errors.

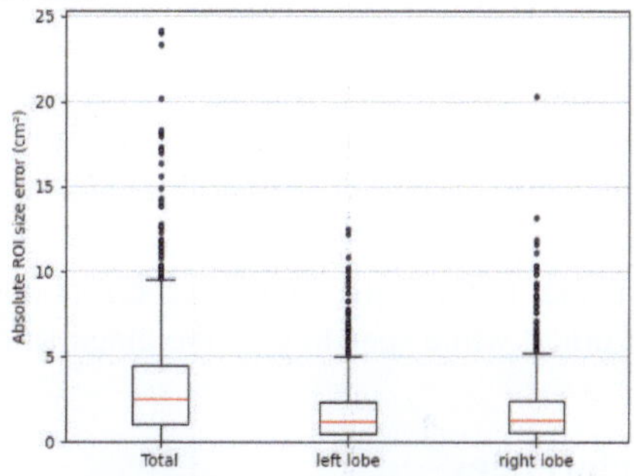

(c) Absolute ROI size errors.

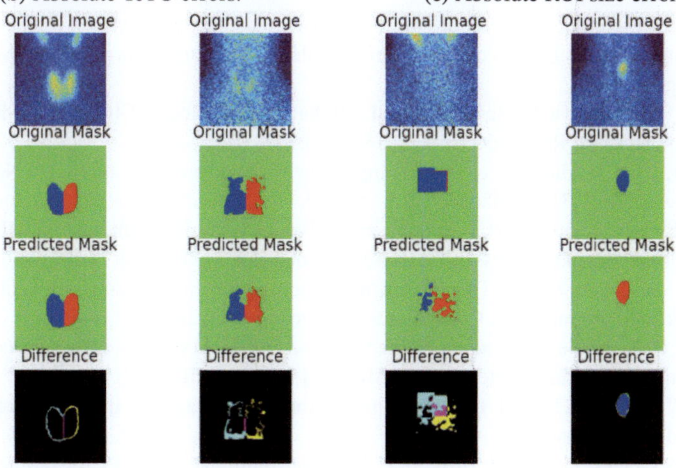

(d) Dice: 0.906. **(e)** Dice: 0.828. **(f)** Dice: 0.151. **(g)** Dice: 0.0.

Fig. 2. Boxplots of the Dice scores (a), absolute TcTU errors (b) and absolute ROI size errors (c). For the Dice scores, "Total" shows the single-class scores, while "left + right" is the average of the left and right lobe scores. For the other two plots, first the results of the total ROI are displayed, followed by the specific results of the left and right lobe. (d) - (g) shows four example scintigrams, their ground truth segmentation, the U-Net segmentation and the difference between both.

Due to the nature of the approach, the medical and ethical risks of it are low. The U-Net does not induce a bias in the medical assistant by providing an automatic diagnosis, but instead simply assists the medical assistant in the time-intensive segmentation of scintigrams and makes it more consistent and accurate. The diagnosis and decision about further treatment is still up to the physician who has much more context and other modalities available, like ultrasound images or blood values. This not only avoids many ethical and regulatory challenges, but also lowers concerns of physicians and increases adoption rate.

A current limitation is the dataset. While the number of samples is large, they only come from a single medical office. A larger dataset incorporating data from multiple offices using different hardware, as well as data from different regions could further improve generalization, considering the variations in iodine sufficiency around the world. Additionally, having multiple expert opinions for many of the scintigrams would reduce the risk of mistakes in the ground truth. This would improve accuracy during training, but would especially allow for the creation of a properly validated evaluation subset.

All in all, the goal of training a network to automatically detect and evaluate thyroids in scintigrams using a U-Net is possible and quite accurate. This could increase the evaluation speed substantially, without quality loss or displacing the physician from the process, taking a time-intensive burden from the physician. The approach has the potential to minimize diagnostic errors due to increased consistency and segmentation accuracy, while speeding up the diagnostic process at the same time.

References

1. Dietlein M, Kopka K, Schmidt M, eds. Nuklearmedizin: Basiswissen und klinische Anwendung. 9., aktualisierte und erweiterte Auflage. Stuttgart: Georg Thieme Verlag, 2024. 1549 pp.
2. Taylor PN, Albrecht D, Scholz A et al. Global epidemiology of hyperthyroidism and hypothyroidism. Nat Rev Endocrinol. 2018;14(5):301–16.
3. Calle S, Choi J, Ahmed S et al. Imaging of the thyroid: practical approach. Neuroimaging Clin N Am. 2021;31(3):265–84.
4. Yu Q, Jiang T, Zhou A et al. Computer-aided diagnosis of malignant or benign thyroid nodes based on ultrasound images. Eur Arch Otorhinolaryngol. 2017;274(7):2891–7.
5. Ma L, Ma C, Liu Y et al. Thyroid diagnosis from spect images using convolutional neural network with optimization. Comput Intell Neurosci. 2019;2019:1–11.
6. Yang P, Pi Y, He T et al. Automatic differentiation of thyroid scintigram by deep convolutional neural network: a dual center study. BMC Med Imaging. 2021;21(1).
7. Qiao T, Liu S, Cui Z et al. Deep learning for intelligent diagnosis in thyroid scintigraphy. J Int Med Res. 2021;49(1).
8. Ronneberger O, Fischer P, Brox T. U-Net: convolutional networks for biomedical image segmentation. Proc MICCAI. 2015:234–41.
9. Kingma DP, Ba J. Adam: a method for stochastic optimization. Proc ICLR. 2014.

Coronary Tree Segmentation and Labelling in X-ray Angiography Images Using Graph Deep Learning

Robin Gayet[1,2], Alaa Abd El Al[2,3], Alexander Meyer[2,3], Anja Hennemuth[1,2,4,5], Matthias Ivantsits[1,2], Antonia Popp[1,2,3]

[1]Institute of Computer-Assisted Cardiovascular Medicine, Deutsches Herzzentrum der Charité, Berlin, Germany
[2]Charité – Universitätsmedizin Berlin, corporate member of Freie Universität Berlin, Humboldt-Universität zu Berlin, and Berlin Institute of Health, Berlin, Germany
[3]Department of Cardiothoracic and Vascular Surgery, Deutsches Herzzentrum der Charité, Berlin, Germany
[4]German Centre for Cardiovascular Research (DZHK), partner site Berlin, Germany
[5]Fraunhofer Institute for Digital Medicine MEVIS, Berlin, Germany
antonia.popp@dhzc-charite.de

Abstract. The significant impact of coronary artery disease on cardiovascular health underscores the need for precise diagnostic methods. The SYNTAX score, based on the locations of stenoses in the coronary tree, provides a quantitative estimation of the disease's complexity, allowing to settle on a treatment strategy. However, expert experience is required for visual localization of stenoses, which would be facilitated by automated labelling of the coronary segments. In this work we represent the connected structure of the coronary tree as a graph, extracted from the angiography image, onto which we apply a graph convolutional network to label the coronary segments according to the SYNTAX score scheme, before creating a multi-class segmentation mask. The method was trained and evaluated using the ARCADE dataset. The segment classification of graph nodes reached an F1-score of 53.68. Our approach achieved a mean F1-score of 45.43 for multi-class segmentation of the image after applying the entire pipeline. Although a baseline nnU-Net model achieves better performance (mean F1-score of 62.53), the results are comparable to other existing approaches and show that graph-based approaches are suitable for the complex task of coronary segment labelling.

1 Introduction

Coronary artery disease (CAD) results from the narrowing of the coronary arteries through atherosclerotic plaque and is a major cause of death [1, 2]. The disease is commonly diagnosed using X-ray coronary angiography (XCA), where the vessel tree is visualized with x-rays during the injection of contrast agent [3]. The best treatment strategy is determined by estimating the CAD complexity using the SYNTAX score methodology [4]. The score is based mainly on the location of stenoses in the coronary tree. To this end, the tree is divided into 25 segments: 17 segments specific to the left and 8 segments to the right coronary artery branch (LCA/RCA). However, since visual assessment of XCA remains a difficult task, automated segmentation and labelling of the coronary arteries would facilitate the interpretation of CAD in XCA images.

C. Palm et al. (Hrsg.), *Bildverarbeitung für die Medizin 2025*, Informatik aktuell,
https://doi.org/10.1007/978-3-658-47422-5_51

In recent years, convolutional neural networks (CNNs) have established as the most popular and best working method for coronary artery segmentation [5]. Several works have been published using CNN-based architectures for automated binary segmentation of coronary vessels in XCA images reaching F1-scores between 82.23 and 86.40 after evaluation on various datasets [6, 7]. The recently published ARCADE dataset with labelled coronary artery segments is a benchmark for the development of models for multi-class segmentation in XCA images [8]. As part of the ARCADE challenge several approaches have been provided using ensemble methods and reaching F1-scores between 42.89 and 44.40 [9, 10]. Labrecque Langlais et al. proposed a 6-algorithm pipeline to estimate the segment and severity of stenoses in XCA images. Their segmentation algorithm labelled only the 11 most present segments and reached an F1-score of 73.39 using the ARCADE dataset [11].

However, the described approaches are based on CNNs and operate on pixel level disregarding the particular topology of the vessel tree. This geometric information can be stored in a graph structure where nodes represent start and end points, bifurcations and samples along the vessel centerline, and are connected by edges to represent the relationship between tree branches. Graph neural networks (GNNs) have only rarely been investigated for coronary segment labelling in 3D coronary CT angiography (CCTA). Hampe et al. propose an approach based on graph attention layers for segment labelling in CCTA volumes [12]. In the semi-automatically extracted vessel graphs each node represents one segment of the coronary tree and contains various geometrical features such as coordinates, radius and tree direction, while edges represent the connectivity between segments. The classification of the graph nodes into 10 segments resulted in an F1-score of 92.40, proving the ability of GNNs to correctly label coronary segments.

So far there are no attempts to investigate GNNs for coronary segment labelling in XCA images. In this work we extract a graph representing the vessel structure shown in XCA images and apply a graph convolutional network (GCN) [13] to label the respective segments by classifying the graph nodes.

2 Materials and methods

Our proposed multi-step method is composed as follows (Fig. 1): First, image classification as showing left or right coronary artery (LCA/RCA) and binary vessel segmentation is performed. The subsequent graph extraction step is decomposed into centerline extraction from the binary mask, followed by the extraction of a graph from the centerline, whose nodes are classified by a GCN according to the SYNTAX score methodology. Finally, a multi-class mask of the coronary artery is obtained by labelling the pixels of the binary mask with the segment class of the associated graph node.

2.1 Data

To fine-tune and evaluate our method we used the ARCADE dataset [8], containing XCA images of 512×512 pixels and their respective multi-class segmentation masks. 959 images represent an LCA branch while the other 541 show an RCA branch. The 25 classes for the coronary segments are distributed as follows among the images: Right coronary artery proximal (540), medial (541), distal (535), posterior descending (451), posterolateral 1 (375), posterolateral 2 (80), posterolateral 3 (87), posterolateral 4 (72), left main (850), left anterior descending proximal (850), medial (500), apical (464), first diagonal (314), add. first diagonal (130), second diagonal (56), add. second diagonal (7), intermediate (93), left circumflex proximal (509), obtuse marginal 1 (179), obtuse marginal 2 (130), distal circumflex (485), left posterolateral 1 (194), left posterolateral 2 (100), left posterolateral 3 (222) and left posterior descending (52).

To fine-tune and evaluate the single models we extended the labels of the ARCADE dataset. For LCA/RCA classification and vessel segmentation, each image was labelled according to the classes present in the respective mask and associated with a binary mask without specific segment labels. For the node classification model, a graph dataset was created by defining positions along the vessel centerline as graph nodes, whose labels are determined according to the corresponding annotation in the multi-label mask.

2.2 Method

2.2.1 LCA/RCA classification. Similar to [9], we trained the YOLOv11m-cls[1] model for LCA/RCA classification using a learning rate of 10^{-2}, the stochastic gradient descent optimizer and the default loss function.

2.2.2 Binary segmentation. For binary vessel segmentation we applied the nnU-Net model [14], a well performing state-of-the-art model in image segmentation which automatically adapts to unseen datasets.

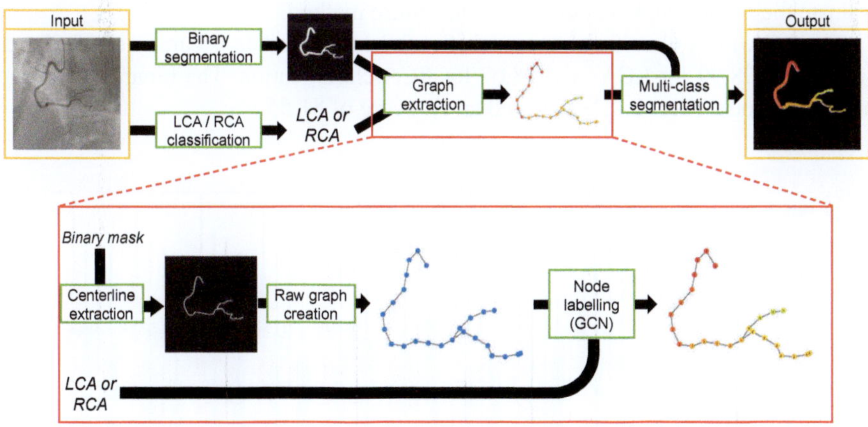

Fig. 1. Our proposed workflow: vessel segmentation of the XCA input image and LCA/RCA classification, graph creation and segment labelling, and pixel labelling in the binary mask. The graph creation consists of vessel centerline extraction, graph definition and node classification using a GCN [13].

[1] ttps://github.com/ultralytics/ultralytics

2.2.3 Graph extraction. The vessel centerline is extracted from the binary vessel mask using Lee's skeletonization algorithm [15] and applying a connected component analysis to keep the largest structure. A graph is created by defining positions along the centerline as nodes, storing their coordinates as features and connecting neighboring nodes with edges. A GCN model [13], provided by the Pytorch Geometric library, is applied to classify the coronary segment depicted by each node. In such a model, one layer allows to aggregate in each node the features of the neighboring nodes. Hence, successive layers yield a larger receptive field. To consider the left/right branch separation in the node-segment assignment, we pursued two approaches in addition to the baseline model: appending an additional node feature depicting the artery branch represented by the graph, and using two separate models for LCA and RCA graphs. The GCN models were trained using the cross-entropy loss, a learning rate of 10^{-3} and the Adam optimizer. After evaluating different parameter settings, the number of features in each hidden layers was set to 20 for every model.

2.2.4 Multi-class segmentation. A region-growing algorithm is applied to label the pixels in the binary vessel mask according to the node classification (Sec. 2.2.2). The positions of the classified graph nodes are considered as seed points and the surrounding pixels are assigned with the respective segment labels by successive dilations of the seed points until all vessel pixels are labelled, resulting in a multi-label segmentation mask.

3 Results

We used 1,000 samples of the ARCADE dataset (Sec. 2.1) for training and 200 for validation of the models of our workflow. The remaining 300 test cases were used to evaluate the models and the outcome of the entire method.

The LCA/RCA classification model (Sec.2.2.1) reached an accuracy of 98.67, and F1-score of 98.99 for LCA- and 98.67 for RCA-classification. The binary vessel segmentation model (Sec. 2.2.2) achieved an F1-score of 81.55.

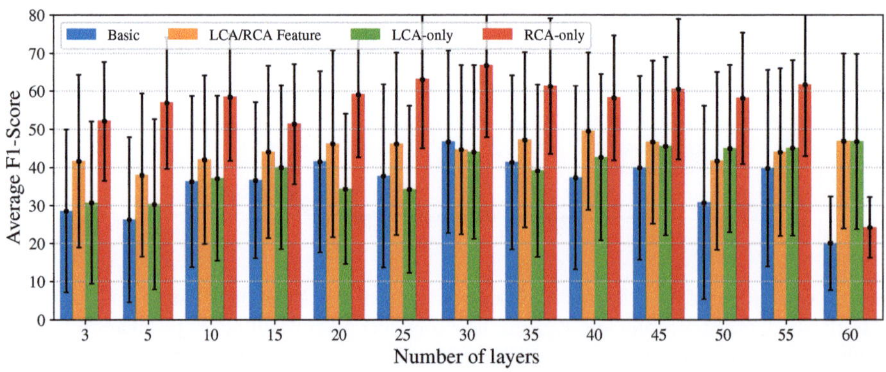

Fig. 2. Average F1-scores and the associated standard deviations with respect to the number of layers in the GCN for graph node classification.

Given that the number of layers in a GCN is directly correlated with its receptive field (Sec. 2.2.3), we investigated the influence of this parameter. Experiments with varying number of hidden layers do not show significant differences if the number of layers is between 10 and 55 (Fig. 2). Based on the respective outcomes, the number of layers were set to 30 for the baseline GCN, 40 for the model with branch feature, 60 for the LCA and 30 for the RCA model. The baseline model, the branch feature model and the combined LCA/RCA models reached F1-scores of 46.71, 49.52 and 53.68 (LCA model: 46.80, RCA model: 66.83).

The evaluation of the multi-class segmentation as outcome of the entire pipeline resulted in F1-scores of 40.44, 41.94 and 45.43 for the basic, LCA/RCA feature and LCA/RCA separate models. For direct comparison an nnU-Net model [14] was trained for multi-class segmentation and achieved an F1-score of 62.53.

4 Discussion

Coronary tree segmentation and segment labelling in XCA images are complex tasks and performance highly depends on the available groundtruth (Fig. 3). Binary vessel segmentation is a prerequisite for successful labelling of the coronary segments (Sec. 2.1). Regarding the vessel segmentation examples shown in Fig. 3, the main segments are detected correctly while smaller segments are missed or detected despite missing annotation in the groundtruth.

In our method, the bottleneck in terms of performance is the graph node classification for segment labelling. Indeed, an nnU-Net model trained for multi-class segmentation achieved better results. Nevertheless, the use of GCNs for coronary segment labelling is a novel approach and might easily benefit from other improvements. For instance, we showed that including enhanced information, such as LCA/RCA classification, improved the results (Fig. 2). Changing the node sampling rate or adding more node features such

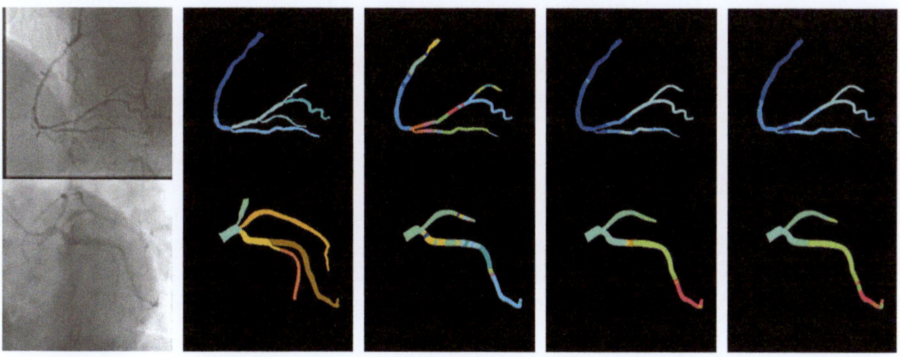

(a) (b) (c) (d) (e)

Fig. 3. (a) Input image; (b) Groundtruth; (c) Basic GCN model; (d) LCA/RCA feature GCN model; (e) LCA/RCA separate models. The segment labelling of the RCA branch (top) is more successful than the segmentation of the more complex LCA branch (bottom).

as local vessel diameter or curvature will be investigated in future work. The number of GCN layers only had a minor impact on the results (Fig. 2). The high class imbalance of segments in the dataset (Sec. 2.1) complicates the training process. The method of Labrecque Langlais et al. [11] surpasses our method using the same dataset, but included only 11 main segments for training and evaluation. Compared to other approaches based on the ARCADE dataset [9, 10], our method achieves comparable results, however, the evaluation methods slightly differ. GCN-based methods yield comparable results for the complex task of coronary segment labelling and encourage further experiments using enhanced features.

References

1. Malakar AK, Choudhury D, Halder B et al. A review on coronary artery disease, its risk factors, and therapeutics. J Cell Physiol. 2019;234(10):16812–23.
2. McCullough PA. Coronary artery disease. Clin J Am Soc Nephrol. 2007;2(3):611–6.
3. Athanasiou LS, Fotiadis DI, Michalis LK. Atherosclerotic plaque characterization methods based on coronary imaging. Academic Press, 2017.
4. Sianos G, Morel MA, Kappetein AP et al. The SYNTAX score: an angiographic tool grading the complexity of coronary artery disease. EuroIntervention. 2005;1(2):219–27.
5. Gharleghi R, Chen N, Sowmya A et al. Towards automated coronary artery segmentation: A systematic review. Comput Methods Programs Biomed. 2022;225:107015.
6. Iyer K, Najarian CP, Fattah AA et al. AngioNet: A convolutional neural network for vessel segmentation in X-ray angiography. Sci Rep. 2021;11(1):18066.
7. Li S, Fan Y. Coronary artery segmentation in X-ray angiography based on deep learning approach. Proc CCC. 2024:7345–50.
8. Popov M, Amanturdieva A, Zhaksylyk N et al. Dataset for automatic region-based coronary artery disease diagnostics using X-ray angiography images. Sci Data. 2024;11(1):20.
9. Ku J, Lee YH, Shin J et al. MPSeg : multi-phase strategy for coronary artery segmentation. arXiv: 2311.10306. 2023.
10. Liu T, Lin H, Katsaggelos AK et al. YOLO-Angio: an algorithm for coronary anatomy segmentation. arXiv: 2310.15898. 2023.
11. Labrecque Langlais É, Corbin D, Tastet O et al. Evaluation of stenoses using AI video models applied to coronary angiography. Digit Med. 2024;7(1):138.
12. Hampe N, Wolterink JM, Collet C et al. Graph attention networks for segment labeling in coronary artery trees. Proc SPIE. 2021;11596:410–6.
13. Kipf TN, Welling M. Semi-supervised classification with graph convolutional networks. arXiv: 1609.02907. 2017.
14. Isensee F, Jaeger PF, Kohl SA et al. nnU-Net: a self-configuring method for deep learning-based biomedical image segmentation. Nat Methods. 2021;18(2):203–11.
15. Lee TC, Kashyap RL, Chu CN. Building skeleton models via 3-D medial surface axis thinning algorithms. CVGIP: Graphical Models and Image Processing. 1994;56(6):462–78.

Abstract: Skeleton Recall Loss

Connectivity Conserving and Resource Efficient Segmentation of Thin Tubular Structures

Yannick Kirchhoff[1,2,3], Maximilian R. Rokuss[1,2], Saikat Roy[1,2], Balint Kovacs[1,4], Constantin Ulrich[1,4], Tassilo Wald[1,2,5], Maximilian Zenk[1,4], Philipp Vollmuth[1,6,7], Jens Kleesiek[8,9], Fabian Isensee[1,5], Klaus Maier-Hein[1,10]

[1]German Cancer Research Center (DKFZ) Heidelberg, Division of Medical Image Computing, Germany
[2]Faculty of Mathematics and Computer Science, Heidelberg University, Germany
[3]HIDSS4Health - Helmholtz Information and Data Science School for Health, Karlsruhe/Heidelberg, Germany
[4]Medical Faculty Heidelberg, Heidelberg University, Heidelberg, Germany
[5]Helmholtz Imaging, German Cancer Research Center, Heidelberg, Germany
[6]Division for Computational Radiology Clinical AI (CCIBonn.ai), Clinic for Neuroradiology, University Hospital Bonn, Bonn, Germany
[7]Medical Faculty Bonn, University of Bonn, Bonn, Germany
[8]Institute for Artificial Intelligence in Medicine (IKIM), University Hospital Essen, Essen, Germany
[9]Cancer Research Center Cologne Essen (CCCE), West German Cancer Center Essen, University Hospital Essen, Essen, Germany
[10]Pattern Analysis and Learning Group, Department of Radiation Oncology, Heidelberg University Hospital

yannick.kirchhoff@dkfz-heidelberg.de

Accurate segmentation of thin tubular structures - e.g., vessels, nerves or roads - is crucial in computer vision. Standard segmentation loss functions, like dice or cross-entropy, focus on volumetric overlap, often neglecting structural connectivity or topology. This can lead to segmentation errors affecting tasks such as flow calculation, navigation, and structural inspection. While topology-focused losses improve results, they often introduce significant computational and memory overheads, making them infeasible for larger volumes as well as multi-class problem. To address this, we propose a novel skeleton recall loss [1], which circumvents intensive GPU-based calculations using inexpensive CPU operations. It outperforms state-of-the-art methods on five public datasets for topology-preserving segmentation, reducing computational overheads by over 90%. Our code is available at GitHub[1].

References

1. Kirchhoff Y, Rokuss MR, Roy S et al. Skeleton recall loss for connectivity conserving and resource efficient segmentation of thin tubular structures. Proc ECCV. 2024:218–34.

[1]https://github.com/MIC-DKFZ/Skeleton-Recall

C. Palm et al. (Hrsg.), *Bildverarbeitung für die Medizin 2025*, Informatik aktuell,
https://doi.org/10.1007/978-3-658-47422-5_52

Unified Framework for Foreground and Anonymization Area Segmentation in CT and MRI Data

Michal Nohel[1,2,3], Constantin Ulrich[1,4,5], Jonathan Suprijadi[1], Tassilo Wald[1,7], Klaus Maier-Hein[1,5,6,7]

[1]German Cancer Research Center (DKFZ), Heidelberg, Division of Medical Image Computing, Germany
[2]Department of Biomedical Engineering, Faculty of Electrical Engineering and Communication, Brno University of Technology, Brno, Czech Republic
[3]University hospital Ostrava, Department of Deputy director for science, research and education
[4]National Center for Tumor Diseases (NCT), NCT Heidelberg, A partnership between DKFZ and University Medical Center Heidelberg
[5]Medical Faculty Heidelberg, University of Heidelberg, Heidelberg, Germany
[6]Pattern Analysis and Learning Group, Department of Radiation Oncology, Heidelberg University Hospital, Heidelberg, Germany
[7]Faculty of Mathematics and Computer Science, Heidelberg University, Germany
constantin.ulrich@dkfz-heidelberg.de

Abstract. This study presents an open-source toolkit to address critical challenges in preprocessing data for self-supervised learning (SSL) for 3D medical imaging, focusing on data privacy and computational efficiency. The toolkit comprises two main components: a segmentation network that delineates foreground regions to optimize data sampling and thus reduce training time, and a segmentation network that identifies anonymized regions, preventing erroneous supervision in reconstruction-based SSL methods. Experimental results demonstrate high robustness, with mean Dice scores exceeding 98.5 across all anonymization methods and surpassing 99.5 for foreground segmentation tasks, highlighting the toolkit's efficacy in supporting SSL applications in 3D medical imaging for both CT and MRI images. The weights and code is available at `https://github.com/MIC-DKFZ/Foreground-and-Anonymization-Area-Segmentation`.

1 Introduction

Deep learning has achieved remarkable success in medical image analysis. Groundbreaking work in segmentation has greatly enhanced treatment planning and monitoring outcomes [1–3], while advances in detection models have improved diagnostic [4]. Despite these advancements, progress in deep learning for medical imaging remains constrained by the scarcity of annotated data, which is essential for training robust models. Self-supervised learning (SSL) offers a solution to this challenge by leveraging vast amounts of unannotated medical images, thus potentially improving all downstream tasks. However, there are two critical limitations hindering the effective use of unannotated medical data within the community.

Firstly, a lot of volume in 3D medical images contains air, which increases training inefficiencies when sampled compared to traditional 2D natural images. This makes

C. Palm et al. (Hrsg.), *Bildverarbeitung für die Medizin 2025*, Informatik aktuell,
https://doi.org/10.1007/978-3-658-47422-5_53

it essential to efficiently filter and use only those parts of the images that contribute valuable information, avoiding unnecessary computational costs. Secondly, data is artificially altered due to privacy concerns; publicly accessible medical datasets are often anonymized, with sensitive areas like the face, ears, and even the top of the head removed or blurred. Such alterations create challenges for deep learning applications, particularly in generative models like GANs, diffusion models, or autoencoders, which rely on original images for accurate supervision. When these images are artificially distorted, networks may receive erroneous signals. For SSL methods focused on reconstruction, identifying and excluding these altered areas from loss calculation becomes especially critical. To improve 3D medical SSL applications, we introduce an open-source toolkit designed to preprocess data for SSL tasks. The toolkit includes two key components: (1) a network that segments all foreground regions within a CT or MR scan, allowing models to selectively sample patches from anatomical regions, thereby reducing training time; and (2) a network that identifies anonymized regions in CT and MRI images, enabling the exclusion of these regions from loss calculations to avoid incorrect supervision signals.

2 Materials and methods

We assembled a diverse collection of CT and MRI images to construct a robust training dataset for anatomical foreground segmentation. This dataset includes the set of publicly available datasets introduced in Tab. 1.

In total, the dataset comprises 3299 3D images: 1899 CT and 1400 MRI scans. The TotalSegmentator MRI dataset was exclusively reserved for testing MRI images, and the MAAL dataset for testing CT images, while the remaining datasets were evenly split 50:50 into training and testing. This resulted in 1483 training and 1816 testing images.

A multi-step approach was applied to obtain anatomical foreground masks for both CT and MRI images. For CT images, the TotalSegmentator tool [3] was utilized in "body mode" to generate initial segmentations, which were manually refined using the MITK [5] and ITK-SNAP [6] software tools to ensure accurate foreground delineation by filling gaps, removing errors, and adding missing regions. On average, correcting a single 3D CT image took only a few minutes. Since TotalSegmentator was only trained on CT images, it did not perform well on MRI images. Therefore, we annotated a smaller subset of images from each dataset using intensity thresholding and manual correction.

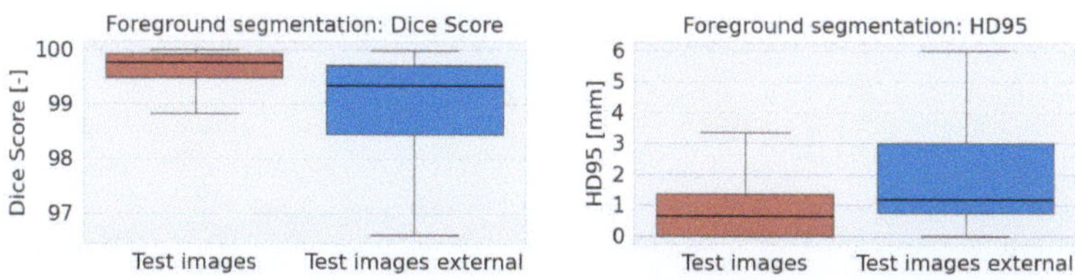

Fig. 1. Boxplot results illustrating the Dice Similarity Coefficient and HD95 for foreground segmentation, shown for both the test portion of the training dataset and the external test dataset.

Tab. 1. Overview of all datasets used for foreground prediction. * A small number of images from the original set of 1,228 CT and 298 MRI were excluded due to file corruption or incompatibility with MITK and ITK-SNAP.

Dataset	# Images	Modalities
LACS [7]	30	cardiac MRI
ACDC [8]	300	cine MRI
AMOS [9]	600	500 CT & 100 MRI (no further information given)
TotSeg [3]	1360*	1092 CT & 268 MRI (no further information given)
HanSeg [10]	84	42 CT & 42 T1w MRI
OASIS3 [11]	860	200 CT, 200 T1w, 200 T2w, 100 Angio & 160 FLAIR
MAAL [12]	65	CT

This initial segmentation process was time-consuming and required significant effort to ensure accurate delineations. Once the initial network was trained on this subset, it was used to predict segmentations for the remaining MRI images, requiring only minor manual refinements, significantly reducing the time to just a few minutes per 3D image. Finally, we trained a nnU-Net on all training data including both modalities, increasing the patch size to 192 × 192 × 192 to reduce inference time and applying z-score normalization to handle CT and MRI images with a single network.

The publicly available OASIS 3 dataset [11] was used as a training dataset for the segmentation of the anonymized facial parts. We selected a total of 1,005 scans of this database, comprising 319 T1-weighted (T1w) images, 329 T2-weighted (T2w) images, 68 angiographic images, 130 FLAIR images, and 159 CT images. These images, originally non-anonymized, were subjected to artificial anonymization using the AFNI (Analysis of Functional NeuroImages) software [13].

AFNI provides three anonymization methods: deface, reface, and reface plus. Deface sets voxel values in the face and ears to zero, reface replaces them with a blurred generic face and blurred ears, and reface plus also applies blurring to the outer skull. Each image was processed with all three methods, resulting in a comprehensive dataset of 3015 anonymized images with corresponding masks and different anonymization schemes.

The dataset was further extended with data from the OpenNeuro dataset collection [14], which is particularly valuable due to its diverse MRI head scans in different acquisition sequences and accessible licensing, making it suitable for SSL training. This

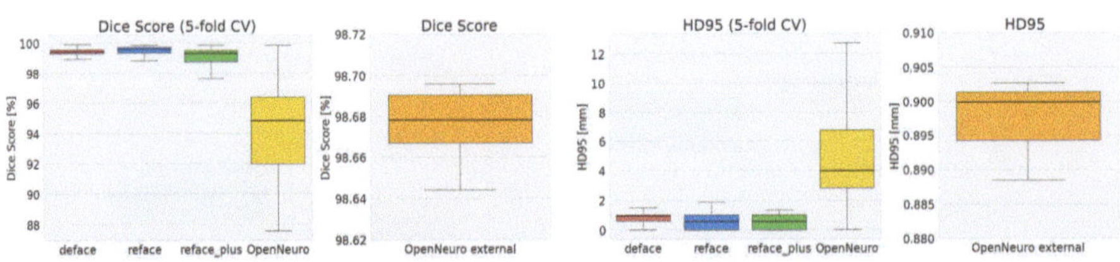

Fig. 2. Boxplot examples illustrating the Dice coefficient and HD95 for segmentation of deface area across different anonymization modes and the external OpenNeuro dataset.

collection employed different anonymization methods, with some datasets providing original deface masks originating from the *Defaced* method [15–18]. There were a total of 107 MRI images in this OpenNeuro dataset, including 78 T1w and 29 T2w images. We then trained a nnU-Net on this dataset and we measured both the Dice score and 95% Hausdorff distance (HD95) on a five-fold cross-validation.

In one dataset within the OpenNeuro collection, 14 images were anonymized through blurring; however, no ground truth masks were provided [19]. To assess the network's performance, we manually annotated these images, which were anonymized following the *Reface Plus* method, blurring the face, skin, and ears. We used this OpenNeuro dataset as an external testing dataset.

The trained model was evaluated on two test datasets: the test splits of the in-distribution training datasets, and the external datasets. The results are presented as boxplots in Fig. 1. On the test split of the training dataset, the model achieved a mean Dice coefficient of 99.56 and a median Dice coefficient of 99.76. The mean Dice coefficient for the external test dataset was 98.57, with a median of 99.34. Regarding HD95, the test portion of the training dataset showed a mean value of 1.38 and a median of 0.67, while the external test dataset yielded a mean HD95 of 2.89 and a median of 1.19. The model performs the task with near-perfect accuracy and demonstrates notable robustness, even on datasets outside the training data distribution.

We employed a 5-fold cross-validation to the model trained for deface segmentation. Results for each anonymization type, as well as for the external dataset with manually created segmentation, are presented in Fig. 2 and Tab. 2. Again, the model solves this task almost perfectly and shows robust performance on the holdout test dataset.

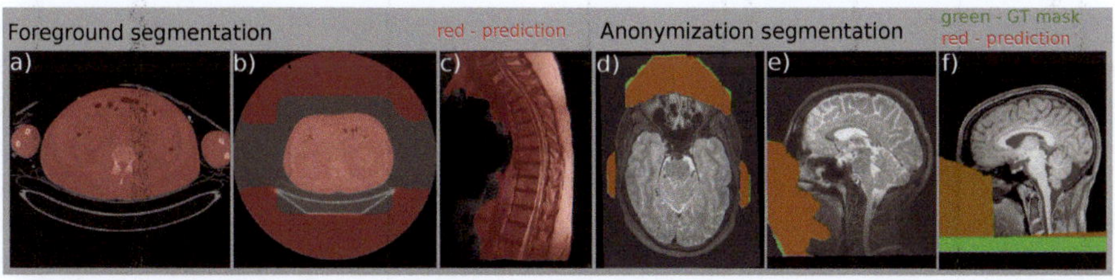

Fig. 3. Example predictions for foreground (FG) segmentation and anonymization segmentation. While in the majority of cases, the FG segmentation is almost perfectly solved (a), we observed a rare failure case for volumes with an artificial boundary between actual air and a region with constant values introduced during image reconstruction (b). Further we observed problems in images without a sharp contrast between the background and surrounding body regions, where even a human would not be able to deliniate the background (c). Lastly, the ground truth masks for the Deface anonymization (green) in the Open Neuro dataset were occasionally ambiguous. While the network accurately predicted the removed portions of the head in the foreground (d-e), we observed in some cases an ambiguity of the anonymization ground truth mask in the background (f).

Tab. 2. Mean, standard dev., and median values of the Dice Similarity Coefficient and HD95 for each anonymization type on the test dataset, including results for the external blurred face dataset.

	Dice Coefficient [%]		HD95 [mm]	
	mean (std)	median	mean (std)	median
Deface	99.05 ± 4.29	99.46	5.08 ± 43.44	1.00
Reface	99.50 ± 0.46	99.63	0.68 ± 3.85	0.59
Reface Plus	99.01 ± 1.92	99.34	0.72 ± 3.43	0.59
OpenNeuro	92.90 ± 7.14	94.88	13.57 ± 29.16	4.03
OpenNeuro - external	98.67 ± 0.05	98.67	0.90 ± 0.01	0.90

3 Discussion

The foreground segmentation network demonstrated robust performance across all test data, achieving near-perfect results, even on external datasets. However, certain edge cases revealed limitations that merit discussion. Specifically, we observed some rare cases as illustrated in Fig. 3 b and c), where the network produced an incorrect prediction. This error, visualized in Fig. 3 b), typically occurred in images with a large field of view lacking foreground content that exceeded the patch size, when there was also a boundary between actual air and a region with constant values—likely introduced during image reconstruction or processing. The network misinterpreted this boundary as foreground.

The deface segmentation network demonstrated highly robust performance across all anonymization types. However, as shown in Fig. 2, the segmentation accuracy for the OpenNeuro is slightly lower. This increased variability arises from ambiguities in the available masks. In defaced cases, we observed instances where the anonymization mask prediction in the foreground was accurate, but the boundaries of the ground truth mask in the background remained ambiguous, leading to mis-segmentation, as illustrated in Fig. 3 f). These failure cases were extremely rare and occurred solely in the background of the volume, presenting no limitations to the toolkit's functionality or intended purpose. At worst, the network might mistakenly sample from the background or omit a small background region in the loss calculation for potential SSL applications. Overall, we have introduced a highly accurate and versatile tool for segmenting anatomical foreground and anonymized regions, providing a valuable resource that particularly benefits SSL methods in medical imaging.

Acknowledgement. This article has been produced with the financial support of the European Union under the LERCO project number CZ.10.03.01/00/22_003/0000003 via the Operational Programme Just Transition.

References

1. Isensee F, Jaeger PF, Kohl SAA et al. nnU-Net: a self-configuring method for deep learning-based biomedical image segmentation. Nat Methods. 2021.
2. Ulrich C, Isensee F, Wald T et al. Multitalent: a multi-dataset approach to medical image segmentation. Proc MICCAI. 2023.

3. Wasserthal J, Breit HC, Meyer MT et al. TotalSegmentator: robust segmentation of 104 anatomic structures in CT images. Radiol: Artif Intell. 2023;5(5).
4. Baumgartner M, Jäger PF, Isensee F et al. nnDetection: a self-configuring method for medical object detection. Proc MICCAI. 2021:530–9.
5. Wolf I, Robert L. Galloway J, Vetter M et al. The medical imaging interaction toolkit (MITK): a toolkit facilitating the creation of interactive software by extending VTK and ITK.
6. Yushkevich PA, Piven J, Hazlett HC et al. User-guided 3D active contour segmentation of anatomical structures: significantly improved efficiency and reliability. NeuroImage. 2006;31(3):1116–28.
7. Tobon-Gomez C, Geers AJ, Peters J et al. Benchmark for algorithms segmenting the left atrium from 3D CT and MRI datasets. IEEE Trans Med Imaging. 2015;34(7):1460–73.
8. Bernard O, Lalande A, Zotti C et al. Deep learning techniques for automatic MRI cardiac multi-structures segmentation and diagnosis: is the problem solved? IEEE Trans Med Imaging. 2018;37(11):2514–25.
9. Ji Y, Bai H, Yang J et al. AMOS: a large-scale abdominal multi-organ benchmark for versatile medical image segmentation. arXiv: 2206.08023. 2022.
10. Podobnik G, Ibragimov B, Tappeiner E et al. HaN-Seg: the head and neck organ-at-risk CT and MR segmentation challenge. Radiother Oncol. 2024;198.
11. LaMontagne P, Benzinger T, Morris J et al. OASIS-3: longitudinal neuroimaging, clinical, and cognitive dataset for normal aging and alzheimer disease. 2019.
12. Landman B, Xu Z, Igelsias JE et al. 2015 MICCAI multi-atlas labeling beyond the cranial vault workshop and challenge. Proc MICCAI. 2015.
13. Cox RW. AFNI: software for analysis and visualization of functional magnetic resonance neuroimages. Comput Biomed Res. 1996;29(3):162–73.
14. Markiewicz CJ, Gorgolewski KJ, Feingold F et al. The OpenNeuro resource for sharing of neuroscience data. eLife. 2021;10.
15. Hanke M, Baumgartner FJ, Ibe P et al. Forrest Gump. OpenNeuro, 2018.
16. Nastase SA, Halchenko YO, Connolly AC et al. Neural responses to naturalistic clips of behaving animals in two different task contexts. Front Neurosci. 2018;12.
17. Strike LT, Hansell NK, Couvy-Duchesne B et al. Genetic complexity of cortical structure: differences in genetic and environmental factors influencing cortical surface area and thickness. Cereb Cortex. 2018;29(3).
18. Hebart MN, Contier O, Teichmann L et al. THINGS-data, a multimodal collection of large-scale datasets for investigating object representations in human brain and behavior. eLife. 2023.
19. di Oleggio Castello MV, Haxby JV, Gobbini MI. Shared neural codes for visual and semantic information about familiar faces in a common representational space. PNAS. 2021;118(45).

Automatic Detection of Bronchoscopes on X-ray Images

Maryam Parvin[1,2], Maximilian Rohleder[1,2], Andreas Maier[1], Holger Kunze[2]

[1]Pattern Recognition Laboratory, Friedrich-Alexander-University, Erlangen
[2]Siemens Healthineers AG, Advanced Therapy, Forchheim
maryam.parvin@fau.de

Abstract. Bronchoscopy is a crucial step in lung cancer diagnosis after observing a nodule in a lung computed tomography (CT) scan. However, it is often a difficult procedure, particularly for less experienced clinicians. We propose a pipeline for the automatic detection of bronchoscopes in x-ray images to support clinicians in lung airway navigation. Segmentation of bronchoscopes, like other tubular structures, is inherently difficult due to their narrow shape and poor image contrast. Our approach employs two preprocessing strategies, contrast limited adaptive histogram equalization (CLAHE) and negative log (NegLog) transform, along with two loss functions: mean squared Error (MSE) and weighted MSE (WMSE), with MSE serving as the baseline. We evaluate on two different datasets, and the model using WMSE as loss function along with CLAHE as preprocessing can predict 99% of the test images with 0.68 mean Dice similarity coefficient (DSC), 0.63 centerline Dice and 3 mm pixel distance. Additionally, we apply random sample consensus (RANSAC) and skeletonization algorithms for post-processing and polyline retrieval and our findings indicate that skeletonization offers a more robust solution for extracting polylines from tubular structures compared to RANSAC.

1 Introduction

Lung cancer is the most frequent cause of cancer-related death in men and it is in the second place for women in Germany [1]. Early detection of lung cancer can considerably improve overall survival rate, and bronchoscopy is a common operation for individuals suspected of having lung cancer [2]. While bronchoscopy is often a challenging procedure for clinicians, having support can enhance the efficiency and safety of the navigation process. Lung airway segmentation is an approach that provides an airway roadmap to guide surgeons during bronchoscopy [3]. In one study, the LungVision system is introduced, integrating real-time fluoroscopy with preoperative CT imaging to assist surgeons [4]. Another method, Naviairway, proposed by Wang et al., utilizes a customized loss function based on Dice loss to improve segmentation accuracy for better detection of fine bronchioles [3].

Another approach to facilitating the bronchoscopy procedure is to detect the location of the bronchoscopes for easier navigation. In this paper, we present a complete deep learning pipeline for detecting bronchoscopes in x-ray images to assist clinicians performing bronchoscopy. Accurate segmentation of tubular structures such as bronchoscopes, blood vessels, or tubular medical instruments is a challenging task due to their thin, tiny structures and poor image contrast [5, 6]. One study proposed an adapted

C. Palm et al. (Hrsg.), *Bildverarbeitung für die Medizin 2025*, Informatik aktuell,
https://doi.org/10.1007/978-3-658-47422-5_54

U-Net model combined with prior information, including an overlay of preoperative 3D segmentation and vesselness features, to segment stents in x-ray fluoroscopy during endovascular aortic repair [7]. Another study introduces soft-clDice, a computationally efficient loss function designed to preserve topology of the structure [6]. In a more recent study, a skeleton-guided 3D convolutional network is proposed and evaluated on airway datasets, introducing a sigmoid-adaptive Tversky loss function, an adaptation of dice loss, to solve gradient imbalance issues caused by the sparse distribution of foreground pixels [5].

In this work, we tackle the issue of class imbalance by implementing a weighted MSE loss function. This function adjusts weights in accordance with the distribution of foreground and background pixels, and we compare its performance against the traditional MSE loss, which serves as our baseline. The main contribution of this work is the development of a pipeline to retrieve parametric information about the shape and position of the bronchoscope in lung x-ray images. Additionally, we evaluate four combinations of loss functions and preprocessing strategies for training the deep learning model, as well as two post-processing algorithms for polyline retrieval from the predicted heatmaps.

2 Methods

2.1 Bronchoscope detection

The overall workflow of the proposed pipeline for bronchoscope detection is illustrated in Fig. 1. After loading the image, preprocessing is applied to improve the contrast of the bronchoscope on the image. The position of the bronchoscope is then returned by a heatmap that has been generated. In a post-processing step, the heatmap is transferred into a parametric description of the position.

To improve the visibility of the bronchoscope, two algorithms are compared. First, CLAHE [8] is used. Alternatively, we apply a negative log transform to the image and subtract the low-pass filtered component, a method referred to as NegLog. In both cases, Z-score normalization is applied to improve model robustness [9].

For retrieving the parametric description of the bronchoscope, we compare polynomial fitting using RANSAC [10] and a Skeletonization method [11]. First, we apply a threshold so that pixels with values below that threshold are set to 0. Thereafter, either of the methods is applied to the mask. The retrieved polylines after applying both methods are shown for two sample predictions in Fig. 2.

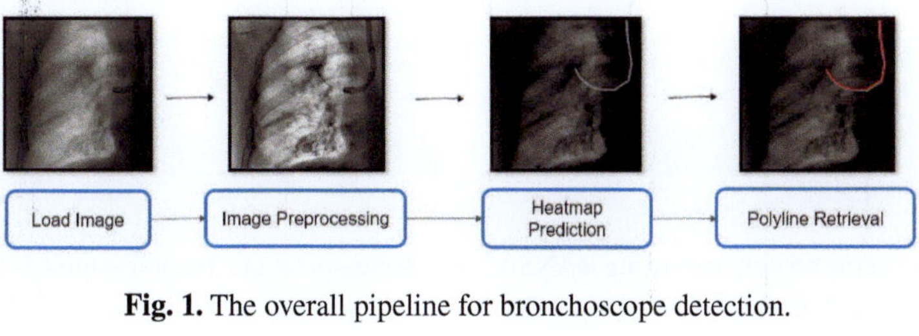

Fig. 1. The overall pipeline for bronchoscope detection.

2.2 Data processing

This retrospective study utilized 161 anonymized cone beam 3D scans collected during bronchoscopic interventions. Each scan comprises 400 projections used to reconstruct a cone-beam computed tomography (CBCT) volume. The bronchoscope and the biopsy needle are annotated manually in a 3D viewer and marked with polylines by a trained medical engineer. The control points of the polylines were projected onto the x-ray images. Inspections validated that the resulting polylines accurately represented the bronchoscope's position on the x-ray projections.

Projections that lacked a marked bronchoscope were excluded from the dataset, resulting in a total of 51,259 projections. The dataset was split 60:20:20 into train, validation and test dataset, ensuring that all projections of a patient belong to one dataset.

As ground truth labels, heatmaps are fed to the network. These heatmaps are generated using a Gaussian distance function, which assigns pixel intensities based on their distance from the curve representing the annotated label coordinates [12].

2.3 Training

We use a well-established deep learning architecture for medical image analysis, the U-Net model [13], with four downsampling and upsampling steps. For training, Adam [14] is used as an optimizer with learning rate 0.001 for 250 epochs. Furthermore, various augmentation strategies including intensity augmentation and geometry augmentations namely changing contrast, translation, rotation, and horizontal flipping have been applied.

We assess various loss functions. For a baseline, we implement the MSE loss. Furthermore, our model incorporates a WMSE loss to address the imbalance between foreground and background pixels in the input images. The WMSE loss is defined as

$$\mathcal{L}_{WMSE}(Y, Y') = \frac{1}{N} \sum_{i=1}^{N} W_i \cdot (Y'_i - Y_i)^2 \tag{1}$$

with Y and Y' denoting the ground truth and predicted heatmaps and N the total number of pixels. The background and foreground weights, $W_{Bg} = \frac{N}{N_{bg}+\epsilon}$ and $W_{Fg} = \frac{N}{N_{fg}+\epsilon}$, are defined based on N_{bg} and N_{fg}, the number of pixels for the background and foreground in the ground truth, and ϵ is a small constant. We apply a transition function $V(Y) = \sin\left(Y \cdot \frac{\pi}{2}\right)$. The final pixel weight W_i is calculated as

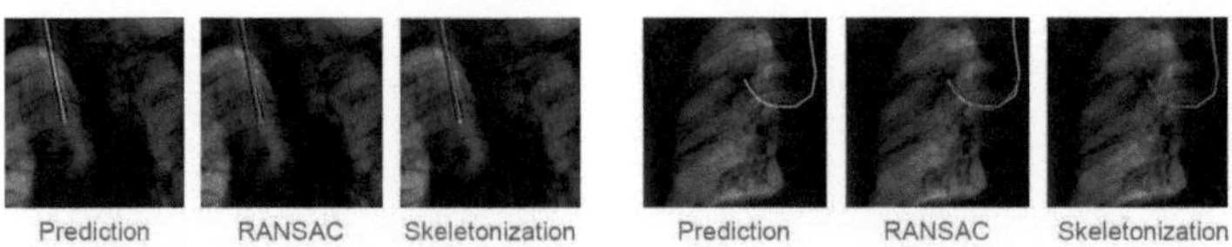

Fig. 2. The retrieved polylines using RANSAC and Skeletonization. The left sample is for straight case and the right sample is for curved case.

Tab. 1. Evaluation results of four combinations of MSE and WMSE loss functions with the preprocessing techniques CLAHE and Negative Log Transform, including All Projections and AP Projections.

Metric	MSE-CLAHE		MSE-NegLog		WMSE-CLAHE		WMSE-NegLog	
	All	AP	All	AP	All	AP	All	AP
DSC								
Mean	0.50	0.65	0.47	0.54	0.58	0.68	0.58	0.65
80th percentile	0.79	0.83	0.76	0.80	0.79	0.83	0.78	0.82
clDice								
Mean	0.46	0.60	0.43	0.49	0.54	0.63	0.53	0.60
80th percentile	0.74	0.79	0.70	0.75	0.76	0.81	0.74	0.79
Pixel distance (mm)								
Mean	3.27	1.27	4.33	0.90	10.60	3.00	10.59	3.22
80th percentile	1.74	0.99	2.01	0.98	7.58	1.30	5.98	1.31
Zero predictions	15%	3%	9%	8%	1%	1%	2%	3%

$$W_i = (1 - V(Y_i)) \cdot W_{Bg} + V(Y_i) \cdot W_{Fg} \tag{2}$$

3 Results

The experiments are conducted with two different loss functions, MSE and WMSE, and two preprocessing approaches, namely CLAHE and Neglog transform. The results are evaluated using both overlap-based metrics such as DSC and a form of distance metric namely pixel distance (PD) following [15]. PD measures how far each pixel in the predicted heatmap is from the nearest ground truth pixel. Additionally, we use the centerline Dice metric (clDice) as described in this article [6]. Due to the high attenuation of lateral projections, we conduct evaluations on the entire test dataset ("All" projections) as well as separately on only the anterior-posterior (AP) projections. The evaluation results for the four different combinations for "All" and "AP" projections are summarized in Tab. 1.

The model using the WMSE loss function with CLAHE preprocessing outperforms the other combinations in terms of both clDice and DSC. In terms of PD, the model with MSE loss and CLAHE preprocessing performs the best in all projections, whereas the MSE-Neglog combination performs better in AP projections. However, both MSE-CLAHE and MSE-Neglog struggle with a higher proportion of test images in both "All" and "AP" projections compared to WMSE-CLAHE. Some of the prediction results of all four combinations, with DSC greater than 0.7 are shown in Fig. 3: the predictions made using WMSE-CLAHE cover nearly all of the bronchoscope topology, while the other combinations miss parts of it. As shown in the ground truth images, the annotation process may have lead to incomplete labeling of the bronchoscope at the borders. Therefore, in the evaluation of AP projections, we disregard area within a certain margin around the border of the test image to account for these inaccuracies. Regarding the post-processing, as shown in the Fig. 2, both RANSAC and Skeletonization perform very well for straight structures. However, RANSAC method mostly struggles for fitting a polyline for curved structures. For quantitative evaluation, we employ the PD metric. While the mean PD for RANSAC is 9.73 mm, deteriored by a small number of bad images, the Skeletonization approach yields a PD of 0 mm.

4 Discussion

In this work, we proposed an efficient pipeline for deriving a parametric line representation of a bronchoscope in fluoroscopy x-ray images. We evaluated the combinations of loss functions and preprocessing methods, showing that the Weighted MSE loss function along with CLAHE preprocessing yields more efficient segmentation in terms of Dice and clDice metrics. Additionally, the pixel distance for the corresponding model in AP projections was a quarter of its value in All projections. We have also retrieved polylines from the predicted heatmaps using both RANSAC and Skeletonization methods, demonstrating that Skeletonization is a more robust approach, particularly for thin and elongated structures like the bronchoscope. However, there are limitations to this work, such as the poor contrast of some images, which could not be fully resolved through preprocessing. Additionally, mispredictions occur where certain bones or connectors are incorrectly segmented as the bronchoscope, as shown in Fig. 3 for WMSE loss function predictions on the right. Finally, the labeling of the bronchoscope on 2D images is incomplete, due to the use of 3D volumes to generate the labels. These errors also pose challenges during post-processing, as they are included in the retrieved polyline. To address these issues in future work, we aim to investigate cropping the input images from the bottom, where no bronchoscope exists according to our prior knowledge, or dynamically cropping according to the position of the annotated coordinates. This approach will prevent the network from being fed unnecessary regions of the image, which might reduce the likelihood of mispredictions. Furthermore, we plan to refine the post-processing step for a more accurate retrieved polyline.

Acknowledgement. This work was supported by Siemens Healthineers, Forchheim.

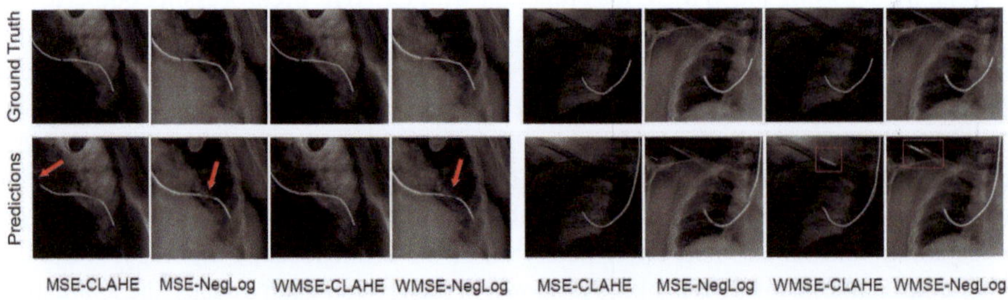

Fig. 3. Prediction results for two example cases comparing four different training strategies.

References

1. Frost N, Griesinger F, Hoffmann H et al. Lung cancer in Germany. J Thorac Oncol. 2022;17(6):742–50.
2. Andolfi M, Potenza R, Capozzi R et al. The role of bronchoscopy in the diagnosis of early lung cancer: a review. J Thorac Dis. 2016;8(11):3329–37.
3. Wang A, Tam TCC, Poon HM et al. NaviAirway: a bronchiole-sensitive deep learning-based airway segmentation pipeline. arXiv: 2203.04294v3. 2023.
4. Pertzov B, Gershman E, Izhakian S et al. The LungVision navigational platform for peripheral lung nodule biopsy and the added value of cryobiopsy. Thorac Cancer. 2021;12:2007–12.
5. Zhu R, Oda M, Hayashi Y et al. Skeleton-guided 3D convolutional neural network for tubular structure segmentation. Int J Comput Assist Radiol Surg. 2024.
6. Shit S, Paetzold JC, Sekuboyina A et al. clDice: a novel topology-preserving loss function for tubular structure segmentation. Proc IEEE CVF CVPR. 2021:16560–9.
7. Breininger K, Albarqouni S, Kurzendorfer T et al. Intraoperative stent segmentation in X-ray fluoroscopy for endovascular aortic repair. Int J Comput Assist Radiol Surg. 2018;13:1221–31.
8. Pizer SM, Amburn EP, Austin JD et al. Adaptive histogram equalization and its variations. Comput Vis Graph Image Process. 1987;39(3):355–68.
9. Kordon F, Lasowski R, Swartman B et al. Improved X-ray bone segmentation by normalization and augmentation strategies. Proc BVM. 2019:104–9.
10. Fischler MA, Bolles RC. Random sample consensus: a paradigm for model fitting with applications to image analysis and automated cartography. Commun ACM. 1981;24(6):381–95.
11. Zhang TY, Suen CY. A fast parallel algorithm for thinning digital patterns. Commun ACM. 1984;27(3):236–9.
12. Kordon F, Stiglmayr M, Maier A et al. A principled representation of elongated structures using heatmaps. Sci Rep. 2023;13:15253.
13. Ronneberger O, Fischer P, Brox T. U-Net: convolutional networks for biomedical image segmentation. Proc MICCAI. 2015:234–41.
14. Kingma DP, Ba J. Adam: a method for stochastic optimization. Proc ICLR. 2015.
15. Maier-Hein L, Reinke A, Jaeger P et al. Metrics reloaded: recommendations for image analysis validation. Nat Methods. 2024;21:195–212.

Automated Segmentation and Analysis of Cone Photoreceptors in Multimodal Adaptive Optics Imaging

Prajol Shrestha[1], Mikhail Kulyabin[1], Aline Sindel[1], Hilde R. Pedersen[2], Stuart Gilson[2], Rigmor Baraas[2], Andreas Maier[1]

[1]Pattern Recognition Lab, FAU Erlangen-Nürnberg, Germany
[2]National Centre for Optics, Vision and Eye Care, USN, Kongsberg, Norway
prajol.shrestha@fau.de

Abstract. Accurate detection and segmentation of cone cells in the retina are essential for diagnosing and managing retinal diseases. In this study, we used advanced imaging techniques, including confocal and non-confocal split detector images from adaptive optics scanning light ophthalmoscopy (AOSLO), to analyze photoreceptors for improved accuracy. Precise segmentation is crucial for understanding each cone cell's shape, area, and distribution. It helps to estimate the surrounding areas occupied by rods, which allows the calculation of the density of cone photoreceptors in the area of interest. In turn, density is critical for evaluating overall retinal health and functionality. We explored two U-Net-based segmentation models: StarDist for confocal and Cellpose for non-confocal modalities. Analyzing cone cells in images from two modalities and achieving consistent results demonstrates the study's reliability and potential for clinical application.

1 Introduction

Cone and rod photoreceptors are the fundamental units of the retina responsible for detecting light. Cones are sensitive to bright light and responsible for color perception. They are densely concentrated in the central fovea within the macula, with their density decreasing rapidly towards the periphery. Rods are sensitive to low light and enable night vision. They are predominantly located in the peripheral regions of the retina [1]. The distribution of photoreceptors varies with eccentricity, allowing the eye to function effectively in different lighting conditions and perceive fine details and a wide range of colors.

Retinal diseases such as age-related macular degeneration, Stargardt disease, and diabetic retinopathy pose significant threats to vision, particularly when they affect cone cells, which are crucial for central and color vision [2]. If these conditions are not diagnosed early, they can lead to severe and often irreversible vision loss. Early detection is essential for effective treatment, allowing interventions that can slow the disease's progression or mitigate its impact on vision. However, detecting these diseases in their early stages is challenging due to the subtle nature of early signs and symptoms and limitations in imaging technologies.

Advanced imaging techniques like adaptive optics scanning light ophthalmoscopy (AOSLO) have become invaluable in addressing retinal diseases. AOSLO provides high-resolution images of the individual photoreceptor cells and supports various modalities, including confocal, non-confocal, and darkfield [3]. The confocal modality reveals the

C. Palm et al. (Hrsg.), *Bildverarbeitung für die Medizin 2025*, Informatik aktuell,
https://doi.org/10.1007/978-3-658-47422-5_55

centers of cone photoreceptors by imaging the functional cone outer segment structure, while the non-confocal modality, most commonly the split detector, reveals rod cells and cone boundaries through the inner segment structure. The darkfield modality highlights the retinal pigment epithelium (RPE) cells, providing additional structural information [4]. The combination of these modalities offers complementary views of the retinal structure, enhancing our ability to study various retinal diseases and conditions.

Conventional method presented in work by Li and Roorda [5] rely on the optical fiber properties of cone photoreceptors and can mislabel rods as cones. Therefore, it needs to be revised by a human expert. Creating a fully automatic method for segmenting and detecting cone and rod areas will significantly increase the possibilities of retinal research. Recently, Kulyabin et al. introduced a method based on deep learning (DL) for automated detection and segmentation of cones in AOSLO images, using the Voronoi algorithm to generate the photoreceptor outlines [6]. However, the method is limited to the range of degrees of eccentricity from the foveal center — 0°, 1°, and 2°. As the size of rods, and consequently rods total area, increases, approximation using the Voronoi algorithm, which uses the centers of cones to generate outlines, becomes less accurate.

In this work, to independently define zones of cones and rods, we investigated different methods for annotating cones for the further training of DL models and calculating photoreceptor densities for a range of 0° - 10° eccentricity from the fovea. Precise segmentation is crucial as it enables a detailed understanding of the shape and area of each cone and helps estimate the areas occupied by rods. U-Net-based models StarDist [7] and Cellpose [8] were used for cell segmentation in confocal and non-confocal modalities [9], respectively. Furthermore, the precise analysis of cones from both modalities was explored to support each other's findings for informed clinical decisions.

2 Materials and methods

In this study, we utilized a semi-automatically labeled dataset of AOSLO images of 11 participants with normal vision, covering an age range of 14 to 65. This diverse sample represents a broad spectrum of healthy retinas, providing valuable insights into retinal structure across different stages of life. We explored various annotation techniques, such as manual annotation and a human-in-the-loop method. After initial manual annotation, we further processed the data by separating regions based on each cone cell's center information using the Voronoi method or using boundary vertices. Additionally, we transformed polygonal annotations into circular shapes using the closest vertex and closest ridge midpoint vertex methods to standardize the representation of cone cells and distinguish them from rods (Fig. 1). In the human-in-the-loop, annotations are automatically predicted, and a human expert makes the necessary corrections.

The dataset was split at the participant level, with 8 participants used for training (272 confocal and 20 non-confocal images) and 3 (96 confocal and 86 non-confocal images) for testing. Due to suboptimal performance simultaneously for all eccentricities, images were further divided into central fovea (0° – 4°) and parafovea (5° – 10°) groups, with further independent training of the models for each of the groups.

Fig. 2 shows the proposed pipeline. For the detection of cone cells in images from confocal modality, we trained the StarDist model [7], which is based on the original

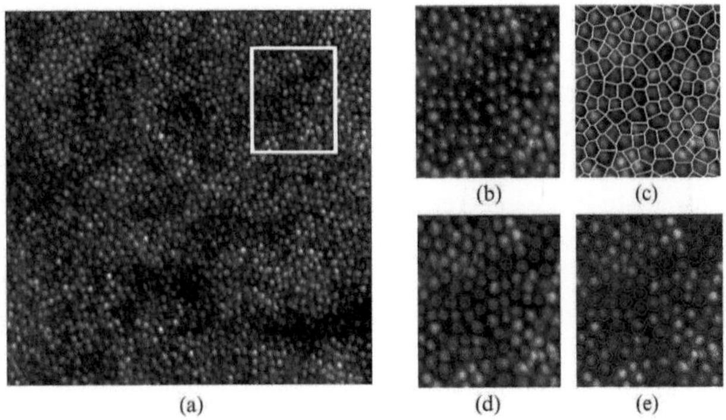

Fig. 1. Annotation of confocal images: original image (a), manually annotated centers (b), Voronoi algorithm (c), circular annotations using midpoint vertices (d), circular annotations using closest vertices (e).

U-Net architecture, utilizing a star-convex polygon for precise localization. To extract the precise shape and location of a cone cell, StarDist evaluates the likelihood of a pixel being the cell center through a predicted probability map and utilizes the predicted distance map to calculate the distance from the center to the cell's boundary. Similarly, for images from non-confocal modality, we trained the Cellpose model [8], which is based on a U-Net with residual blocks and an image style transfer. The Cellpose model generates a vector flow field using the predicted horizontal and vertical gradients of the image, and by tracking this field, pixels belonging to each cone cell are grouped and further refined with the predicted binary map to extract the exact shapes of the cells.

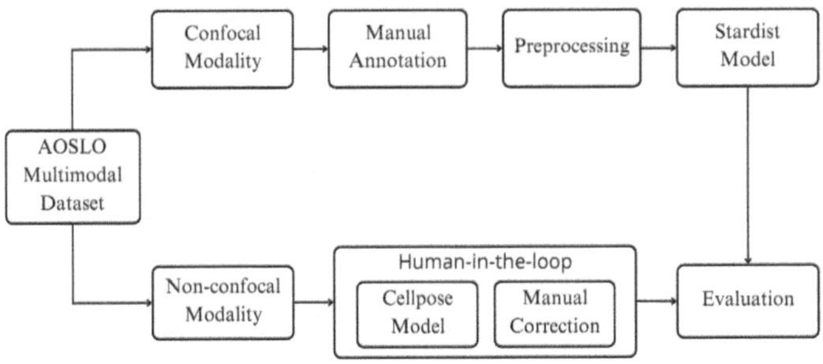

Fig. 2. Pipeline for processing multimodal AOSLO dataset, incorporating images of confocal and non-confocal modalities with manual and semi-automated annotation steps.

3 Results

The StarDist model was trained on confocal images over 600 epochs with 100 steps per epoch, using an ADAM optimizer with a learning rate of 0.0003, a batch size of 4, and a patch size of 64 × 64 pixels. For non-confocal images, we utilized the Cellpose GUI to generate initial annotations automatically, followed by manual adjustments to refine the annotations. These refined annotations were used to train the model iteratively. Each training group consisted of 5 to 10 non-confocal images, trained for 200 epochs using stochastic gradient descent, a learning rate of 0.1, and a weight decay of 0.0001.

Tab. 1. Evaluation metrics for segmentation models on confocal and non-confocal images.

Modality	Annotation Type	Eccentricity					
		Central fovea		Parafovea		All	
		IoU	Dice	IoU	Dice	IoU	Dice
Non-confocal	Human-in-the-loop	**0.52**	**0.68**	**0.54**	**0.70**	**0.50**	**0.67**
Confocal	Closest vertex	**0.67**	**0.80**	**0.78**	**0.88**	**0.69**	**0.81**
Confocal	Closest ridge midpoint	0.48	0.61	0.58	0.70	0.53	0.64
Confocal	Manual	0.61	0.74	0.69	0.81	0.63	0.86

Both models were trained on a single NVIDIA RTX 2080Ti GPU. IoU and the Dice score were used to evaluate the segmentation performance, ensuring alignment between predicted outputs and actual cell boundaries.

Tab. 1 shows the experiment results. The predicted segmentation masks from both models were evaluated with the IoU and Dice metrics, using the ground truth masks. For confocal images with the closest vertex annotation style, the central fovea segmentation achieved an IoU of 0.67 and a Dice score of 0.80, while parafovea segmentation performed better, with an IoU of 0.78 and a Dice score of 0.88. In contrast, the model performed less effectively with other annotation styles. For non-confocal images, the results were lower, with IoU of 0.52 and a Dice score of 0.68 for the central fovea and IoU of 0.54 and a Dice score of 0.70 for the parafovea. Additionally, there was a strong correlation between the predicted and ground truth masks, as confirmed by a Pearson correlation coefficient of 0.850 and a Spearman correlation coefficient of 0.847.

Fig. 3 presents the predictions on confocal images using the StarDist model, with predictions for central fovea and parafovea. Fig. 4 displays parafovea predictions on non-confocal images using the Cellpose model. These predictions appear promising, with only minor quantitative errors, indicating the strong performance of both models in segmenting and detecting the cells.

To compute the density of cones d and the mean cone area $\bar{A}$ according to predicted cone centers and mask, we applied (1) and (2)

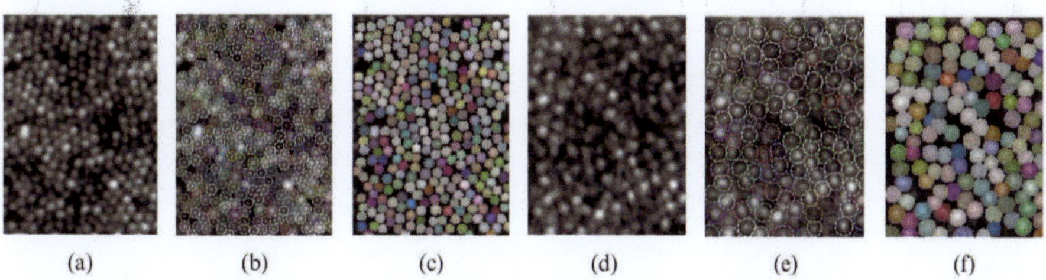

Fig. 3. StarDist model results on confocal images. Central fovea: original image (a), predicted centers and boundaries (b), segmentation masks (c). Parafovea: original image (d), predicted centers and boundaries (e), segmentation masks (f).

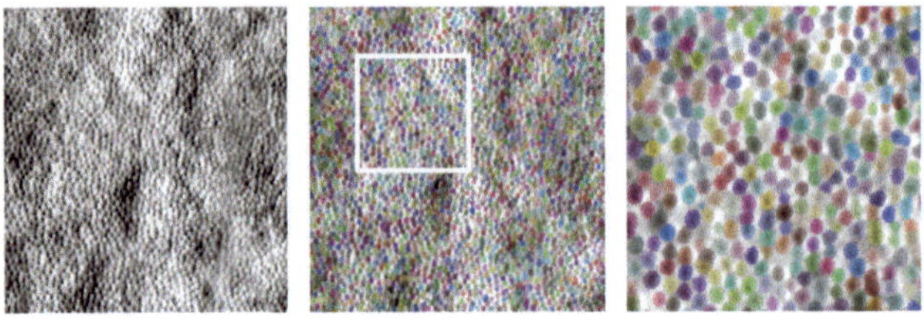

(a) (b) (c)

Fig. 4. Cellpose model results on non-confocal images in parafovea: original image (a), predicted masks (b), zoomed-in highlighted area within the white box (c).

$$d = \frac{N}{h \times w \times \left(\frac{\mu}{s_f}\right)^2} \tag{1}$$

$$\bar{A} = \frac{\sum(p \times \mu^2)}{N} \tag{2}$$

where N is the total number of cones, h and w are the height and the width of the area in pixels, μ denotes the spatial resolution (microns per pixel), s_f is the scaling factor, and p represents the pixel count per cone. The density values are fitted (Fig. 5) according to the asymmetric power function [4].

Fig. 5 highlights the distribution of cone inner segment areas as a function of eccentricity, providing a clear visualization of the variation in average cone sizes. This analysis is crucial for understanding the spatial organization of the retina by isolating cones from rods, resulting in a more precise evaluation of cone photoreceptors and contributing to a more accurate assessment of retinal health.

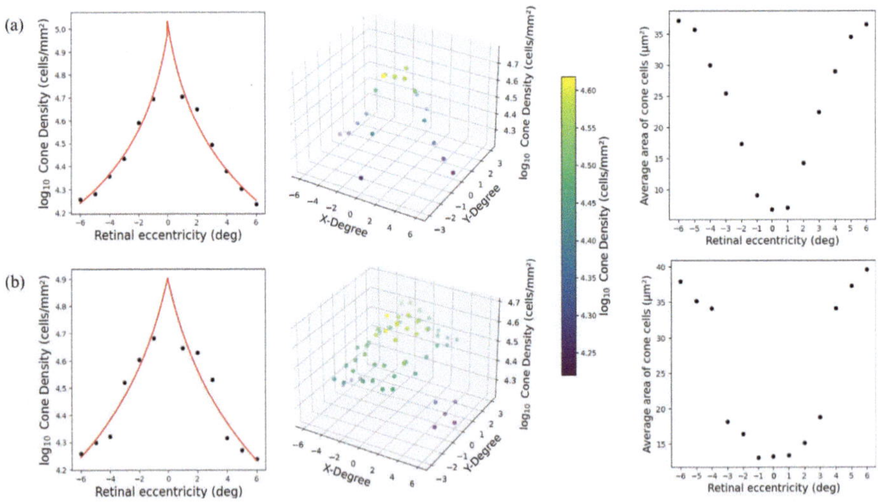

Fig. 5. Visualizations of cone density and average cone area as a function of eccentricity: cone density fitted with asymmetric power function, volumetric cone density, average cone area computed using confocal modality (a) and non-confocal modality (b) images from the same participant.

4 Discussion

We proposed an automated approach to segment cone photoreceptors and measure their density and inner segment area as a function of eccentricity in multimodal AOSLO images, isolating cones from rods using DL models for a detailed understanding of retinal structure. Our findings align with earlier studies on how cone density changes with distance from the fovea. Additionally, we observed that the cones' average inner segment area is smaller near the fovea, where the cone density is highest, and gradually increases as we move further away [9]. This trend is significant, as it provides insights into the spatial organization of cones, which can be helpful in conditions like Stargardt disease. We generated detailed cone density maps, allowing us to analyze how cone distribution relates to other retinal features. The models perform well in segmenting cone boundaries. However, detecting cones in low-contrast areas or where cones are tightly packed is more challenging, particularly within the central fovea. Variations in image quality, such as noise or motion blur, can also affect the results. As with many automated methods, improving the prediction is challenging, particularly when the boundaries are unclear, leading to differences in ground truth generation. To address this, we are using active learning with human feedback to increase the quality and consistency of ground truth and predictions. Furthermore, integrating novel SOTA models such as SAM (Segment Anything Model) is a potential improvement in handling more complex issues.

References

1. Kolb H, Fernandez E, Nelson R. Webvision: the organization of the retina and visual system. University of Utah Health Sciences Center, 1995.
2. Pedersen HR, Gilson S, Hagen LA et al. Multimodal in-vivo maps as a tool to characterize retinal structural biomarkers for progression in adult-onset Stargardt disease. Frontiers Ophthalmol. 2024;4.
3. Roorda A, Duncan JL. Adaptive optics ophthalmoscopy. Annu Rev Vis Sci. 2015;1(1):19–50.
4. Baraas RC, Pedersen HR, Knoblauch K et al. Human foveal cone and RPE cell topographies and their correspondence with foveal shape. Vis Sci. 2022;63(2):8.
5. Li K, Roorda A. Automated identification of cone photoreceptors in adaptive optics retinal images. JOSA A. 2007;24(5):1358–63.
6. Kulyabin M, Sindel A, Pedersen H et al. Generalist segmentation algorithm for photoreceptors analysis in adaptive optics imaging. arXiv: 2408.14810. 2024.
7. Schmidt U, Weigert M, Broaddus C et al. Cell detection with star-convex polygons. Proc MICCAI. 2018:265–73.
8. Pachitariu M, Stringer C. Cellpose 2.0: how to train your own model. Nat Methods. 2022;19:1634–41.
9. Scoles D, Sulai YN, Langlo CS et al. In vivo imaging of human cone photoreceptor inner segments. Investi Ophthalmol Vis Sci. 2014;55(7):4244–51.

Comprehensive Dataset of Coarse Tumor Annotations for The Cancer Genome Atlas Breast Invasive Carcinoma

Sweta Banerjee[1], Christof A. Bertram[2], Jonas Ammeling[3], Viktoria Weiss[2], Thomas Conrad[4], Robert Klopfleisch[4], Christopher Kaltenecker[5], Katharina Breininger[6], Marc Aubreville[1]

[1]Flensburg University of Applied Sciences, Flensburg, Germany
[2]University of Veterinary Medicine, Vienna, Austria
[3]Technische Hochschule Ingolstadt, Ingolstadt, Germany
[4]Freie Universität Berlin, Berlin, Germany
[5]Medical University of Vienna, Vienna, Austria
[6]Julius-Maximilians-Universität Würzburg, Würzburg, Germany
sweta.banerjee@hs-flensburg.de

Abstract. Automated tumor segmentation of histologic images is crucial for the development of computer-assisted diagnostic workflows aiming at accurate prognostication. We present a dataset of coarse annotations of over 1,000 high-resolution breast tumor images from The cancer genome atlas breast invasive carcinoma (TCGA-BRCA) repository, each annotated with binary segmentation masks that delineate coarse tumor areas. Additionally, a subset of 20 images includes fine-grained annotations, providing precise delineation of tumor boundaries beyond the broader outlines used in coarse annotations. Initial evaluations using U-Net and DeepLabv3 models show promising segmentation performance. On a held-out, coarsely annotated test set, U-Net achieved an average intersection over union (IoU) score of 0.795, while DeepLabv3 scored 0.783. On the finely annotated subset of this test set, U-Net reached an average IoU of 0.746, with DeepLabv3 slightly outperforming at 0.765. The public availability of this dataset aims to support research in automated tumor analysis, advancing diagnostic workflows and thereby ultimately improving breast cancer management.

1 Introduction

Despite significant improvements in treatment choices, breast cancer continues to rank among the leading causes of mortality for women [1]. Improving curative outcomes requires early detection and precise diagnosis of malignancy and prospective tumor growth patterns [2]. Multiple factors are evaluated by a pathologist during the histopathologic assessment of tumor tissue. In the case of breast cancer, the grading scheme includes the count of mitotic figures–a crucial marker of tumor aggressiveness and proliferation – or the assessment of nuclear pleomorphism and tubule formation [3]. It has been shown that there is a high inter-rater disagreement between pathologists in this assessment, impacting the reproducibility of the findings [4]. Deep learning-based computer vision algorithms can help experts address this issue. Since all of those prognostic criteria must be assessed within the tumor area, the precise delineation of the tumor is of great importance.

C. Palm et al. (Hrsg.), *Bildverarbeitung für die Medizin 2025*, Informatik aktuell,
https://doi.org/10.1007/978-3-658-47422-5_56

For example, evaluating the tumor grade requires identifying the areas with the highest mitotic activity; yet, surrounding tissues like the epidermis can contain a significant number of mitotic figures. These extra-tumoral detections are unrelated to the tumor behavior and can result in erroneous evaluations if they are not thoroughly separated. In addition, a detailed examination of important tumor-related variables, such as size and margin characteristics, is made possible by accurate tumor area annotations. These measures are essential for clinical decision making because they affect tumor classification, surgical procedure planning, and ultimately treatment outcome. Understanding the biological function and response of the tumor to treatment is further aided by the capacity to assess spatial heterogeneity within the tumor [5].

The performance of deep learning algorithms hinges on the availability of large and diverse data sets. One of the most well-known large-scale histopathology datasets in the domain of breast cancer is the The cancer genome atlas-breast invasive carcinoma (TCGA-BRCA) dataset [6], encompassing 1,093 total cases of breast cancer along with anonymized clinical patient records and digitized histological slides (whole slide images, WSIs). Despite its importance and popularity, the dataset lacks explicit tumor region labels, which are crucial for many analyses. While selected regions of interest were previously annotated [7], this is not true for the entire WSIs. For researchers and physicians who want to gain valuable information about tumor pathology, the lack of tumor region labels poses a serious obstacle.

Fine-grained annotation of WSIs is a labor-intensive and costly task, which involves assessment of the tumor at various magnification levels during the annotation. For many downstream tasks (e.g., region selection for mitotic count assessment, tumor micro-environment analysis, tumor growth pattern analysis), a fine-grained delineation is, however, not necessary, and coarse annotations, which can be carried out by a pathologist within a much shorter time frame, are fully sufficient. Moreover, algorithmic approaches have been developed that make use of coarse annotations by incorporating assumptions about uncertainty [8].

In this work, we propose a new dataset of coarse tumor area annotations for 1,039 WSIs, corresponding to 1,039 cases, of the TCGA-BRCA dataset to close this gap. We provide baseline experiments to show the quality of the dataset and its potential limitations. To enable evaluation of algorithmic approaches towards automatic refinement of those annotations, we also provide fine-grained annotations for a randomly selected subset of 20 WSIs.

We provide polygon tumor annotations as well as the derived binary tumor masks in our Github repository[1]. By making this resource available, we intend to further advance the field of breast cancer research and eventually improve treatment outcome.

2 Materials and methods

2.1 Dataset description

The dataset created in this work comprises coarse binary segmentation annotations of the publicly available TCGA-BRCA dataset using the WSIs with Hematoxylin & Eosin-staining [6].

[1] `https://github.com/DeepMicroscopy/TCGA-BRCA-TumorArea-Coarse`

Tab. 1. Dataset Statistics.

Dataset features	Mean	Std. dev.	25th percentile	75th percentile
Polygon annotations per slide	1.601	1.445	1.000	2.000
Points per polygon	803.338	571.386	343.000	1121.250
Tumor area (mm^2)	103.390	73.979	47.735	141.979

Of the 1,093 cases with WSIs in the TCGA-BRCA database, we included 1,039 WSIs (corresponding to the same number of cases) in the dataset. The 54 WSIs were excluded due to low spatial resolution of less than $0.25\mu m/px$ (N=23), extremely poor tissue quality in most parts of the WSI with loss of cellular details (N=11), absence of breast cancer in the WSI (N=8), non-breast tissue (N=6), out-of-focus in most of the WSI (N=1), extensive air bubbles obscuring the underlying tissue (N=3), and IHC staining (N=2).

Annotations were created by a board-certified pathologist. For all 1,039 included WSIs, coarse annotations were created using the Exact software platform [9]. For this, the pathologist examined the WSI at various magnifications to confirm the neoplastic tissue and subsequently zoomed out until the entire tumor tissue was visible in the viewing window. At this low magnification, the tumor area was coarsely delineated by polygon annotations aiming at spending 5 minutes on average for each of the 1,039 WSIs. Most of the slides were annotated using a single polygon annotation (see Tab. 1). In 80 WSIs, there were large non-neoplastic tissue areas within the annotations, which were delineated by a second annotation class in order to exclude them for the binary mask. Furthermore, for 20 WSIs of this dataset, to be used in the test set, fine annotations

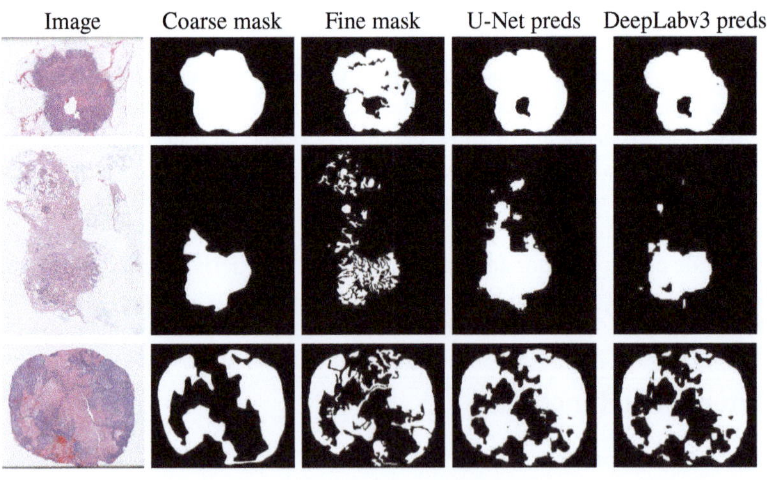

Fig. 1. Examples of segmentation results. Each row shows a histology image, the corresponding coarse and fine ground truth masks, and segmentation predictions from U-Net and DeepLabv3 models.

were created, featuring more precise delineation around tumor regions compared to the broader outlines used in the coarse annotations. The annotations software SlideRunner [10] was used as in this software the magnification and location of the WSI can be changed while the polygon annotation tool is active, which enabled a more accurate placement of the polygon annotation points. The time investment for the fine annotations was on average 20 minutes per WSI.

To promote transparency and facilitate research, annotations are publicly available both as annotation polygons and as coarse and fine image masks[2].

2.2 Technical validation

For technical validation of the dataset, we trained a segmentation model on the 16× downsampled images of the dataset. Images were downsampled to balance computational efficiency with the retention of tumor-relevant features, ensuring that cell-level details were maintained for segmentation accuracy [11]. We trained two architectures for the segmentation into tumor and background classes: U-Net [12] and DeepLabv3 [13], both with a ResNet18 encoder pre-trained on ImageNet, with a 5-fold cross-validation setting. From the final set of annotated images, 103 images were held out as the test set. Of the remaining images, 20% were randomly assigned to the validation set, while the remaining 80% were used for training. Despite being a few years old, U-Net remains highly effective for medical segmentation [14]. We trained the networks on image patches sized 256 × 256 pixels. Patch sampling was employed to capture various regions within each WSI, with 30 patches randomly sampled from tumor and background areas to avoid class imbalance and ensure robust learning. Data augmentation included random horizontal and vertical flips, 90-degree rotations, brightness and contrast adjustments, elastic transformations, Gaussian blurring, and affine transformations (scaling, slight rotations, and shearing) to simulate variability in tissue morphology and staining. We used the Adam optimizer and trained the networks with a combination of binary cross-entropy and Dice loss. The initial learning rate was set to 10^{-6} with a triangular cyclic schedule ranging from 10^{-6} to 10^{-4} to stabilize learning. We trained the models with a batch size of 2 for 100 epochs for each fold. No weight decay was applied, and hyperparameters were optimized based on preliminary runs using validation intersection over union (IoU) as the selection metric. For each fold, we saved the best model based on the validation IoU and used it to perform an ensembled sliding window inference on both the coarse and fine annotations from the held-out test sets, using a window size of 512 and an overlap of 256.

3 Results

On the coarsely annotated held-out set (103 cases), U-Net achieved an intersection over union (IoU) of 0.795, while on the finely annotated held-out set (20 cases), it achieved an IoU of 0.746. Similarly, DeepLabv3 achieved IoU scores of 0.783 and 0.765 on the coarsely and finely annotated sets, respectively. In addition to evaluating

[2] `https://github.com/DeepMicroscopy/TCGA-BRCA-TumorArea-Coarse`

Tab. 2. Results of our baseline experiments. Values indicate mean ± standard deviation.

Model	Val IoU	Val F1	Test IoU		Test F1	
			Coarse	Fine	Coarse	Fine
U-Net	0.760±0.05	0.853±0.04	0.795±0.19	0.746±0.13	0.868±0.17	0.847±0.09
DeepLabv3	0.767±0.03	0.859±0.03	0.783±0.20	0.765±0.12	0.858±0.18	0.861±0.08

IoU, we calculated the F1 scores for U-Net and DeepLabv3 to assess the balance between precision and recall. U-Net achieved an F1 score of 0.868 and DeepLabv3 scored 0.858 on the coarsely annotated test set, while on the finely annotated test set, U-Net achieved 0.847 and DeepLabv3 achieved 0.861. The detailed results are provided in Tab. 2. Fig. 1 presents examples of segmentations from both U-Net and DeepLabv3.

4 Discussion

This study introduces a novel dataset of coarse tumor annotations for the TCGA-BRCA, addressing an important gap in accessible tumor region labels for breast cancer research. Our initial segmentation models, U-Net and DeepLabv3, performed comparably, with IoU scores of 0.795 and 0.783 respectively, demonstrating the utility of our dataset in training models for tumor segmentation.

As visible in Fig. 1, the coarseness of the annotated masks does reproduce in its predictions, which can be interpreted as the networks learning the distinctive style of the annotations. Larger gaps in the tumor, e.g., due to tissue rupture, which were partially omitted in the coarse annotations, are correctly predicted by the utilized models (see first row of Fig. 1). We tie this to the receptive field of the networks, limiting their ability to overfit to the coarseness of annotations.

While the coarseness of predictions might limit some applications, we hypothesize that many downstream tasks, which require tumor segmentation as a preprocessing task (e.g., tumor area estimation, mitotic hotspot detection), will not be impacted significantly by it. There are also effective algorithmic approaches that leverage coarse masks to achieve high-quality results, addressing potential limitations in fine detail [8].

Compared to existing breast cancer datasets, which often lack explicitly labeled tumor regions, this dataset provides valuable annotations for the entire WSIs of the popular TCGA-BRCA dataset. By providing annotated tumor regions, this dataset can assist in automating key diagnostic workflows, such as calculating tumor burden or identifying hotspot mitotic areas, potentially saving pathologists' time by requiring fewer corrections of false model predictions.

Acknowledgement. The authors would like to acknowledge support by the German Research Foundation (DFG), project number 520330054, and the Austrian Science Fund (FWF), project number I 6555-B.

References

1. Sung H, Ferlay J, Siegel RL et al. Global cancer statistics 2020: GLOBOCAN estimates of incidence and mortality worldwide for 36 cancers in 185 countries. CA Cancer J Clin. 2021;71(3):209–49.
2. Tubiana M, Pejovic MH, Koscielny S et al. Growth rate, kinetics of tumor cell proliferation and long-term outcome in human breast cancer. Int J Cancer. 1989;44(1):17–22.
3. Fitzgibbons PL, Connolly JL. Protocol for the examination of resection specimens from patients with invasive carcinoma of the breast. CAP guidelines. 2023;4.8.1.0.
4. Meyer JS, Alvarez C, Milikowski C et al. Breast carcinoma malignancy grading by Bloom-Richardson system vs proliferation index: reproducibility of grade and advantages of proliferation index. Modern Pathol. 2005;18(8):1067–78.
5. O'Connor JP, Rose CJ, Waterton JC et al. Imaging intratumor heterogeneity: role in therapy response, resistance, and clinical outcome. Clin Cancer Res. 2015;21(2):249–57.
6. Lingle W, Erickson B, Zuley M et al. The Cancer Genome Atlas Breast Invasive Carcinoma Collection (TCGA-BRCA)(Version 3)[Data set]. Cancer Imag Arch. 2016.
7. Amgad M, Elfandy H, Hussein H et al. Structured crowdsourcing enables convolutional segmentation of histology images. Bioinformatics. 2019;35(18):3461–7.
8. Zheng H, Zhuang Z, Qin Y et al. Weakly supervised deep learning for breast cancer segmentation with coarse annotations. Proc MICCAI. 2020:450–9.
9. Marzahl C, Aubreville M, Bertram CA et al. EXACT: a collaboration toolset for algorithm-aided annotation of images with annotation version control. Sci Rep. 2021;11(1):4343.
10. Aubreville M, Bertram C, Klopfleisch R et al. Sliderunner: a tool for massive cell annotations in whole slide images. Proc BVM. 2018:309–14.
11. Sirinukunwattana K, Alham NK, Verrill C et al. Improving whole slide segmentation through visual context-a systematic study. Proc MICCAI. 2018:192–200.
12. Ronneberger O, Fischer P, Brox T. U-net: convolutional networks for biomedical image segmentation. Proc MICCAI. 2015:234–41.
13. Chen LC. Rethinking atrous convolution for semantic image segmentation. arXiv: 1706.05587. 2017.
14. Isensee F, Wald T, Ulrich C et al. nnU-Net revisited: a call for rigorous validation in 3d medical image segmentation. Proc MICCAI. 2024:488–98.

Abstract: Neural Cellular Automata Learn and Predict on Low-Power Devices

Nick Lemke, Mirko Konstantin, Henry Krumb, John Kalkhof, Anirban Mukhopadhyay

Darmstadt University of Technology, Karolinenplatz 5, 64289 Darmstadt, Germany
nick.lemke@gris.informatik.tu-darmstadt.de

Various deep-learning architectures have been proposed for medical image analysis in recent times. For example, the U-Net-based models, not to forget the nnU-Net framework, set the current gold standard in medical image segmentation. More recently, vision transformers have been adopted for medical image processing, improving accuracy even further. Despite the architectural differences between the just-named and other well-known architectures, they all have one thing in common: The excessive number of parameters. A novel architecture that is different in this regard, is the neural cellular automaton (NCA). Inspired by Conway's Game of Life, it is a cellular automaton, but with rules learned by a neural network instead of hand-crafted rules. As such simple rules in emergent systems can lead to complex behavior, NCAs need less than 100 thousand parameters, which is less than 100× smaller than a comparable U-Net. Despite their small size, the segmentation quality of NCAs is comparable to the models mentioned above and in some cases even outperforming them. In our recent work, we investigate training and inference with NCAs on device classes that have not been considered within the medical imaging community so far. Specifically, we found that NCAs can be trained on smartphones, for which we developed a method for unsupervised fine-tuning of pre-trained NCAs. Going one layer below phones, we found that NCA inference can be implemented on even cheaper hardware, such as a $10 ESP32-S3 microcontroller. An NCA running on the ESP32-S3 segments a 32×32 capsule endoscopy image in three seconds with a maximum power draw of 0.7 Watts. The microcontroller itself is the size of a common capsule endoscope, so future capsule endoscopes could perform on-device segmentation. Our findings on NCAs and specifically their trainability on cheap hardware could benefit low- and middle-income countries, that do not have the financial capacities to buy expensive hardware for training and deployment of deep learning models. Also, the unsupervised fine-tuning of segmentation models will benefit small doctor's offices that cannot buy a big GPU machine capable of fine-tuning a segmentation model tailored for the local x-ray machine. We believe that NCAs will drive future research on medical image analysis thanks to their lightweight nature, their robustness towards artifacts, and their prediction quality [1].

References

1. Kalkhof J, Ranem A, Mukhopadhyay A. Unsupervised training of neural cellular automata on edge devices. Proc MICCAI. 2024:498–507.

C. Palm et al. (Hrsg.), *Bildverarbeitung für die Medizin 2025*, Informatik aktuell,
https://doi.org/10.1007/978-3-658-47422-5_57

Abstract: Nuclear Pleomorphism in Canine Cutaneous Mast Cell Tumors

Andreas Haghofer[1,2], Eda Parlak[3], Alexander Bartel[4], Taryn A. Donovan[5], Charles-Antoine Assenmacher[6], Pompei Bolfa[7], Michael J. Dark[8], Andrea Fuchs-Baumgartinger[3], Andrea Klang[3], Kathrin Jäger[9], Robert Klopfleisch[4], Sophie Merz[10], Barbara Richter[3], Yvonne Schulman[11], Hannah Janout[1,2], Jonathan Ganz[12], Josef Scharinger[2], Marc Aubreville[12,13], Stephan M. Winkler[1], Matti Kiupel[13], Christof A. Bertram[3],

[1]University of Applied Sciences Upper Austria, Hagenberg, Austria
[2]Johannes Kepler University, Linz, Austria
[3]University of Veterinary Medicine Vienna, Vienna, Austria
[4]Freie Universität Berlin, Berlin, Germany
[5]The Schwarzman Animal Medical Center, New York, USA
[6]University of Pennsylvania, Philadelphia, PA, USA
[7]Ross University School of Veterinary Medicine, Basseterre, St. Kitts
[8]University of Florida, Gainesville, FL, USA
[9]Laboklin GmbH & Co. KG, Bad Kissing, Germany
[10]IDEXX Vet Med Labor GmbH, Kornwestheim, Germany
[11]Heska, an Antech Company, Loveland, CO, USA
[12]Technische Hochschule Ingolstadt, Ingolstadt, Germany
[13]Hochschule Flensburg, Flensburg, Germany
Christof.Bertram@vetmeduni.ac.at

In histological preparations of tumors, an important criterion for evaluation of malignancy is the variation of nuclear size (anisokaryosis), which is traditionally estimated by pathologists. To improve reproducibility, nuclear size measurements (morphometry) can be performed. In this study [1] we developed a segmentation-based nuclear morphometry algorithm and compared its prognostic value with pathologist's estimates (routine method) and manual morphometry (gold standard method). The three methods were assessed in 96 canine cutaneous mast cell tumors with known patient survival. Estimates by 11 pathologists resulted in highly variable sensitivity (Sen) and specificity (Sp) ranging from Sen = 0%, Sp = 98.8% to Sen = 92.3%, Sp = 31.3%. Manual morphometry of 100 nuclei resulted in a high AUC of 0.839 , however, an average time investment of 17.5 minmakes this method impractical. Automated morphometry resulted in an AUC of 0.943 and is a promising solution for addressing the shortcomings of the other methods.

References

1. Haghofer A, Parlak E, Bartel A et al. Nuclear pleomorphism in canine cutaneous mast cell tumors: comparison of reproducibility and prognostic relevance between estimates, manual morphometry, and algorithmic morphometry. Vet Pathol. 2024:Epub ahead of print.

C. Palm et al. (Hrsg.), *Bildverarbeitung für die Medizin 2025*, Informatik aktuell,
https://doi.org/10.1007/978-3-658-47422-5_58

Abstract: Leveraging Image Captions for Selective Whole Slide Image Annotation

Jingna Qiu[1], Marc Aubreville[2,3], Frauke Wilm[1,4], Mathias Öttl[1,4], Jonas Utz[1], Maja Schlereth[1], Katharina Breininger[1,5]

[1]Department AI in Biomedical Engineering, FAU Erlangen-Nürnberg, Erlangen, Germany
[2]Technische Hochschule Ingolstadt, Ingolstadt, Germany
[3]Flensburg University of Applied Sciences, Flensburg, Germany
[4]Pattern Recognition Lab, FAU Erlangen-Nürnberg, Erlangen, Germany
[5]Center for AI and Data Science, Universität Würzburg, Würzburg, Germany
jingna.qiu@fau.de

Obtaining dense annotations for histopathological whole-slide images (WSI), such as segmentation masks or mitotic figure identification, is a labor intensive process due to the large image size and the extensive manual effort required for annotation. Identifying informative regions in WSIs for annotation while leaving other regions unlabeled can significantly reduce the annotation effort. These selected annotation regions should contain valuable training information that allows proper model training without significantly impacting performance compared to full annotation. In addition, they can help train an initial model to further identify valid annotation regions that improve the model or to speed up manual annotation by suggesting references. Our paper introduces prototype sampling, a method to improve annotation efficiency by detecting WSI regions that are relevant to certain histopathological tasks. Specifically, through keyword search or text-to-image retrieval, we identify a set of prototypes for each class in the task from a public image-caption database and then select WSI regions that are similar to these prototypes for annotation. We evaluated our method in two histopathological tasks, breast cancer metastasis segmentation and mitotic figure detection. Our results show that the annotation regions selected by prototype sampling are rich in useful training information and thus can achieve higher model performance compared to state-of-the-art methods, especially when the annotation budget is extremely limited. For both tasks, prototype sampling approaches full annotation performance by annotating less than 20% of the area. An inspection of selected regions shows that the performance advantage of prototype sampling stems from its ability to recognize authentic class samples, suggesting its specific benefit in identifying annotation samples for underrepresented classes. The source code is available[1] [1].

References

1. Qiu J, Aubreville M, Wilm F et al. Leveraging image captions for selective whole slide image annotation. Proc MICCAI. 2024:207–17.

[1]https://github.com/DeepMicroscopy/Prototype-sampling

C. Palm et al. (Hrsg.), *Bildverarbeitung für die Medizin 2025*, Informatik aktuell,
https://doi.org/10.1007/978-3-658-47422-5_59

Abstract: Würstchen

An Efficient Architecture for Large-scale Text-to-image Diffusion Models

Pablo Pernias[1], Dominic Rampas[1], Mats L. Richter[2], Christopher J. Pal[3,4], Marc Aubreville[5,6]

[1]Luma AI, Inc.
[2]H Company Inc.
[3]Mila, Quebec AI Institute
[4]Polytechnique Montr eal, Canada CIFAR AI Chair
[5]Flensburg University of Applied Sciences
[6]Technische Hochschule Ingolstadt
marc.aubreville@hs-flensburg.de

We introduce Würstchen , a novel architecture for text-to-image synthesis that combines competitive performance with unprecedented cost-effectiveness for large-scale text-to-image diffusion models. A key contribution of our work is to develop a latent diffusion technique in which we learn a detailed but extremely compact semantic image representation used to guide the diffusion process. This highly compressed representation of an image provides much more detailed guidance compared to latent representations of language and this significantly reduces the computational requirements to achieve state-of-the-art results. Our approach also improves the quality of text-conditioned image generation based on our user preference study. The training requirements of our approach consists of 24,602 A100-GPU hours - compared to Stable Diffusion 2.1's 200,000 GPU hours. Our approach also requires less training data to achieve these results. This makes it ideally suited for image generation in domains where data is comparatively scarce, such as many medical imaging modalities. Furthermore, our compact latent representations allows us to perform inference over twice as fast, slashing the usual costs and carbon footprint of a state-of-the-art (SOTA) diffusion model significantly, without compromising the end performance. In a broader comparison against SOTA models our approach is substantially more efficient and compares favorably in terms of image quality. We believe that this work motivates more emphasis on the prioritization of both performance and computational accessibility [1].

References

1. Pernias P, Rampas D, Richter ML et al. Würstchen: an efficient architecture for large-scale text-to-image diffusion models. Proc ICLR. 2024.

C. Palm et al. (Hrsg.), *Bildverarbeitung für die Medizin 2025*, Informatik aktuell,
https://doi.org/10.1007/978-3-658-47422-5_60

Enhancing Zero-shot Learning in Chest X-ray Diagnostics using BioBERT for Textual Representation

Prakhar Bhardwaj, Sheethal Bhat, Andreas Maier

Fakultät für Pattern Recognition, FAU Erlangen-Nürnberg
prakhar.bhardwaj@fau.de

Abstract. Accurate diagnosis of pulmonary diseases from chest X-rays remains a challenging task, especially due to the scarcity of labeled data. In this work, we propose an enhanced zero-shot learning framework that integrates BioBERT—a pre-trained model for biomedical text representation—into a contrastive learning pipeline for medical imaging diagnostics. Our method leverages the synergy between textual radiology reports and image data by combining BioBERT with a CLIP-based architecture. To address the lack of textual data in standard datasets, we generate synthetic radiology reports for each pathology, aiming to mimic the complexity of actual clinical descriptions. Through extensive experiments, we demonstrate significant improvements in disease classification accuracy and generalization, particularly in zero-shot inference scenarios. Our analysis also reveals how similarities in pathology descriptions can lead to misclassifications, emphasizing the importance of nuanced textual representations. This work establishes a zero-shot learning method in medical imaging, highlighting the potential of BioBERT in enhancing automated diagnostic systems for chest X-rays.

1 Introduction

The integration of artificial intelligence (AI) into medical imaging has revolutionized diagnostic practices, especially in fields like radiology. Chest X-rays (CXRs) are one of the most widely used diagnostic tools, essential for detecting a range of thoracic diseases such as pneumonia, pulmonary edema, and pleural effusion [1]. Despite their importance, the interpretation of CXRs remains a complex task that often requires significant expertise due to subtle patterns and overlapping pathologies. AI-driven systems, particularly those based on deep learning, have shown promise in assisting radiologists by improving diagnostic accuracy, reducing errors, and speeding up the analysis process [2]. Studies have demonstrated that AI models can match or even surpass human performance in detecting pathologies in CXRs with high accuracy in some cases. However, the success of these models depends heavily on the availability of large, well-annotated datasets, which are often difficult to obtain in medical imaging.

A key challenge in medical AI systems is the labor-intensive process of data annotation [3]. Annotating medical images, especially CXRs, requires skilled radiologists, making the process time-consuming and costly. As a result, there is a growing need for methods that can leverage large-scale, unlabeled data.

Self-supervised learning has emerged as a powerful technique to overcome the challenges of data annotation. By utilizing unlabeled data, self-supervised models generate

C. Palm et al. (Hrsg.), *Bildverarbeitung für die Medizin 2025*, Informatik aktuell,
https://doi.org/10.1007/978-3-658-47422-5_61

labels through pretext tasks, enabling them to learn meaningful representations without human supervision. Momentum contrast (MoCo) [4] and other contrastive learning methods have been particularly successful in learning robust image representations in the absence of labeled data. Additionally, models like contrastive language-image pre-training (CLIP) [5] have shown significant potential in zero-shot learning by aligning visual and textual representations in a shared embedding space. However, the generic text encoders used in CLIP models are often not optimized for domain-specific language, such as the highly specialized vocabulary found in medical reports.

To address this gap, we propose an enhanced framework that integrates BioBERT [6], a pre-trained language model specifically designed for biomedical text mining, into the CLIP architecture as shown in Fig. 1. Due to the lack of textual reports in standard CXR datasets, we generate synthetic radiology reports for each pathology to train the text encoder effectively. By replacing the general text encoder in CLIP with BioBERT and incorporating synthetic reports, we aim to improve the alignment between textual radiology reports and CXR images, especially for underrepresented diseases.

The main contributions of this work are as follows:

- *Enhanced zero-shot learning model:* We integrate BioBERT into the CLIP architecture to improve text-image alignment for medical diagnostics, allowing for accurate zero-shot classification of diseases from CXRs.
- *Synthetic radiology reports:* We generate synthetic reports for each pathology to address the absence of textual data in standard datasets, enabling the training of the text encoder.
- *Analysis of misclassifications:* We investigate how similarities in pathology descriptions can lead to misclassifications, highlighting the importance of nuanced textual representations in distinguishing between conditions.

By combining domain-specific textual representation with self-supervised learning techniques, our method provides a scalable solution for improving diagnostic accuracy in medical imaging, particularly in resource-constrained settings where labeled data is scarce.

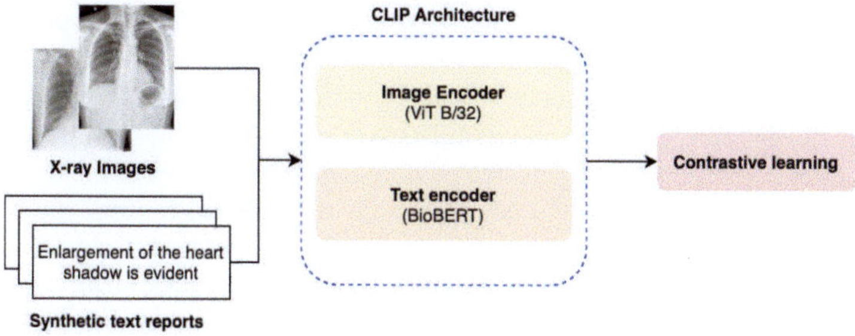

Fig. 1. Proposed CLIP model with X-ray images and sythetic reports as inputs and ViT B/32 as image encoder and BioBERT as text encoder.

Tab. 1. Example pathologies and corresponding synthetic report texts.

Pathology	Synthetic Report Text
Cardiomegaly	Enlargement of the heart shadow is evident
Atelectasis	Partial collapse or incomplete inflation of the lung is noted.
Infiltration	Diffuse infiltration, likely of inflammatory or infectious nature
Pneumothorax	Presence of air or gas in the pleural cavity
Emphysema	Abnormal enlargement of air spaces is evident
Effusion	Excess fluid in the pleural cavity is noted

2 Materials and methods

2.1 Dataset

To evaluate the performance of our proposed zero-shot learning model, we utilize the NIH Chest X-ray Dataset [7], which comprises 112,120 chest X-ray images annotated for 14 thoracic diseases. However, this dataset does not include corresponding radiology reports, which are essential for training text-image alignment models like CLIP. The dataset was split into training (80%), validation (10%), and testing (10%) sets. Images were resized to 224×224 pixels, and pixel intensity values were normalized to ensure consistency.

To overcome the absence of textual reports, we generate synthetic text reports for each pathology. These synthetic reports are designed to mimic the structure and language of actual radiology reports, capturing essential details and terminology associated with each condition.

2.2 Implementation details

Our model architecture is based on the CLIP framework with modifications to the text encoder and image learning pipeline. Since the NIH Chest X-ray Dataset does not provide textual reports, we create synthetic text reports to enable the training of the text encoder. These synthetic reports are constructed by combining standardized descriptions of each pathology, inspired by the language and structure of actual radiology reports found in datasets like MIMIC-CXR [8].

For each pathology, we generate a set of synthetic reports that include common phrases and terminologies used by radiologists to describe that condition. Tab. 1 presents examples of synthetic reports for selected pathologies. While these synthetic reports may not capture the full variability and complexity of real clinical reports, they provide a starting point for training the text encoder to align textual and visual representations.

We integrate BioBERT [6], a pre-trained language model specifically designed for biomedical text mining, into the CLIP architecture as the text encoder. BioBERT is fine-tuned on the synthetic reports to improve its understanding of biomedical language and its alignment with the visual features extracted from the chest X-ray images. The model is trained using the NIH chest X-ray dataset, augmented with the synthetic text reports. The training process involves optimizing the shared embedding space for both image and text encoders. We use a batch size of 32 and a learning rate of 0.001. The BioBERT

Tab. 2. Comparison of AUC Scores for different pathologies, showing baseline with different text encoders: Transformer and BioBERT with varying token lengths and Data Distribution.

Pathology	# Images	% of Data	Transformer (77)	BioBERT (128)	BioBERT (512)
Pneumonia	1,431	1.3%	0.770	0.387	**0.778**
Infiltration	19,894	17.7%	0.730	0.759	**0.816**
Cardiomegaly	2,772	2.5%	**0.940**	0.609	0.716
Edema	2,303	2.1%	0.890	0.745	**0.930**
Pleural Thickening	3,385	3.0%	**0.740**	0.443	0.455
Class-wise average			**0.806**	0.588	0.739
Weighted average			**0.765**	0.689	**0.769**

text encoder's parameters are updated during training to ensure robust representation of biomedical language.

The model's performance is evaluated on both multi-label classification (for seen diseases) and zero-shot classification (on unseen diseases). The primary evaluation metrics include the area under the receiver operating characteristic (AUROC) [9], to measure the model's ability to generalize to both seen and unseen pathologies, highlighting the impact of BioBERT integration on the zero-shot learning task.

3 Results

The integration of BioBERT into the CLIP-based framework significantly impacted the model's performance in medical image-text matching tasks, particularly in terms of the area under the curve (AUC) scores for various pathologies. By replacing the original CLIP text encoder with BioBERT, a model pre-trained on biomedical text, the system was better able to handle the domain-specific language and context-dependent nuances found in radiology reports. One of the most important modifications introduced by this change was the increase in the processed sequence length from 77 tokens (as in the original CLIP model) to 512 tokens, allowing the model to capture more details from the radiology reports.

Tab. 2 presents a comparison of AUC scores for different pathologies using the original Transformer-based text encoder with a 77-token limit and BioBERT with token limits of 128 and 512, along with the data distribution for each pathology. The results show a clear improvement in performance with the use of BioBERT, particularly when the token limit is extended to 512 tokens, enabling the model to leverage the full content of radiology reports.

The use of BioBERT had a noticeable effect on the model's ability to classify certain pathologies. There was a substantial improvement in the AUC score for Pneumonia, increasing from 0.387 with a 128-token length to 0.778 with a 512-token length. The AUC score for Infiltration rose from 0.759 to 0.816, and for Edema from 0.745 to 0.930 when increasing the token length to 512. These improvements indicate that the additional textual information allowed for better feature alignment and prediction accuracy, particularly for pathologies with complex descriptions. However, the AUC score for Pleural Thickening showed only a slight improvement, from 0.443 to 0.455, and Cardiomegaly experienced a decline from 0.940 with the Transformer to 0.716 with BioBERT (512 tokens). The modest gain and decline suggest limitations due to the synthetic report texts and data distribution. Pleural Thickening's synthetic reports often consisted solely of the label itself, limiting the model's ability to exploit BioBERT's capabilities fully. Cardiomegaly, being only 2.5% of the dataset, suffered from underrepresentation, restricting the model's ability to learn comprehensive representations for this condition.

The results indicate that increasing the token length from 77 to 512 tokens significantly improves the model's performance in most cases. By allowing BioBERT to process longer sequences, the model better aligned text descriptions with corresponding image features, leading to improved classification outcomes across several pathologies. We also calculated the class-wise and weighted average AUC scores to provide a comprehensive evaluation. The class-wise average AUC improved from 0.588 with BioBERT (128 tokens) to 0.739 with BioBERT (512 tokens), while the weighted average AUC increased from 0.689 to 0.769. The weighted average offers a more accurate reflection of real-world performance, emphasizing the model's improved accuracy on more prevalent conditions in the dataset.

Our experiments revealed that some pathologies share similar textual descriptions, leading to potential misclassifications due to overlapping language used to describe different conditions. For example, pathologies like Pneumothorax and Pleural Effusion both involve abnormalities in the pleural cavity and may include similar terms such as "air," "fluid," or "pleural space" in their descriptions. This overlap can make it challenging for the model to distinguish between these conditions based solely on text representations. A correlation study of the synthetic report texts showed significant textual overlap between certain pairs of diseases, such as Edema and Effusion, which may cause the model to misclassify images if it relies heavily on shared textual features rather than focusing on discriminative visual cues.

4 Discussion

The integration of BioBERT as the text encoder in the CLIP-based framework significantly improved the model's performance in several chest X-ray classification tasks, particularly for conditions like Pneumonia, Infiltration, and Edema. The increase in AUC scores, especially when using a 512-token length, highlights the benefits of processing the full content of radiology reports. This approach enabled better feature alignment by capturing the subtleties and context-specific information inherent in clinical language.

However, our reliance on synthetic reports introduces limitations. While synthetic reports provide a consistent and controlled set of textual descriptions, they lack the variability and complexity of actual clinical reports. Real radiology reports often contain nuanced language, variations in terminology, and additional contextual information that can influence the model's understanding. Adapting our method to use actual text reports, such as those available in the MIMIC-CXR dataset, could further improve the model's performance by providing richer and more diverse textual data. We also observed that for Cardiomegaly and Pleural Thickening, the performance worsened with increasing context length. This decline can be attributed to specific characteristics of the dataset and the nature of the synthetic reports used for these pathologies. As Cardiomegaly represents only 2.5% of the data distribution, making it one of the least represented classes and in the case of Pleural Thickening, the synthetic reports generated were minimalistic, often consisting solely of the label itself without additional descriptive context. As a result, increasing the token length does not provide BioBERT with meaningful additional information to enhance its understanding of this condition.

Our findings also highlight that the similarity in pathology descriptions can lead to misclassification. The overlap in textual features between certain conditions emphasizes the importance of incorporating more detailed and discriminative textual and visual features. Techniques such as attention mechanisms or incorporating additional clinical context could help the model focus on the most relevant features and improve classification accuracy.

Overall, our study demonstrates that integrating domain-specific language models like BioBERT into vision-language frameworks can enhance zero-shot learning in medical imaging. By leveraging more accurate textual representations and addressing issues such as class imbalance and insufficient textual variability, we can develop models that perform better in clinical settings. Future work should focus on utilizing actual clinical reports, improving synthetic text generation, and exploring methods to better distinguish between similar pathologies.

References

1. Meedeniya D, Kumarasinghe H, Kolonne S et al. Chest X-ray analysis empowered with deep learning: a systematic review. Appl Soft Comput. 2022;126:109319.
2. Pesapane F, Codari M, Sardanelli F. Artificial intelligence in medical imaging: threat or opportunity? Radiologists again at the forefront of innovation in medicine. Eur Radiol Exp. 2018;2:35.
3. Pierre K, Haneberg AG, Kwak S et al. Applications of artificial intelligence in the radiology roundtrip: process streamlining, workflow optimization, and beyond. Semin Roentgenol. 2023;58(2):158–69.
4. He K, Fan H, Wu Y et al. Momentum contrast for unsupervised visual representation learning. Proc IEEE CVF CVPR. 2020.
5. Radford A, Kim JW, Hallacy C et al. Learning transferable visual models from natural language supervision. Proc ICML. 2021.
6. Lee J, Yoon W, Kim S et al. BioBERT: a pre-trained biomedical language representation model for biomedical text mining. Bioinformatics. 2020;36(4):1234–40.
7. Wang X, Peng Y, Lu L et al. ChestX-Ray8: hospital-scale chest X-ray database and benchmarks on weakly-supervised classification and localization of common thorax diseases. Proc IEEE CVPR. 2017:3462–71.
8. Johnson AEW, Pollard TJ, Berkowitz SJ et al. MIMIC-CXR, a de-identified publicly available database of chest radiographs with free-text reports. Sci Data. 2019;6:317.
9. Fawcett T. An introduction to ROC analysis. Pattern Recognit Lett. 2006;27(8):861–74.

Abstract: Simulation-informed Learning for Time-resolved Angiographic Contrast Agent Concentration Reconstruction

Noah Maul[1,2], Annette Birkhold[2], Fabian Wagner[1], Mareike Thies[1], Maximilian Rohleder[1,2], Philipp Berg[3,4], Markus Kowarschik[2], Andreas Maier[1]

[1]Pattern Recognition Lab, Friedrich-Alexander-Universität Erlangen-Nürnberg, Germany
[2]Siemens Healthineers AG, Forchheim, Germany
[3]Research Campus STIMULATE, University of Magdeburg, Germany
[4]Department of Medical Engineering, University of Magdeburg, Germany
noah.maul@fau.de

Three-dimensional digital subtraction angiography (3D-DSA) is a well-established X-ray-based technique for visualizing vascular anatomy. Recently, four-dimensional DSA (4D-DSA) reconstruction algorithms have been developed to enable the visualization of volumetric contrast flow dynamics through time-series of volumes. This reconstruction problem is ill-posed mainly due to vessel overlap in the projection direction and geometric vessel foreshortening, which leads to information loss in the recorded projection images. However, knowledge about the underlying fluid dynamics can be leveraged to constrain the solution space. In our work, we implicitly include this information in a neural network-based model that is trained on a dataset of image-based blood flow simulations. The model predicts the spatially averaged contrast agent concentration for each centerline point of the vasculature over time, lowering the overall computational demand. The trained network enables the reconstruction of relative contrast agent concentrations with a mean absolute error of 0.02 ± 0.02 and a mean absolute percentage error of $5.31 \pm 9.25\%$. Moreover, the network is robust to varying degrees of vessel overlap and vessel foreshortening. Our approach demonstrates the potential of the integration of machine learning and blood flow simulations in time-resolved angiographic contrast agent concentration reconstruction[1] [1].

References

1. Maul N, Birkhold A, Wagner F et al. Simulation-informed learning for time-resolved angiographic contrast agent concentration reconstruction. Comput Biol Med. 2024;182:109178.

---

[1]The concepts and information presented are based on research and are not commercially available.

C. Palm et al. (Hrsg.), *Bildverarbeitung für die Medizin 2025*, Informatik aktuell,
https://doi.org/10.1007/978-3-658-47422-5_62

U-Net and GAN for Virtual Contrast in Breast MRI

How Do They Compare to Real Contrast Images?

Aju George[1], Hannes Schreiter[1], Julian Hossbach[1,2], Tri-Thien Nguyen[1,2], Ihor Horishnyi[1], Chris Ehring[1], Shirin Heidarikahkesh[1], Lorenz A.Kapsner[1,3], Frederik B.Laun[1], Michael Uder[1], Sabine Ohlmeyer[1], Sebastian Bickelhaupt[1,4], Andrzej Liebert[1]

[1]Institute of Radiology, Uniklinikum Erlangen, FAU Erlangen-Nürnberg, Erlangen, Germany
[2]Pattern Recognition Lab, FAU Erlangen-Nürnberg, Erlangen Germany
[3]Lehrstuhl für Medizinische Informatik, FAU Erlangen-Nürnberg, Erlangen Germany
[4]German Cancer Research Center, Heidelberg, Germany
aju.george@fau.de

Abstract. Multiparametric MRI with gadolinium-based contrast agents demonstrates high sensitivity for detecting lesions in the breast, particularly in women with denser breast tissue. However, its use is limited by increased costs, time and contraindications in certain patients. This study explores a pix2pix generative adversarial network (GAN) to create virtual contrast-enhanced (vCE) MRI from un-enhanced T1w, T2w, and DWI sequences and compares it with a U-Net model. The vCE GAN achieved an SSIM of 80.75 and PSNR of 21.90, while the vCE U-Net scored 87.39 and 24.39, respectively. A multi-reader Turing test showed that 45.89% of vCE GAN images were rated as real, comparable to 45.09% for true CE images. In contrast, 47.25% of vCE U-Net images were rated as real.

1 Introduction

Breast cancer accounts for 31% of all cancer diagnoses in women, making it the most prevalent cancer among females. The 5-year survival rate is 99% for localized breast cancer but drops significantly to 30% for distant-stage breast cancer [1]. The early wide spread screening with mammography has reduced the mortality rate significantly [2], but it fails to detect significant amount of breast cancer especially in women with high amount of Fibro-glandular tissue (FGT) [3].

Apart from mammography, multiparametric MRI scans, including contrast-enhanced (CE) imaging with gadolinium-based contrast agents (GBCA), have high sensitivity in detecting breast lesions, particularly in women with dense breast tissue [4]. Although GBCA are generally considered safe, their use requires intravenous access and physician supervision, resulting in higher costs and longer examination times, and its use is limited in patients with severe renal impairment and pregnant individuals [5].

In recent years several publications aimed at creating virtual contrast-enhanced (vCE) images in breast MRI without using GBCA through deep learning techniques [6–12]. Most of these approaches have utilized encoder-decoder [11, 12] or U-NET-based architectures [6, 10] to synthesize vCE from either T1-weighted (T1w) images or a combination of multiple imaging sequences, such as T1w, T2-weighted (T2w), and

C. Palm et al. (Hrsg.), *Bildverarbeitung für die Medizin 2025*, Informatik aktuell,
https://doi.org/10.1007/978-3-658-47422-5_63

diffusion-weighted imaging (DWI). While these methods have shown promising results, incorporating adversarial training strategies can enhance the network's ability to capture more in-depth information and details such as generative adversarial networks (GANs) [13]. Several previous publications in the area of vCE breast MRI focused on GAN-based models [7–9] however, these studies primarily rely on either T1w or a combination of T1w and T2w scans for vCE synthesis, without utilizing DWI scans, despite evidence indicating that including DWI can significantly improve the vCE image quality [14].

This study aims to generate 2nd time point of CE T1w subtraction image (further referring as CE) synthetically from un-enhanced sequences, including T1w, T2w, and three DWI scans, using a pix2pix GAN [15]. The results of the proposed method are further compared with the images from a previous vCE U-Net implementation [6], and a multi-reader Turing test were performed to evaluate the visual appearance of the synthetic images.

2 Materials and methods

2.1 Datasets

In this IRB-approved retrospective study, a dataset of clinical breast examinations acquired between 2017 and June 2022 at the University Clinic Erlangen with two 3 Tesla scanners (Siemens Healthineers MAGNETOM Vida and Skyra) was used. The dataset (n = 2126, mean age 49 ± 12 years) included T1w, T2w, dynamic contrast-enhanced (DCE) imaging, and DWI with b-values of 50, 750, and 1500 s/mm^2 acquisitions. The dataset was split into training (n = 1615), validation (n = 256), and test (n = 255) sets. For training, all slices from each subject were used, resulting in multiple samples per subject. Preprocessing was performed according to Liebert et al. [14], including field-of-view (FoV) resampling, z-dimension alignment, z-score intensity normalization, intensity clamping, and rescaling. This resulted in an in-plane resolution of (280 × 448) and an average of 109 slices per subject.

2.2 Neural network and training

Both vCE U-Net and vCE GAN were trained for 100 epochs. The vCE U-Net was trained in accordance to Schreiter, et al. [6] using a combination of L1 and structural similarity index measure (SSIM) loss [16]. Fig. 1 depicts the overall architecture of the vCE GAN model. The loss function for generator (G) in vCE GAN is given in Eq. 1, where x represents the input sequences and y denotes the ground truth CE image

$$\mathcal{L}_G(x, y) = \lambda_1(\mathcal{L}_{\text{L1}}(G(x), y) + \mathcal{L}_{\text{SSIM}}(G(x), y)) + \lambda_2\mathcal{L}_{\text{BCE}}(D(G(x), x), 1) \quad (1)$$

The discriminator (D) minimizes the Binary cross entropy (BCE) Loss between the label smoothed target (real: *1*, fake: *0*) and the predicted label for CE or the vCE image given by $\mathcal{L}_D(x, y, G(x)) = \mathcal{L}_{\text{BCE}}(D(G(x), x), \mathit{0}) + \mathcal{L}_{\text{BCE}}(D(y, x), \mathit{1})$.

The model was trained with a batch size of n = 48 slices on an NVIDIA A100 (40 GB) GPU. Both the G and D were optimized using the ADAM optimizer, with a learning rate of 1×10^{-4} for the G and a learning rate of 1×10^{-3} for the D.

2.3 Performance evaluation

The performance of the models was evaluated quantitatively using SSIM, peak signal-to-noise ratio (PNSR), normalized root mean square error (NRMSE) and median symmetric accuracy (MEDSYMAC). Additionally, a multi-reader Turing test was conducted to gain qualitative insights into the model's performance. For the study, single slices from the test dataset, representing real CE images and generated vCE GAN and vCE U-Net images, were split into three sessions, ensuring that each session contained a mix of real and generated images without overlapping cases from different image types. Four experienced readers: one radiologist (R2) with 9 years of experience, one research scientist (R4) with three years of experience in breast MRI and two medical students with 1.5 years (R3) and 2 months (R1) of experience in MRI research, independently participated in the Turing test to assess whether the images appeared real or synthetic.

3 Results

The vCE U-Net outperformed the vCE GAN in most quantitative performance metrics, except for MEDSYMAC, as shown in Tab. 1. However, a comparison of the CE, vCE U-Net and vCE GAN images (Fig. 2) shows that, the vCE GAN image (Fig. 2 C) achieved better structural details compared to vCE U-Net (Fig. 2 B). Both models rarely create false positive enhancement in regions with appearance similar to cysts in the original

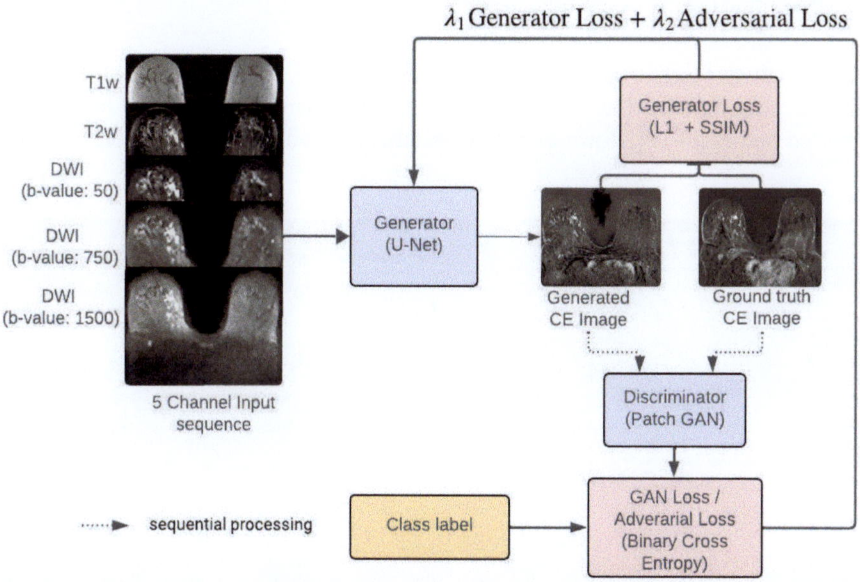

Fig. 1. Overview of the vCE GAN architecture for generating CE images. In this architecture, the U-Net similar to Schreiter, et al [6] was used as the generator. A patchGAN [17] was used as the discriminator, similar to the approach in pix2pix networks [15].

Tab. 1. Metrics values for vCE.

Model	SSIM (↑)	PSNR [dB] (↑)	NRMSE (↓)	MEDSYMAC (↓)
vCE GAN	80.75 ± 3.21	21.90 ± 1.79	0.12 ± 0.01	0.012 ± 0.01
vCE U-Net	87.39 ± 2.37	24.39 ± 1.85	0.09 ± 0.01	0.019 ± 0.01

image (subject 2 Fig. 2). However, intensity enhancement was lower in the vCE GAN image (Fig. 2 F) than the vCE U-Net image (Fig. 2 E). In terms of FGT and the MR image artifacts appearance, the vCE GAN images exhibited a more inhomogeneous appearance than the vCE U-Net images, making it appear more realistic and closer to the ground truth in perception.

The summarized results of the Turing test are given in Tab. 2 and exemplary cases with reader ratings from the Turing test are shown in Fig. 3. In the Turing test classification results for subject 4, all readers demonstrated high inter-reader agreement for the vCE U-Net images compared to the vCE GAN images, likely due to the U-Net's ability to produce sharper and more homogeneous images. However the similarity in inhomogeneity in the CE (Fig. 3 A) and vCE GAN (Fig. 3 C) images of subject 4 led to mix opinions among readers, a pattern also observed in subject 6. In subject 5 the CE image (Fig. 3 D) exhibited low signal areas, resulting in 2 out of 4 readers classifying as fake. Conversely, all readers agreed that vCE GAN image (Fig. 3 F) appeared real, as it did not contain low-signal areas unlike the CE image.

4 Discussion

The quantitative performance metrics of the proposed vCE GAN network generally showed values on the low end or below the performance levels noted in previously reported studies [9–12]. However, the model still achieved higher SSIM scores compared

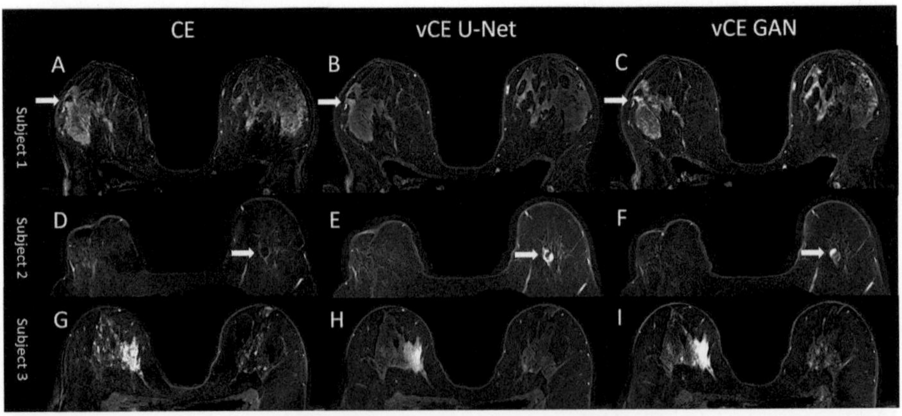

Fig. 2. Comparison of CE, vCE U-Net and vCE GAN from 3 subjects. For subject 2 an enhancement of a cyst like structure can be noted in the left breast (white arrows).

Tab. 2. Multi-reader Turing test results, showing the percentage of images each reader classified as 'real' for each image type.

	R1	R2	R3	R4	Average	Total
CE	42.10 %	50.00 %	34.37 %	53.9 %	45.09 %	256
vCE U- Net	37.50 %	57.81 %	36.71 %	57.0 %	47.25 %	256
vCE GAN	40.23 %	50.78 %	38.67 %	53.9 %	45.89 %	256

to the two previous GAN based studies [7, 8]. Even when compared to the vCE U-Net trained on the in-house data set [6], the quantitative performance of the vCE GAN network was notably lower.

The visual qualitative evaluation in a Turing test showed a more realistic appearance of the vCE GAN which proves the general need for visual evaluations of such images. The reduced accuracy of the readers for the CE and vCE GAN image classification compared to the cleaner vCE U-Net suggests that the real or learned artifacts are seen as indicator for fake images. The adversarial training strategies enabled the vCE GAN model to produce images with image distortions and artifacts in a similar style, as seen in CE images (Fig. 2 A, D & G). This shows that distinguishing real and fakes is a challenging task. However, since vCE U-Net was trained with only data consistency losses, it seemed to be unable to create these unpredictable effects in its reconstructions (Fig. 2 E & H, Fig. 3 H). The missing MR artifacts might explains why R1 & R3 were more critical in classifying vCE U-Net as real, while R2 & R4 were potentially more convinced the quantitatively better image quality.

This study is not without limitations. The data were collected from a single site, and the lesion enhancement was not assessed. Addressing these limitations in future research could improve the robustness and generalizability of the results.

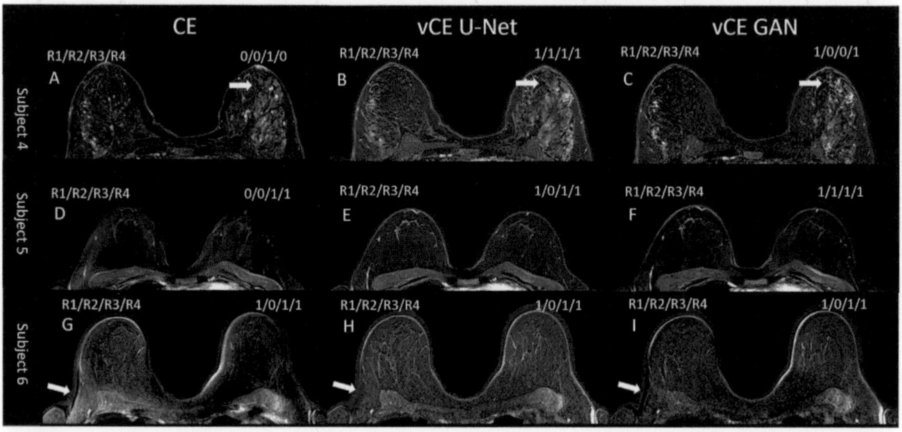

Fig. 3. Comparison of CE, vCE U-Net and vCE GAN of 3 subjects. Classification by multiple readers is indicated in each image, with '0' for 'fake' and '1' for 'real'. In subject 6 an artifact can be noted in the right breast (white arrows) in the CE and vCE GAN images.

References

1. Siegel RL, Miller KD, Wagle NS et al. Cancer statistics. CA Cancer J Clin. 2023;73(1).
2. Tabár L, Vitak B, Chen THH et al. Swedish two-county trial: impact of mammographic screening on breast cancer mortality during 3 decades. Radiology. 2011;260(3):658–63.
3. Wanders JO, Holland K, Karssemeijer N et al. The effect of volumetric breast density on the risk of screen-detected and interval breast cancers: a cohort study. Breast Cancer Res. 2017;19:1–13.
4. Heywang SH, Fenzl G, Hahn D et al. MR imaging of the breast: comparison with mammography and ultrasound. J Comput Assist Tomogr. 1986;10(4):615–20.
5. Chung M, Calabrese E, Mongan J et al. Deep learning to simulate contrast-enhanced breast MRI of invasive breast cancer. Radiology. 2022;306(3):e213199.
6. Schreiter H, Eberle J, Kapsner LA et al. Virtual dynamic contrast enhanced breast MRI using 2D U-Net architectures. medRxiv. 2024:2024–8.
7. Müller-Franzes G, Huck L, Tayebi Arasteh S et al. Using machine learning to reduce the need for contrast agents in breast MRI through synthetic images. Radiology. 2023;307(3):e222211.
8. Wang P, Nie P, Dang Y et al. Synthesizing the first phase of dynamic sequences of breast MRI for enhanced lesion identification. Front Oncol. 2021;11:792516.
9. Kim E, Cho HH, Kwon J et al. Tumor-attentive segmentation-guided gan for synthesizing breast contrast-enhanced mri without contrast agents. IEEE J Transl Eng Health Med. 2022;11:32–43.
10. Sikka D, Zhu N, Liu C et al. Predicting gadolinium contrast enhancement for structural lesion analysis using DeepContrast.
11. Chung M, Calabrese E, Mongan J et al. Deep learning to simulate contrast-enhanced breast MRI of invasive breast cancer. Radiology. 2022;306(3):e213199.
12. Zhang T, Han L, D'Angelo A et al. Synthesis of contrast-enhanced breast MRI using T1- and multi-b-value DWI-based hierarchical fusion network with attention mechanism. Proc MICCAI. 2023:79–88.
13. Goodfellow I, Pouget-Abadie J, Mirza M et al. Generative adversarial networks. Proc ACM. 2020;63(11):139–44.
14. Liebert A, Schreiter H, Kapsner LA et al. Impact of non-contrast enhanced imaging input sequences on the generation of virtual contrast-enhanced breast MRI scans using neural networks. medRxiv. 2024:2024–5.
15. Isola P, Zhu JY, Zhou T et al. Image-to-image translation with conditional adversarial networks. Proc IEEE CVPR. 2017:1125–34.
16. Wang Z, Bovik AC, Sheikh HR et al. Image quality assessment: from error visibility to structural similarity. IEEE Trans Image Process. 2004;13(4):600–12.
17. Li C, Wand M. Precomputed real-time texture synthesis with markovian generative adversarial networks. Proc ECCV III. 2016:702–16.

Abstract: Client Security Alone Fails in Federated Learning

2D and 3D Attack Insights

Santhosh Parampottupadam[1,2], Ralf Floca[1], Dimitrios Bounias[1,2], Benjamin Hamm[1,2], Saikat Roy[1], Sinem Sav[3], Maximilian Zenk[1,2], Klaus Maier-Hein[1,2,4]

[1]German Cancer Research Center (DKFZ), Division of Medical Image Computing, Heidelberg, Germany
[2]Medical Faculty Heidelberg, Heidelberg University, Heidelberg, Germany
[3]Department of Computer Engineering, Bilkent University, Turkey
[4]Pattern Analysis and Learning Group, Department of Radiation Oncology, Heidelberg University Hospital, 69120 Heidelberg, Germany
santhosh.parampottupadam@dkfz-heidelberg.de

Federated learning (FL) plays a vital role in boosting both accuracy and privacy in the collaborative medical imaging field. The importance of privacy increases with the diverse security standards across nations and corporations, particularly in healthcare and global FL initiatives. Current research on privacy attacks in federated medical imaging focuses on sophisticated gradient inversion attacks that can reconstruct images from FL communications. These methods demonstrate potential worst-case scenarios, highlighting the need for effective security measures and the adoption of comprehensive zero-trust security frameworks. Our paper introduces a novel method for performing precise reconstruction attacks on the private data of participating clients in FL settings using a malicious server. We conducted experiments on brain tumor MRI and chest CT data sets, implementing existing 2D and novel 3D reconstruction techniques. Our results reveal significant privacy breaches: 35.19% of data reconstructed with 6 clients, 37.21% with 12 clients in 2D, and 62.92% in 3D with 12 clients. This underscores the urgent need for enhanced privacy protections in FL systems. To address these issues, we suggest effective measures to counteract such vulnerabilities by securing gradient, analytic, and linear layers. Our contributions aim to strengthen the security framework of FL in medical imaging, promoting the safe advancement of collaborative healthcare research. The original paper was accepted at the MICCAI workshop and is available here [1].

References

1. Parampottupadam S, Floca R, Bounias D et al. Client security alone fails in federated learning: 2D and 3D attack insights. Proc MICCAI EMERGE. 2024.

C. Palm et al. (Hrsg.), *Bildverarbeitung für die Medizin 2025*, Informatik aktuell,
https://doi.org/10.1007/978-3-658-47422-5_64

Abstract: Selective Reduction of CT Data for Self-supervised Pre-training Improves Downstream Classification Performance

Daniel Wolf[1,2], Tristan Payer[1], Catharina S. Lisson[2], Christoph G. Lisson[2], Meinrad Beer[2], Michael Götz[‡2], Timo Ropinski[‡1]

[1]Visual Computing Research Group, Institute of Media Informatics, Ulm University, Germany
[2]Experimental Radiology Research Group, Department for Diagnostic and Interventional Radiology, Ulm University Medical Center, Germany
daniel.wolf@uni-ulm.de

Self-supervised pre-training of deep learning models with contrastive learning is a widely used technique in image analysis. As shown in our previous work [1] contrastive pre-training has strong potential on medical images. However, further research is necessary to incorporate the particular characteristics of these images. We hypothesize that the similarity of medical images hinders the success of contrastive learning in the medical imaging domain. To this end, in our publication [2] we investigate different strategies based on deep embedding, information theory, and hashing in order to identify and reduce redundancy in medical pre-training datasets. The effect of these different reduction strategies on contrastive learning is evaluated on two pre-training datasets and several downstream classification tasks. In all of our experiments, dataset reduction leads to a considerable performance gain in downstream tasks, e.g., an AUC score improvement from 0.78 to 0.83 for the COVID CT Classification Grand Challenge, 0.97 to 0.98 for the OrganSMNIST Classification Challenge and 0.73 to 0.83 for a brain hemorrhage classification task. Furthermore, pre-training is up to nine times faster due to the dataset reduction. In conclusion, the proposed approach highlights the importance of dataset quality and provides a transferable approach to improve contrastive pre-training for classification downstream tasks on medical images.

References

1. Wolf D, Payer T, Lisson CS et al. Self-supervised pre-training with contrastive and masked autoencoder methods for dealing with small datasets in deep learning for medical imaging. Sci Rep. 2023;13(1):20260.
2. Wolf D, Payer T, Lisson CS et al. Less is more: selective reduction of CT data for self-supervised pre-training of deep learning models with contrastive learning improves downstream classification performance. Comput Biol Med. 2024;183:109242.

[‡]These authors contributed equally the least to this work.

C. Palm et al. (Hrsg.), *Bildverarbeitung für die Medizin 2025*, Informatik aktuell,
https://doi.org/10.1007/978-3-658-47422-5_65

Abstract: Death by Retrospective Undersampling

Caveats and Solutions for Learning-Based MRI Reconstructions

Junaid R. Rajput[1,2], Simon Weinmueller[1], Jonathan Endres[1], Peter Dawood[1], Florian Knoll[3], Andreas Maier[2], Moritz Zaiss[1]

[1]Institute of Neuroradiology, University Hospital Erlangen, Erlangen, Germany
[2]Pattern Recognition Lab Friedrich-Alexander-University Erlangen-Nürnberg
[3]Department of Artificial Intelligence in Biomedical Engineering Friedrich Alexander University of Erlangen–Nuernberg, Erlangen, Germany
junaid.rajput@fau.de

This study challenges the validity of retrospective undersampling in MRI data science by analysis via an MRI physics simulation. We demonstrate that retrospective undersampling, a method often used to create training data for reconstruction models, can inherently alter MRI signals from their prospective counterparts. This arises from the sequential nature of MRI acquisition, where undersampling post-acquisition effectively alters the MR sequence and the magnetization dynamic in a non-linear fashion. We show that even in common sequences, this effect can make learning-based reconstructions unreliable. Our simulation provides both, (i) a tool for generating accurate prospective undersampled datasets for analysis of such effects, or for MRI training data augmentation, and (ii) a differentiable reconstruction operator that models undersampling correctly. The provided insights are crucial for the development and evaluation of AI-driven acceleration of diagnostic MRI tools [1].

References

1. Rajput JR, Weinmueller S, Endres J et al. Death by retrospective undersampling - caveats and solutions for learning-based MRI reconstructions. Proc MICCAI. 2024:233–41.

C. Palm et al. (Hrsg.), *Bildverarbeitung für die Medizin 2025*, Informatik aktuell,
https://doi.org/10.1007/978-3-658-47422-5_66

Two-stage Approach for Low-dose and Sparse-angle CT Reconstruction using Backprojection

Tim Selig[1], Patrick Bauer[2], Jürgen Frikel[3], Thomas März[1], Martin Storath[4], Andreas Weinmann[1]

[1]Hochschule Darmstadt, Fachbereich Mathematik und Naturwissenschaften, Schöfferstraße 3, 64295 Darmstadt, Germany
[2]LIST3N, University of Technology of Troyes, 12 Rue Marie Curie, 10300 Troyes, France
[3]OTH Regensburg, Faculty of Computer Science and Mathematics, Galgenbergstr. 32, 94053 Regensburg, Germany
[4]Technische Hochschule Würzburg-Schweinfurt, Fakultät Angewandte Natur- und Geisteswissenschaften and Institute of Digital Engineering, Ignaz-Schön-Straße 11, 97421 Schweinfurt, Germany
tim.selig@h-da.de

Abstract. This paper presents a novel two-stage approach for computed tomography (CT) reconstruction, focusing on sparse-angle and low-dose setups to minimize radiation exposure while maintaining high image quality. Two-stage approaches consist of an initial reconstruction followed by a neural network for image refinement. In the initial reconstruction, we apply the backprojection (BP) instead of the traditional filtered backprojection (FBP). This enhances computational speed and offers potential advantages for more complex geometries, such as fan-beam and cone-beam CT. Additionally, BP addresses noise and artifacts in sparse-angle CT by leveraging its inherent noise-smoothing effect, which reduces streaking artifacts common in FBP reconstructions. For the second stage, we fine-tune the DRUNet proposed by Zhang et al. to further improve reconstruction quality. We call our method BP-DRUNet and evaluate its performance on a synthetically generated ellipsoid dataset alongside the well-established LoDoPaB-CT dataset. Our results show that BP-DRUNet produces competetive results in terms of PSNR and SSIM metrics compared to the FBP-based counterpart, FBP-DRUNet, and delivers visually competitive results across all tested angular setups.

1 Introduction

Computed tomography (CT) is vital for medical imaging but exposes patients to ionizing radiation during image reconstruction. To minimize this exposure, configurations such as low-dose CT and sparse-angle CT are employed [1]. While these approaches reduce radiation exposure, they also introduce noise and artifacts that degrade image quality. This work focuses on reconstructing CT images from a limited number of projections obtained with reduced radiation exposure.

The mathematical model for CT is given by the Radon transform, for which several analytical inversion formulas exist [2]. The most well-known is the filtered backprojection (FBP) formula, in which the data is first filtered and then backprojected to reconstruct the desired object [2]. An analytically equivalent approach, that reverses the

C. Palm et al. (Hrsg.), *Bildverarbeitung für die Medizin 2025*, Informatik aktuell,
https://doi.org/10.1007/978-3-658-47422-5_67

order of filtering and backprojection is known as backprojection filtration (BPF) [2, 3]. The numerical implementation of FBP has advantages over the implementation of BPF, which is why FBP is used as the standard reconstruction technique in CT [4]. For further details, we refer to [4–6].

In recent years convolutional neural networks (CNNs), have proven to effectively reduce artifacts and noise in medical image reconstruction [7]. In CT imaging, two-stage approaches that combine initial reconstruction using FBP with image enhancement via U-Net-type CNNs have become popular [8–10].

In this work, we investigate a two-stage approach consisting of backprojection (BP) and a U-Net. This method offers several advantages: BP is easier to implement and computationally more efficient than FBP, particularly when dealing with large datasets. While FBP is well suited in uniform, parallel-beam geometries, its performance declines in more complex geometries like fan-beam or cone-beam CT. In contrast, BP is adaptable and can efficiently accommodate various geometries. In the second stage, we employ the DRUNet model [11], originally designed for removing Gaussian noise from natural grayscale images. Here, DRUNet is trained on pairs of BP images and high-quality reconstructions. We refer to this two-stage method as BP-DRUNet.

We compare BP-DRUNet with an analogous FBP-based two-stage process described in [12], referred to here as FBP-DRUNet. While both methods utilize the same network architecture, they are trained for different objectives. The FBP-DRUNet learns to reduce noise and streaking artifacts that are generated in FBP reconstructions [13, 14]. In addition, the BP-DRUNet has to learn the spatial filtering, which is applied to the backprojected CT data.

We evaluate the performance of BP-DRUNet and FBP-DRUNet on two distinct datasets. First, we generate a custom ellipsoid dataset to simulate CT data, introducing Poisson noise in the sinogram domain and varying the number of projection angles. Second, we use the LoDoPaB-CT dataset [15], which contains over 40,000 pairs of human chest CT images acquired under low-dose parallel-beam conditions. To simulate a sparse-angle setting, we reduce the number of projections in the sinogram domain.

Our experiments and their qualitative and quantitative evaluation reveal that the proposed BP-based two-stage approach BP-DRUNet achieves comparable or even improved performance in low-dose and sparse-angle CT reconstructions, which are practically relevant CT scenarios. Therefore, it is a valid alternative to FBP-based two-stage approaches which offers additional advantages as mentioned above. In particular, it can be more easily extended to more complex imaging scenarios.

2 Materials and methods

2.1 Reconstruction framework

The projection data is reconstructed through a two-stage process: an initial reconstruction followed by a U-Net for image enhancement. In the first stage, we derive the input data for the U-Net using two variations: either BP or the traditional FBP utilizing the Ram-Lak filter. For the second stage, we employ DRUNet, a U-Net introduced by Zhang et al. [11], originally pretrained for Gaussian noise removal on natural grayscale images. We adapt its pretrained weights for low-dose and sparse-angle CT reconstruction. Specifically, we fine-tune a DRUNet on BP images to mitigate blurring artifacts. For comparison, we also fine-tune a DRUNet on FBP images, as described in [12].

2.2 Implementation details

In the training process, we minimize the loss between the output of BP-DRUNet or FBP-DRUNet and their corresponding GT images. To achieve this, we utilize the ADAM optimizer [16] and use the following loss function:

$$L = L_{MAE} + \alpha(1 - SSIM) + \lambda\|\theta\|_2^2, \quad (1)$$

This loss function combines Mean Absolute Error (MAE) and the Structural Similarity (SSIM) [17], by following the ideas of [9]. Incorporating SSIM in the loss function ensures that our optimization process doesn't merely focus on minimizing pixel-wise differences but also considers perceptually significant changes [18]. The parameter α regulates the influence of the SSIM term and is tailored individually for each dataset, determined experimentally. To maintain stability, we apply L_2 regularization with a coefficient $\lambda = 10^{-5}$. Initially, the learning rate is set to 10^{-4} and is halved every 32 epochs. Each model is trained for 320 epochs. For data augmentation we rotate every input and ground truth images in all four compass directions. Additionally, we apply Gaussian noise augmentation as follows: initially in its original state, and subsequently, with the addition of 1% Gaussian noise to the input images.

2.3 Datasets

2.3.1 Ellipsoid dataset. Our synthetically generated ellipsoid dataset comprises 1224 training, 216 validation and 120 test images. Each image is standardized to dimensions of 512×512 pixels. Within each image, the number of ellipsoids varies randomly, ranging from 4 to 9, inclusively. The center coordinates of these ellipsoids are randomly chosen, with the constraint of maintaining a minimum distance of 100 pixels from the image borders. Moreover, the radii of each ellipsoid are independently selected, with horizontal and vertical radii varying randomly between 50 and 150 pixels. Additionally, each ellipsoid undergoes a random rotation. Finally the resulting images are scaled in the range from 0 to 1 to obtain the ground truth (GT) images.

Our goal is to generate realistic noisy projection data from the GT images. First, we use the Operator Discretization Library (ODL) with the `astra_cuda` backend [19] to create projection data in parallel-beam geometry. In the second step, we focus on modeling the noise associated with photon generation, attenuation, and detection. This entire process can be modeled by a Poisson distribution [15]. We essentially follow the algorithm proposed by Leuschner et al. in [15]. The noise level is determined by the mean photon count per detector bin N_0, measured without attenuation. Following [15], we select $N_0 = 2^{12}$ and to explore a different noise setting, we additionally evaluate $N_0 = 2^{14}$. (A higher N_0 value means lower noise.) We utilize 30 and 90 equidistant projection angles, spanning a 180-degree rotation.

2.3.2 LoDoPaB-CT Dataset. The LoDoPaB-CT dataset, as detailed in [15], comprises an extensive collection of over 40,000 pairs of human chest CT images alongside their corresponding simulated low-dose measurements. For the training process of our models, we followed the default dataset split recommended by Leuschner et al. in [15], with distinct sets containing 35,820 training samples, 3,522 validation samples, and 3,553 test samples. The projection data within the LoDoPaB-CT dataset contains low-dose measurements obtained from 1000 projection angles spanning a 180-degree range. To construct a sparse-angle and low-dose dataset, we thin the sinogram while maintaining equidistant projection angles. This results in projection data with 100 projection angles.

3 Results

Fig. 1 visualizes the outputs of BP-DRUNet and FBP-DRUNet on a sample from the custom ellipsoid dataset (90 equally spaced views, $N_0 = 2^{14}$). Fig. 2 shows the analogous results on a sample from the LoDoPaB-CT test dataset, reconstructed with 100 equally spaced views. The visual quality of BP-DRUNet and FBP-DRUNet are comparable. The other noise and view configurations (not presented in this paper) have shown similar performance, making the displayed images representative of the overall performance.

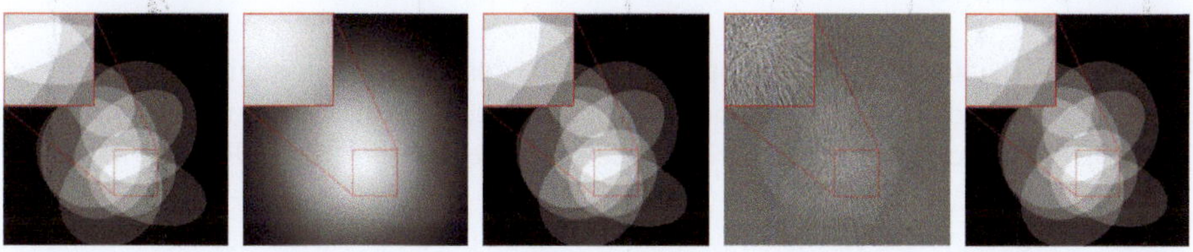

(a) GT. **(b)** BP. **(c)** BP-DRUNet. **(d)** FBP. **(e)** FBP-DRUNet.

Fig. 1. Reconstruction outputs from BP-DRUNet and FBP-DRUNet, alongside their respective BP and FBP input reconstructions and the corresponding ground truth (GT) image. The test sample is taken from our custom ellipsoid dataset, generated using 90 equally spaced projection angles with additional noise, characterized by a mean photon count per detector bin without attenuation ($N_0 = 2^{14}$).

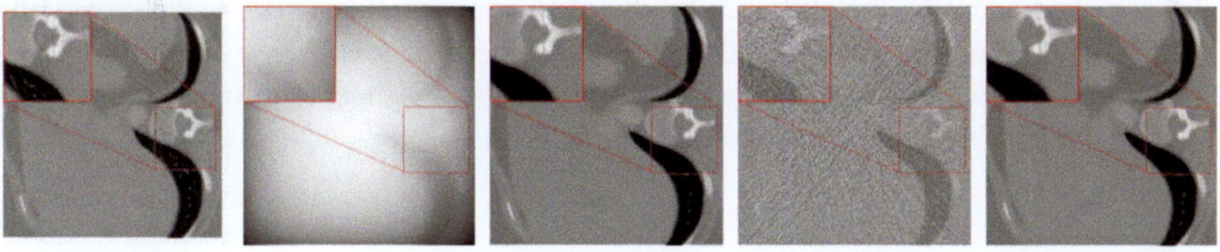

(a) GT. **(b)** BP. **(c)** BP-DRUNet. **(d)** FBP. **(e)** FBP-DRUNet.

Fig. 2. Reconstruction outputs from BP-DRUNet and FBP-DRUNet, alongside their respective BP and FBP input reconstructions and the corresponding ground truth (GT) image. The test sample is taken from the LoDoPaB-CT test dataset, generated using 100 equally spaced projection angles.

Tab. 1. PSNR and SSIM metrics evaluated on the custom ellipsoid test dataset for BP-DRUNet and FBP-DRUNet, assessed for 30 and 90 views, along with varying noise levels characterized by the mean photon count per detector bin without attenuation $N_0 \in \{2^{12}, 2^{14}\}$.

Method	Views	N_0	PSNR	SSIM
BP-DRUNet	30	2^{12}	33.558 ± 2.920	0.9645 ± 0.0227
FBP-DRUNet			33.243 ± 2.799	0.9622 ± 0.0275
BP-DRUNet	90	2^{12}	34.888 ± 2.989	0.9721 ± 0.0183
FBP-DRUNet			34.788 ± 2.733	0.9690 ± 0.0281
BP-DRUNet	30	2^{14}	35.151 ± 2.835	0.9728 ± 0.0226
FBP-DRUNet			34.788 ± 2.904	0.9689 ± 0.0350
BP-DRUNet	90	2^{14}	36.660 ± 3.069	0.9787 ± 0.0266
FBP-DRUNet			35.819 ± 3.499	0.9718 ± 0.0355

The metrics used for evaluation are Peak Signal-to-Noise Ratio (PSNR) and SSIM. Tab. 1 illustrates that BP-DRUNet slightly surpasses FBP-DRUNet on the custom ellipsoid dataset across different angular setups and noise levels. This confirms our qualitative findings and indicates that BP-DRUNet is a competitive alternative for low-dose and sparse-angle CT reconstruction.

4 Conclusion

We presented a novel two-stage approach for low-dose and sparse-angle CT reconstruction. This method utilizes BP for the initial reconstruction, differing from the commonly used FBP. The second stage features a specific U-Net architecture (DRUNet) for image enhancement.

BP-DRUNet yields consistently better results on the ellipsoid dataset across different projection angles and noise levels in terms of PSNR and SSIM metrics. These quantitative results demonstrate that BP-DRUNet effectively mitigates noise and artifacts in low-dose and sparse-angle CT images. Qualitatively, both methods yielded strong visual results. Overall, these findings suggest that BP-DRUNet is a promising alternative to conventional FBP-based methods for low-dose and sparse-angle CT applications, offering a robust solution to minimize radiation exposure while maintaining image quality.

Future work will focus on extending the quantitative evaluation, assessing additional datasets, and adapting the approach to other CT configurations, such as fan-beam and cone-beam geometries, where traditional FBP is not a viable option for initial reconstruction. A specific point requiring further investigation is that preliminary experiments suggest the BP-DRUNet produces inferior results on the ellipsoid dataset in a noise-free setting.

Acknowledgement. T. S., T. M. and A. W. acknowledge support by the Hessian Ministry of Higher Education, Research, Science, and the Arts and funding from the EUt+/h-da. M. S. acknowledges support of the Bavarian State Ministry of Economic Affairs, Regional Development and Energy (DIK-2105-0044 / DIK0264). A. W. acknowledges support of Deutsche Forschungsgemeinschaft (DFG) under project number 514177753.

References

1. Hu Z, Gao J, Zhang N et al. An improved statistical iterative algorithm for sparse-view and limited-angle CT image reconstruction. Sci Rep. 2017;7(1).
2. Natterer F. The Mathematics of Computerized Tomography. Society for Industrial and Applied Mathematics, 2001.
3. Xia D, Cho S, Pan X. Backprojection-filtration reconstruction without invoking a spatially varying weighting factor. Med Phys. 2010;37(3):1201–9.
4. Herman GT. Fundamentals of Computerized Tomography. Springer London, 2009.
5. Zeng G, Gullberg G. Can the backprojection filtering algorithm be as accurate as the filtered backprojection algorithm? Proc IEEE NSS. 1994;3:1232–6.
6. Wang Z, Cai J, Guo W et al. Backprojection Wiener deconvolution for computed tomographic reconstruction. Plos One. 2018;13(12):e0207907.
7. Litjens G, Kooi T, Bejnordi BE et al. A survey on deep learning in medical image analysis. Med Image Anal. 2017;42:60–88.
8. Mazandarani FN, Babyn P, Alirezaie J. UNeXt: a low-dose CT denoising UNet model with the modified ConvNeXt block. Proc IEEE ICASSP. 2023:1–5.
9. Xiong L, Li N, Qiu W et al. Re-UNet: a novel multi-scale reverse U-shape network architecture for low-dose CT image reconstruction. Med Biol Eng Comput. 2024;62:701–12.
10. Liu T, Chaman A, Belius D et al. Learning multiscale convolutional dictionaries for image reconstruction. IEEE Trans Comput Imaging. 2022;8:425–37.
11. Zhang K, Li Y, Zuo W et al. Plug-and-play image restoration with deep denoiser prior. IEEE Trans Pattern Anal Mach Intell. 2022;44(10):6360–76.
12. Selig T, März T, Storath M et al. Low-dose CT image reconstruction by fine-tuning a UNet pretrained for Gaussian denoising for the downstream task of image enhancement. arXiv: 2403.03551. 2024.
13. Borg L, Jørgensen JS, Frikel J et al. Analyzing reconstruction artifacts from arbitrary incomplete X-ray CT data. SIAM J Imaging Sci. 2018;11(4):2786–814.
14. Frikel J, Quinto ET. Characterization and reduction of artifacts in limited angle tomography. Inverse Probl. 2013;29:125007.
15. Leuschner J, Schmidt M, Baguer DO et al. LoDoPaB-CT, a benchmark dataset for low-dose computed tomography reconstruction. Sci Data. 2021;8:109.
16. Kingma DP, Ba J. Adam: a method for stochastic optimization. arXiv: 1412.6980. 2014.
17. Wang Z, Bovik A, Sheikh H et al. Image quality assessment: from error visibility to structural similarity. IEEE Trans Image Proc. 2004;13(4):600–12.
18. Setiadi DRIM. PSNR vs SSIM: imperceptibility quality assessment for image steganography. Multimed Tools Appl. 2020;80(6):8423–44.
19. Aarle W van, Palenstijn WJ, De Beenhouwer J et al. The ASTRA toolbox: a platform for advanced algorithm development in electron tomography. Ultramicroscopy. 2015;157:35–47.

Learned Shift-variant CBCT Reconstruction Weights for Non-continuous Trajectories

Chengze Ye, Linda-Sophie Schneider, Yipen Sun, Mareike Thies, Andreas Maier

Pattern Recognition Lab, FAU Erlangen-Nürnberg
chengze.ye@fau.de

Abstract. The differentiable shift-variant filtered back-projection neural network provides an efficient solution for the reconstruction of cone-beam computed tomography (CBCT) data with arbitrary source trajectories. This data-driven approach enables the automatic estimation of trajectory-specific redundancy weights, which are difficult to calculate in practice. The objective of this study is to learn redundancy weights tailored for non-continuous trajectories. The experimental results using random and random nearest-neighbor reordered (RNNR) trajectories show that the model achieves effective image reconstruction, even with non-continuous trajectories. A quantitative analysis of the reconstruction results demonstrates minimal variation in performance metrics across different random seeds, which highlights the model's robustness and stability. Furthermore, the model's consistency across random and RNNR trajectories demonstrates that a data-driven approach to learning redundancy weights is not strictly dependent on trajectory ordering. This marks a significant improvement over traditional analytic method. The approach provides a flexible and effective alternative for CBCT imaging in scenarios with non-continuous or even unordered trajectories, opening new possibilities for imaging applications.

1 Introduction

Cone beam computed tomography (CBCT) represents a crucial imaging technique in the domain of interventional medicine, offering the capacity to capture three-dimensional images through the utilisation of a cone-shaped X-ray beam. With the advent of robotic C-arm systems in recent years, imaging has moved beyond simple circular orbits. These advanced machines can now follow highly customizable, non-circular source detector paths, offering greater flexibility in capturing anatomical structures. This flexibility not only accelerates data collection but also significantly improves image quality by reducing distortions caused by metal implants.The Feldkamp-Davis-Kress (FDK) algorithm is one of the most commonly used algorithm for the CBCT reconstruction. However, this method is unable to handle non-circular trajectories. Consequently, iterative reconstruction algorithms have emerged as the principal solution for addressing the reconstruction challenges associated with non-circular trajectory CBCT. These algorithms optimize the image incrementally to gradually approximate the true data; however, this process is not only time-consuming but also demands significant computational resources, leading to overall inefficiencies in reconstruction.

To address these limitations, Defrise and Clack [1] proposed a shift-variant filtered back-projection (FBP) algorithm that markedly accelerates the reconstruction speed for

C. Palm et al. (Hrsg.), *Bildverarbeitung für die Medizin 2025*, Informatik aktuell,
https://doi.org/10.1007/978-3-658-47422-5_68

non-circular trajectory CBCT. Nevertheless, this approach still necessitates the recalculation of the filter for each specific trajectory geometry. This process is both complex and computationally intensive, representing a significant bottleneck in the reconstruction workflow.

Our previous research [2] extend the shift-variant FBP algorithm by the integration of known operators, resulting in the creation of a differentiable neural network tailored to shift-variant FBP for CBCT reconstruction. In this method, the orbit-related part of the filter defined from Defrise and Clack's algorithm are estimated through a data-driven training process.

This study experimentally validates the robustness of the differentiable shift-variant FBP neural network. We evaluate its capability to achieve stable image reconstructions using random and random nearest-neighbor reordered (RNNR) trajectories. We want to know whether this model has the potential to overcome the requirement of continuous trajectories. This adaptability could significantly expand the scope of applications for CBCT technology.

2 Materials and methods

2.1 Shift-variant FBP algorithm

The shift-variant FBP algorithm, proposed by Defrise and Clack [1], has been developed to reconstruct CBCT data with any specific trajectory. This algorithm allows for the simultaneous acquisition and processing of projections, thereby considerably accelerating the reconstruction process. The reconstruction formula is as follows

$$f(x) = \int_{\Lambda} d\lambda \int_{S^2/2} d\theta - \frac{1}{4\pi^2} \mid a'(\lambda) \cdot \theta \mid \frac{1}{n(\theta, \lambda)} \times \delta'((x - a(\lambda)) \cdot \theta) S(\theta, \lambda) \quad (1)$$

In this formula, $\lambda \in \Lambda$ refers to the parameter defining the source position $a(\lambda)$, while $\theta \in S^2$, where S^2 represents the set of all unit vectors in $\mathbb{R}^3$. The function $S(\theta, \lambda)$ is Grangeat's intermediate function, which connects cone-beam projections to the first derivative of the Radon transform. Additionally, $n(\theta, \lambda)$ denotes the number of intersections between the trajectory $a(\Lambda)$ and the plane orthogonal to θ, passing through the point $a(\lambda)$ along the trajectory.

In equation (1), the function $n(\theta, \lambda)$ exhibits discontinuities, which can result in artifacts during discrete implementations. In order to resolve this issue, Defrise and Clack replaced the crofton symbol $\frac{1}{n(\theta,\lambda)}$ with a smooth, differentiable function

$$M(\theta, \lambda) = \frac{\mid a'(\lambda) \cdot \theta \mid^m c(\lambda)}{\sum_{\alpha=1}^{n(\theta,\lambda)} \mid a'(\lambda_\alpha) \cdot \theta \mid^m c(\lambda_\alpha)} \quad (2)$$

where m is a positive integer greater than 2, $c(\lambda)$ is a smooth function that is equal to one across almost the entire interval Λ, except near the interval boundaries, where it tends toward 0.

Nevertheless, the practical calculation of equation (2) presents a number of challenges. For instance, selecting an appropriate parameter m for a given trajectory geometry requires experiments. Furthermore, computing the gradient of the trajectory $a'(\lambda)$ for discontinuous orbits is impossible.

2.2 Differentiable shift-variant FBP neural network

Our previous work [2] presents a method for CBCT reconstruction from arbitrary orbits, which employs the differentiable shift-variant FBP model. This approach is based on the known operator learning to transform the original formula into a neural network representation, thereby converting (1) into (3)

$$f(x) = A_{3d}^T w_d A_{2d}^T D w_{\text{red}} w_{\text{sino}} D A_{2d} w_{\cos} g(x, y, \lambda) \quad (3)$$

The first step in this formula is the application of a cosine weight $w_{\cos}$ to the projection $g(x, y, \lambda)$, which is then followed by a 2D Radon transform A_{2d}. Subsequent to this, differentiation D is applied in the sinogram domain, along with the application of a weight w_{sino}, which leads to the computation of Grangeat's intermediate function.

The factors $\frac{1}{n(\theta,\lambda)}$ and $\mid a'(\lambda) \cdot \theta \mid$ in equation (1) are associated with the trajectory geometry and can be interpreted as redundancy weight w_{red}. This redundancy weight is applied in the sinogram domain and is treated as a trainable parameter, thereby enabling optimization during the training process. Subsequently, a second differentiation D is performed, and the data is backprojected into the detector coordinate system using A_{2d}^T; after this, the weight in the detector coordinate system w_d is applied to obtain the filtered projections. Ultimately, the reconstruction volume $f(x)$ is achieved through a 3D backprojection A_{3d}^T. A neural network architecture can then be constructed based on this (Fig. 1).

The differentiable nature of this pipeline allows it to learn the redundancy weights based on the provided trajectory geometries in a data-driven manner. In this approach, only the redundancy weights are treated as trainable parameters, while the rest of the implementation adheres to a differentiable version of the original algorithm [1]. The following section will present the experiments conducted to analyse the potential and robustness of this reconstruction pipeline.

2.3 Experiments

2.3.1 Geometry configuration. To examine the stability and robustness of the differentiable shift-variant FBP model in the reconstruction of non-continuous trajectories, we devised a geometric configuration with an exceptionally intricate trajectory, based on the precise geometric parameters of the clinical C-arm system, Artis zeego (Siemens AG, Forchheim, Germany). These parameters are detailed in our previous work [3].

This trajectory is founded upon a spherical surface, with the presumption that the scanned object is situated at the sphere's center. The source points are positioned on a

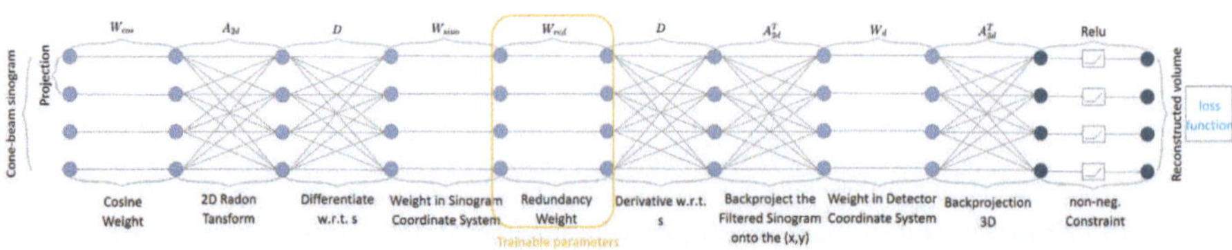

Fig. 1. Differentiable shift-variant FBP neural network architecture [3].

surface close to the central plane of the sphere. Within the spherical zone, 400 source points were randomly selected and distributed uniformly across the surface, resulting in the formation of a discontinuous random trajectory. Based on the initial random trajectory, starting from the first point, we applied the nearest neighbor algorithm to reorder these points, generating a more continuous RNNR trajectory, as shown in Fig. 2.

2.3.2 Data preparation. To ensure the reliability of the experimental results, five distinct random seeds were employed to construct random trajectories, which were subsequently generated into corresponding RNNR trajectories. The model was trained using a simulated dataset, after which its performance was evaluated using real medical data. For each trajectory, 30 simulated data samples were generated using the methods from paper [3]. Of these, 24 were employed for training purposes, while the remaining 6 were used for validation. To facilitate evaluation, 5 samples from the Pancreatic-CT-CBCT-SEG dataset [4] were utilized. Specifically, we employed cone beam forward projection from the PyroNN software [5], maintaining the same trajectory geometry as the training data to generate the sinograms, which were then used as input for the model.

2.3.3 Implementation details. The neural network architecture was developed using PyTorch 2.1.1 and trained on an Nvidia A40 GPU. In order to implement the 2D Radon transform, 2D backprojection, and 3D cone-beam backprojection, operators from the PyroNN framework [5] were employed. To guarantee that the learned redundancy weights are adequately smooth and do not introduce artifacts into the reconstruction results, a Gaussian filter layer was incorporated after the redundancy weight layer. The sigma value was set to 20, and the kernel size was 121. Prior to the training process, the redundancy weight layer was randomly initialized with values distributed uniformly between -1 and 0. The total loss is comprised of two components: mean squared error (MSE) loss and structural similarity index (SSIM) loss, weighted by 5^{-3}. Prior to calculating the loss, both the reconstructed output and the reference are normalized to the range $[0, 1]$. For parameter updates, the AdamW optimizer was employed in conjunction with the one-cycle learning rate policy, which adjusted the learning rate cyclically between 0.2 and 2 over 500 epochs, enhancing the training performance.

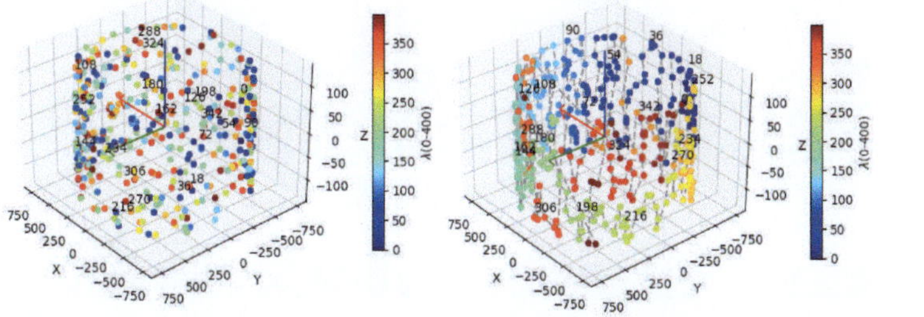

(a) **(b)**

Fig. 2. (a) Random trajectory. (b) RNNR trajectory.

Tab. 1. Comparison of image quality metrics for different trajectory categories.

	Random trajectory			RNNR trajectory		
	MSE ↓	PSNR (dB) ↑	SSIM ↑	MSE ↓	PSNR (dB) ↑	SSIM ↑
Seed 0	0.105 ± 0.016	35.88 ± 1.27	0.921 ± 0.009	0.105 ± 0.016	35.95 ± 1.26	0.923 ± 0.008
Seed 1	0.103 ± 0.017	36.08 ± 1.28	0.924 ± 0.006	0.102 ± 0.017	36.19 ± 1.28	0.924 ± 0.006
Seed 2	0.106 ± 0.018	35.84 ± 1.24	0.921 ± 0.007	0.106 ± 0.017	35.82 ± 1.25	0.920 ± 0.007
Seed 3	0.102 ± 0.017	36.15 ± 1.25	0.926 ± 0.006	0.104 ± 0.016	35.94 ± 1.24	0.924 ± 0.006
Seed 4	0.104 ± 0.017	36.00 ± 1.24	0.922 ± 0.006	0.102 ± 0.067	36.13 ± 1.24	0.925 ± 0.007
Overall	0.104 ± 0.017	35.98 ± 1.26	0.923 ± 0.007	0.104 ± 0.017	36.01 ± 1.26	0.923 ± 0.007

3 Results

The performance of the trained model was evaluated across a range of trajectory categories, with the results presented in Tab. 1. For each trajectory category, the five samples generated as described in section 2.3.2 were used to test and calculate the mean and standard deviation of MSE, peak signal-to-noise ratio (PSNR), and SSIM. The model demonstrated minimal variation in these metrics across different random seeds, indicating that the reconstruction quality remains consistent regardless of the random seed used to construct trajectories. This consistency serves to highlight the robustness and stability of the model. Additionally, the RNNR trajectories demonstrated a slight enhancement in performance compared to the random trajectories. Nevertheless, this improvement was slight, thereby confirming that the data-driven approach for estimating redundancy weights is not strictly dependent on trajectory ordering. Fig. 3 further illustrates this by providing a visualization of the reconstructed results, offering a qualitative perspective on the images across both random and nearest-neighbor trajectories.

Our previous work [2] employed a continuous sinusoidal trajectory geometry for the purposes of training and testing the model. The resulting MSE was 0.0904 ± 0.0149, PSNR was 37.20 ± 1.34, and SSIM was 0.9591 ± 0.0051. In comparison to the data presented in the table 1, these findings demonstrate that the model exhibits a better

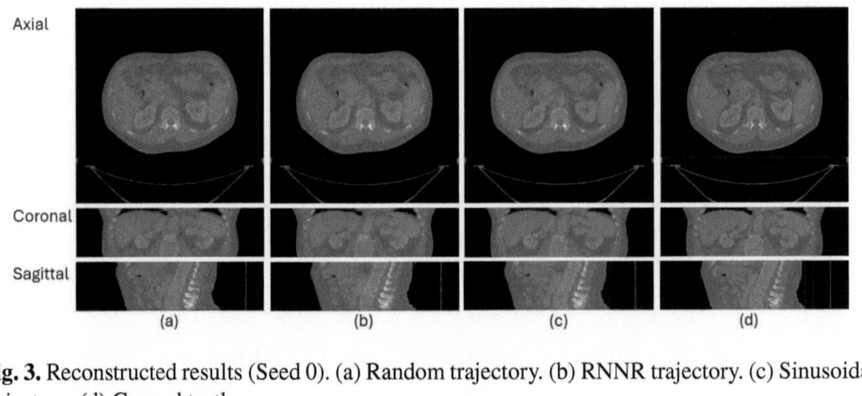

Fig. 3. Reconstructed results (Seed 0). (a) Random trajectory. (b) RNNR trajectory. (c) Sinusoidal trajectory. (d) Ground truth.

performance for continuous trajectories in comparison to non-continuous ones. Furthermore, as illustrated in Fig. 3, the comparison clearly demonstrates that the discontinuities in the trajectory results in artifacts.

4 Discussion

In this study, we conducted experiments using designed random and RNNR trajectories to demonstrate that the differentiable shift-variant FBP model overcomes the limitations of redundancy weight estimation in the traditional shift-variant FBP algorithm, which relies on trajectory continuity. The model is optimized directly based on the reconstruction target, thereby enabling robust image reconstruction even in the presence of non-continuous or even unordered trajectories. However, this may entail a certain degree of compromise in terms of accuracy. Furthermore, the experimental findings suggest that the nearest neighbor algorithm does not offer significant continuity for random trajectories. Future research will investigate the potential of alternative trajectory optimization algorithms to enhance model performance. Consequently, the differentiable shift-variant FBP model provides an effective alternative in scenarios where trajectory continuity cannot be guaranteed, significantly expanding the scope for application in imaging.

Acknowledgement. The authors gratefully acknowledge the scientific support and HPC resources provided by the Erlangen National High Performance Computing Center (NHR@FAU) of the FAU Erlangen-Nürnberg.

References

1. Defrise M, Clack R. A cone-beam reconstruction algorithm using shift-variant filtering and cone-beam backprojection. IEEE Trans Med Imaging. 1994;13(1):186–95.
2. Ye C, Schneider LS, Sun Y et al. Deep learning computed tomography based on the Defrise and Clack algorithm. arXiv: 2403.00426. 2024.
3. Ye C, Schneider LS, Sun Y et al. DRACO: differentiable reconstruction for arbitrary CBCT orbits. arXiv: 2410.14900. 2024.
4. Hong J, Reyngold M, Crane C et al. Breath-hold CT and cone-beam CT images with expert manual organ-at-risk segmentations from radiation treatments of locally advanced pancreatic cancer [Data set]. The Cancer Imaging Archive. 2021.
5. Syben C, Michen M, Stimpel B et al. PYRO-NN: Python reconstruction operators in neural networks. Med Phys. 2019;46(11):5110–5.

Self-supervised 3D Vision Transformer Pre-training for Robust Brain Tumor Classification

Danilo Weber Nunes[1,2], David Rauber[1], Christoph Palm[1,2]

[1]Regensburg Medical Image Computing (ReMIC), Ostbayerische Technische Hochschule Regensburg (OTH Regensburg), Regensburg, Germany
[2]Regensburg Center of Health Sciences and Technology (RCHST), OTH Regensburg, Regensburg, Germany
danilo.webernunes@oth-regensburg.de

Abstract. Brain tumors pose significant challenges in neurology, making precise classification crucial for prognosis and treatment planning. This work investigates the effectiveness of a self-supervised learning approach–masked autoencoding (MAE)–to pre-train a vision transformer (ViT) model for brain tumor classification. Our method uses non-domain specific data, leveraging the ADNI and OASIS-3 MRI datasets, which primarily focus on degenerative diseases, for pre-training. The model is subsequently fine-tuned and evaluated on the BraTS glioma and meningioma datasets, representing a novel use of these datasets for tumor classification. The pre-trained MAE ViT model achieves an average F1 score of 0.91 in a 5-fold cross-validation setting, outperforming the nnU-Net encoder trained from scratch, particularly under limited data conditions. These findings highlight the potential of self-supervised MAE in enhancing brain tumor classification accuracy, even with restricted labeled data.

1 Introduction

Brain tumors, although relatively uncommon, represent a critical category of neurological disorders. In recent years, significant progress has been made in brain tumor segmentation from MRI scans, driven by advances in collaborative data initiatives like the BraTS Challenge [1] and methodological improvements. However, the accurate classification of different brain tumor types remains a less explored area despite its crucial role in determining prognosis and treatment strategies.

Most existing research on tumor classification has relied on the 2D brain tumor dataset from figshare [2], which contains contrast-enhanced T_1-weighted (T_1-Ce) MRI slices of gliomas, meningiomas, and pituitary tumors. This dataset's exclusive focus on 2D slices with visible tumors simplifies the classification, as models are tasked with minimal localization effort. However, classifying tumors within 3D MRI data poses additional challenges. The additional spatial dimension adds complexity, requiring models to handle large volumes of non-tumorous tissue with sparse tumor regions.

The scarcity of large-scale, MRI-based datasets specifically designed for brain tumor classification has limited the development of pre-trained models for this purpose. As a result, most deep learning approaches lack robust pre-trained architectures optimized to distinguish tumor types, particularly under limited-data conditions.

C. Palm et al. (Hrsg.), *Bildverarbeitung für die Medizin 2025*, Informatik aktuell,
https://doi.org/10.1007/978-3-658-47422-5_69

In this work, we propose that self-supervised pre-trained Vision Transformers (ViTs) are effective tumor classifiers, even when pre-training is conducted on data from other medical domains. We employ masked autoencoding (MAE) [3], a self-supervised learning (SSL) technique, to pre-train a ViT model [4] on the ADNI [5] and OASIS-3 [6] datasets, which primarily focus on degenerative neurological diseases rather than tumors. This approach enables the model to learn generalized representations, which we hypothesize will be transferable to the task of tumor classification.

To assess our approach, we fine-tune and test our model on the BraTS Glioma [1] and Meningioma [7] datasets to classify between the two tumors, marking the first use of these datasets for this purpose. Our work contributes to the field by demonstrating the potential of self-supervised pre-trained ViTs for brain tumor classification, advancing the use of deep learning in scenarios where large, labeled datasets are limited.

2 Materials and methods

This section describes the datasets in more detail, followed by a presentation of the network architectures and the training procedures.

2.1 Data

This work utilizes four distinct datasets, with the ADNI and OASIS-3 datasets serving as sources for model pre-training. Both datasets focus primarily on neurodegenerative diseases, particularly Alzheimer's disease (AD), and also include individuals categorized as cognitively normal (CN) and those with mild cognitive impairment (MCI) in the case of ADNI. The OASIS-3 dataset further extends its cohort to include individuals diagnosed with vascular dementia (VD). Skull stripping was the only preprocessing step. While these datasets offer various imaging modalities, only T_1-weighted sequences were used, as they provide high-quality images and resemble the target modality, T_1-Ce.

For the fine-tuning and evaluation of the pre-trained model, we incorporated data from the BraTS glioma and the recently released meningioma datasets to perform tumor classification. Given that T_1-Ce is the standard imaging modality for preoperative evaluation due to its ability to delineate tumor location, size, heterogeneity, and vascularity [8],

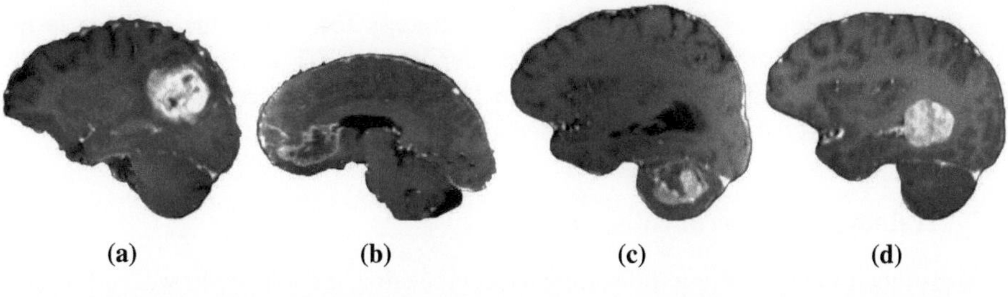

(a) (b) (c) (d)

Fig. 1. Example of gliomas (a,b) [1] and meningiomas (c,d) [7] tumors in the sagittal plane. A meningioma with heterogeneous contrast uptake similar to a glioma is presented in (c). A more common meningioma with homogeneous contrast uptake is depicted in (d) for comparison.

Tab. 1. Summary of the datasets utilized in this work and the modalities provided by them.

Dataset	MRI examinations	Modalities used	Used for
ADNI [5]	9303	T_1	Pre-training
OASIS-3 [6]	4110	T_1	Pre-training
BraTS Adult Glioma [1]	1470	T_1-Ce	Fine-tuning
BraTS Adult Meningioma [7]	1141	T_1-Ce	Fine-tuning

this modality was selected for the classification task. While gliomas and meningiomas differ in typical morphology and anatomical location, certain meningiomas can resemble gliomas in appearance, potentially complicating diagnosis and increasing the risk of misdirected treatment strategies. Fig. 1 illustrates an example where gliomas and meningiomas exhibit similar contrast enhancement patterns, underscoring the challenge of relying solely on anatomical features for diagnosis.

The final dataset used in this work comprises 16,024 MRI examinations aggregated from the four datasets. Tab. 1 provides a breakdown of the contributions of each dataset detailing their respective roles in pre-training and classification.

2.2 Network architectures

We compared our proposed model against a CNN-based architecture, selecting the encoder of a 3D nnU-Net model [9], known for its effectiveness in MRI segmentation. After the bottleneck, average pooling and flattening operations were applied, followed by a fully connected (FC) layer for classification, resulting in 6.1 M trainable parameters.

Our model is primarily based on the ViT architecture [4] incorporating a global pooling mechanism via a learnable token added to the start of the sequence, followed by an FC layer. Following [3], we adapted a fixed 2D sinusoidal-cosine positional encoding (PE) to the 3D case rather than the learnable PE in the original ViT. To adapt the model for 3D tasks, we used a $16 \times 16 \times 16$ patch size and stacked 8 transformer modules, each with 12 attention heads and an embedding size of 768. While this architecture is larger than the nnU-Net encoder, containing 60.6 M parameters, only the last three Transformer layers (21.3 M parameters) were fine-tuned for this task. Preliminary experiments confirmed that the large patch-to-embedding ratio was suitable for classification and reduced memory demands during training.

For pre-training, we used the MAE SSL strategy [3], where the encoder is the ViT architecture described above. The decoder, also a ViT and symmetrical to the encoder, brings the total parameter count to 121 M. Only the encoder is fine-tuned for classification, and the decoder is discarded after pre-training.

2.3 Training and experimental setup

Two distinct training configurations were used. In the first, the ViT model was pre-trained with an SSL approach using MAE [3]. Here, 75 % of image patches were masked, and the model learned to reconstruct them by minimizing the mean squared error (MSE).

This model was trained for 1000 epochs on 80 % of the patients from the combined ADNI and OASIS-3 datasets, with the remaining 20 % reserved for validation.

Data augmentation techniques included Z-Score normalization to all volumes while keeping background voxels at 0 and random flipping along the left-right and anterior-posterior axes. Additionally, random-sized regions were selected, and if smaller than $128 \times 128 \times 128$, padding was applied. Augmentations were applied with a 50 % probability. The model was trained with a base learning rate (LR) of 1.5×10^{-4}, using cosine decay with 40 warm-up epochs as the LR scheduler and a batch size of 54. AdamW served as the optimizer, with $\beta_1 = 0.9$, $\beta_2 = 0.95$, and a weight decay of 0.05.

The second training configuration involved supervised training on the combined BraTS glioma and meningioma datasets. Both the nnU-Net encoder and the MAE pre-trained ViT models were trained in this setup. Preliminary experiments showed that fine-tuning only the last three layers of the MAE pre-trained ViT was sufficient. As the pre-training approach was applicable only to transformer-based models, all variants of the nnU-Net encoder model were trained from scratch. To comprehensively evaluate the models' ability to differentiate between tumor types, a patient-wise 5-fold cross-validation scheme was used, and the best result per fold was presented.

To examine model performance under data constraints, training data was progressively reduced by randomly sampling N % of the original training patients while maintaining a consistent validation set. Both models were trained on identical patient subsets in each fold. The augmentation steps used during self-supervised pre-training were also applied in this configuration, with the additional step of rescaling voxel intensities. This was achieved by multiplying each voxel v by a random factor between -0.1 and 0.1, following the transformation $v = v \times (1 + \text{factor})$.

Despite conducting a hyperparameter search, both models followed a similar training recipe. They were trained for 300 epochs with a base LR of 1.0×10^{-6}, employing the oneCycle LR scheduler, which used a linear annealing strategy and no warm-up epochs. The Adam optimizer, with $\beta_1 = 0.9$ and $\beta_2 = 0.95$, was used with label smoothing set to 0.1. Minor hyperparameter variations included weight decay and batch size, where the nnU-Net encoder used a weight decay of 0.001 and a batch size of 6, while the MAE pre-trained ViT employed a weight decay of 0.0001 and a batch size of 8.

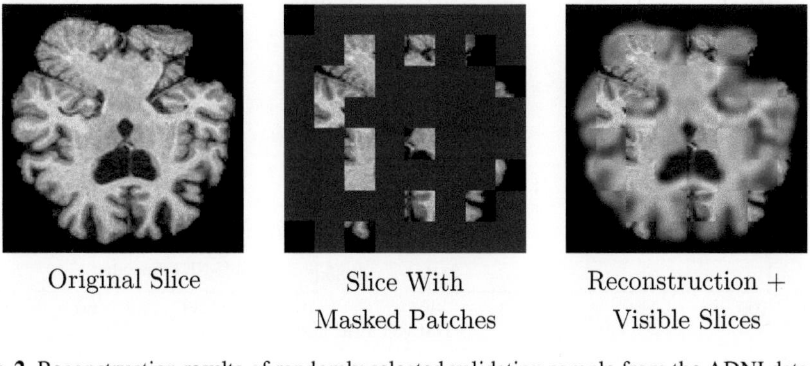

Fig. 2. Reconstruction results of randomly selected validation sample from the ADNI dataset.

3 Results

The SSL reconstruction results demonstrate that, despite being trained on only 25 % of each image, the MAE pre-trained ViT model effectively captures the underlying brain structures. The model quite accurately reconstructs brain slices, even those with varying shapes and complex anatomical details, as shown in Fig. 2 (ADNI dataset). Notably, these reconstructions are generated exclusively on masked patches, producing a composite image that combines visible and reconstructed regions.

In the supervised training setup, the nnU-Net encoder achieved a mean F1 score of 0.88 ± 0.02 and a mean AUC ROC of 0.94 ± 0.02. In comparison, the MAE pre-trained ViT outperformed these benchmarks, achieving a mean F1 score of 0.91 ± 0.01 and a mean AUC ROC of 0.97 ± 0.01. These metrics indicate a notable improvement relative to the same ViT model trained from scratch, which exhibited substantially lower results, with a mean F1 score of 0.80 ± 0.01 and an AUC ROC of 0.87 ± 0.02.

Fig. 3 presents the performance trend as training data volume decreases. Both networks show an expected positive correlation between the amount of available training data and F1 score, with the nnU-Net Encoder model demonstrating a slightly higher Spearman correlation of $\rho = 0.88$ than the MAE pre-trained ViT model with $\rho = 0.82$, both statistically significant with $p < 0.05$.

Interestingly, the MAE pre-trained ViT model maintained competitive performance even under limited data conditions. When trained on only 60 % of the available data, it matched the nnU-Net Encoder model trained on the full dataset, achieving an F1 score of 0.88 ± 0.01 and AUC ROC of 0.94 ± 0.01. This highlights the MAE pre-trained ViT's robustness and efficiency in data-limited scenarios.

4 Discussion

This work introduces a novel approach to utilizing the BraTS glioma and meningioma datasets, demonstrating the versatility and efficiency of self-supervised ViTs in brain tumor classification. By repurposing the BraTS glioma and meningioma datasets for

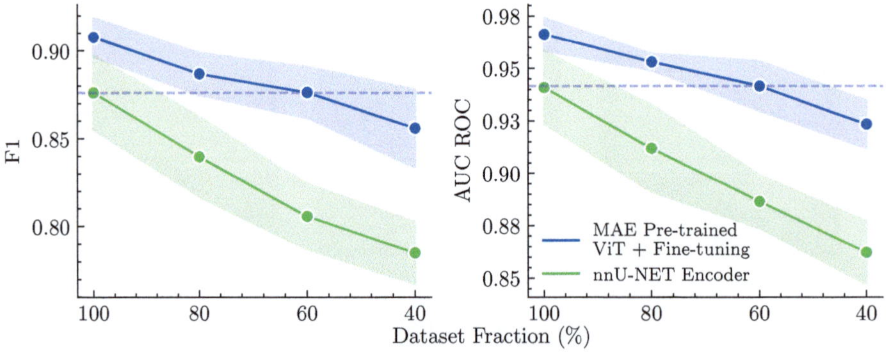

Fig. 3. Effect on models' performance (F1 score and AUC ROC) as the training dataset is reduced.

tumor classification rather than segmentation, we established results in one of the most comprehensive 3D tumor classification datasets to date.

The results show that our pre-trained transformer-based model achieved robust classification performance, outperforming the encoder section of the widely used nnU-Net trained from scratch. These findings suggest that SSL pre-training enhances model performance despite originating from a different modality (T_1 rather than T_1-Ce). By facilitating the use of larger architectures that would otherwise overfit due to limited data, SSL pre-training enables models to capture generalized features effectively, sustaining performance in data-scarce environments and surpassing smaller models.

Future research will explore expanding the pre-training datasets used and incorporating a broader range of modalities (e.g., different MRI weightings) to improve versatility and robustness in classification tasks. We will also investigate how various modalities impact model performance. Additionally, we plan to explore the benefits of scaling model architectures further, examining how larger, pre-trained transformer-based models can push the boundaries in brain tumor classification, segmentation, and other complex medical image computing tasks.

References

1. Menze BH, Jakab A, Bauer S et al. The multimodal brain tumor image segmentation benchmark (BRATS). IEEE Trans Med Imaging. 2014;34(10):1993–2024.
2. Cheng J, Huang W, Cao S et al. Enhanced performance of brain tumor classification via tumor region augmentation and partition. PLoS One. 2015;10(10):e0140381.
3. He K, Chen X, Xie S et al. Masked autoencoders are scalable vision learners. Proc IEEE CVF CVPR. 2022:16000–9.
4. Dosovitskiy A, Beyer L, Kolesnikov A et al. An image is worth 16x16 words: transformers for image recognition at scale. Proc ICLR. 2021.
5. Jack Jr CR, Bernstein MA, Fox NC et al. The Alzheimer's disease neuroimaging initiative (ADNI): MRI methods. J Magn Reson Imaging. 2008;27(4):685–91.
6. LaMontagne PJ, Benzinger TL, Morris JC et al. OASIS-3: longitudinal neuroimaging, clinical, and cognitive dataset for normal aging and Alzheimer disease. MedRxiv. 2019:2019–12.
7. LaBella D, Khanna O, McBurney-Lin S et al. A multi-institutional meningioma MRI dataset for automated multi-sequence image segmentation. Sci Data. 2024;11(1):496.
8. Huang RY, Bi WL, Griffith B et al. Imaging and diagnostic advances for intracranial meningiomas. Neuro Oncol. 2019;21(Supplement_1):i44–i61.
9. Isensee F, Jäger PF, Full PM et al. nnU-Net for brain tumor segmentation. arXiv: 2011.00848. 2020.

Abstract: Evolutionary Normalization Optimization Boosts Semantic Segmentation Network Performance

Luisa Neubig, Andreas M. Kist

Department Artificial Intelligence in Biomedical Engineering, Friedrich-Alexander-Universität Erlangen-Nürnberg (FAU), Germany
luisa.e.neubig@fau.de

Normalization methods play a critical role in the performance and generalization of deep neural networks for semantic segmentation, particularly in medical imaging. While batch normalization (BN) is widely used, its limitations, such as reduced performance with small batch sizes, have led to alternative normalization methods, such as instance normalization (IN), layer normalization (LN), group normalization (GN), and filter response normalization (FRN). However, most segmentation networks apply a single normalization method uniformly, without optimizing layer- or task-specific configurations. This study introduces an evolutionary normalization method search (evoNMS), a novel approach that leverages neural architecture search to optimize the use of normalization methods at each layer of a U-Net architecture for medical image segmentation. Using an evolutionary algorithm, evoNMS explores various combinations of normalization techniques (BN, IN, GN, FRN, LN.) across the encoder-decoder architecture. By selecting the best configurations based on segmentation metrics such as the Dice coefficient, intersection over union and Hausdorff distance (HD95), the performance will be iteratively improved over generations. We evaluated evoNMS on 11 biomedical segmentation datasets, including those from the Medical Segmentation Decathlon, BAGLS, and Kvasir-SEG, and compared its performance with the state-of-the-art (nnU-Net) and U-Nets with fixed normalization strategies. Our key findings show that evoNMS outperforms or matches state-of-the-art architectures across multiple datasets. In particular, IN and GN have emerged as the most effective methods for many datasets, with evoNMS discovering patterns of normalization dependence on specific encoder and decoder layers. The study also revealed that IN normalization in the latent space and no normalization method in the last layer is the best configuration across multiple datasets; however, the most effective configuration is highly task- and modality-dependent [1].

References

1. Neubig L, Kist AM. Evolutionary normalization optimization boosts semantic segmentation network performance. Proc MICCAI. 2023:703–12.

C. Palm et al. (Hrsg.), *Bildverarbeitung für die Medizin 2025*, Informatik aktuell,
https://doi.org/10.1007/978-3-658-47422-5_70

Integration of Key-value Attention into Pure and Hybrid Transformers for Semantic Segmentation

DeShin Hwa, Tobias Holmes, Klaus Drechsler

BMI Lab, Aachen University of Applied Sciences
holmes@fh-aachen.de

Abstract. While CNNs were long considered state of the art for image processing, the introduction of Transformer architectures has challenged this position. While achieving excellent results in image classification and segmentation, Transformers remain inherently reliant on large training datasets and remain computationally expensive. A newly introduced Transformer derivative named KV Transformer shows promising results in synthetic, NLP, and image classification tasks, while reducing complexity and memory usage. This is especially conducive to use cases where local inference is required, such as medical screening applications. We endeavoured to further evaluate the merit of KV Transformers on semantic segmentation tasks, specifically in the domain of medical imaging. By directly comparing traditional and KV variants of the same base architectures, we provide further insight into the practical tradeoffs of reduced model complexity. We observe a reduction in parameter count and multiply accumulate operations between 5 % and 10 % , while achieving similar performance from most of the KV variant models when directly compared to their QKV implementation.

1 Introduction

1.1 Motivation

Convolutional neural networks (CNNs) have long been the state of the art for image classification and segmentation, particularly in medical imaging. However, CNNs have limitations in capturing long-range dependencies and global context due to their reliance on local receptive fields and convolutional kernels. This can lead to a loss of global information. Vision transformers (ViTs) [1], derived from transformers [2] used in NLP, address these issues with self-attention mechanisms that capture long-range dependencies and spatial relationships more effectively. However, transformers and ViTs remain more computationally expensive than traditional CNNs due to the quadratic complexity of the self-attention mechanism and the absence of weight-sharing, unlike CNNs, which use convolutional kernels. To this end, Borji [3] proposed the KV Transformer to investigate the possibility of reducing model complexity while retaining performance by omitting one of the vectors used in the attention mechanism. This is especially beneficial in resource-constrained settings like medical screenings, where efficient inference is preferable. Thus, we endeavour to assess the performance of KV attention in pure and hybrid Transformer models and for medical image segmentation tasks.

C. Palm et al. (Hrsg.), *Bildverarbeitung für die Medizin 2025*, Informatik aktuell,
https://doi.org/10.1007/978-3-658-47422-5_71

1.2 Related work

First introduced in 2017 by Vaswani et al. [2], transformers revolutionized the field of natural language processing (NLP) and subsequently computer vision through their novel use of self-attention mechanisms. Dosovitskiy et al. [1] adapted the Transformer architecture to image classification tasks by splitting input images into fixed-size patches. Each patch is flattened into a vector and then linearly projected into a higher-dimensional representation using a linear transformation defined as: $Z = WP + b$ where P is the flattened patch vector, W is the weight matrix, b is the bias vector, and Z is the resulting high-dimensional representation. To address the lack of spatial inductive bias inherent in transformers compared to CNNs, positional embeddings are added to preserve the arrangement of the patches. Once the patches are embedded, they are fed into a standard transformer encoder, which applies self-attention mechanisms. The output of the self-attention layer can be computed using

$$\text{Attention}(Q, K, V) = \text{softmax}\left(\frac{QK^T}{\sqrt{d_k}}\right) V \tag{1}$$

where Q, K, and V are the query, key, and value matrices respectively, and d_k is the dimensionality of the keys. Finally, the patch representations are processed through a multi-layer perceptron (MLP) head to convert the high-dimensional transformer outputs back into task-specific predictions. For image classification, the prepended class token is processed by the MLP head to produce a single class prediction. In 2020, Zheng et al. [4] introduced segmentation transformer (SETR), with a purely ViT-based encoder for semantic segmentation (Fig. 1a). Semantic segmentation is achieved by use of a convolutional decoder with progressive upsampling (PUP). Herein, the high dimensional feature maps that are output from the transformer encoder are reconstructed into the dimension of the input image. The output of the encoder is a token sequence with a shape of $z_L \in \mathbb{R}^{N\times C}$ where C is the feature dimension. This sequence is first reshaped into a feature map of shape $z_L \in \mathbb{R}^{\frac{H}{16}\times\frac{W}{16}\times C}$ and subsequently sent through four convolution layers, which each perform a 2× upsampling operation. The resulting feature map has the shape of the input image and a depth equal to the number of classes to be segmented $(H \times W \times C)$ (Fig. 2). In traditional transformers, the self-attention mechanism computes three components, queries (Q), keys (K), and values (V), dynamically for every token in the sequence, thereby determining the importance of each token relative to others. Borji [3] expands on the original transformer architecture and its various derivates by investigating whether the inclusion of queries, keys, and values are required in order to achieve competitive performance. The self attention mechanism in a standard transformer is given by Eq 1. The weight matrices $W_q, W_k,$ and W_v are the parameters responsible for projecting the input X into an output tensor of dimension d, with $Q = XW_q, K = XW_k,$ and $V = XW_v$. This formulation relies on computing the dot product between each token in the query (Q) and the corresponding token in the key (K). The approach proposed by Borji [3] modifies this by replacing Q with K, such that

$$\text{Attention}(K, V) = \text{softmax}\left(\frac{KK^T}{\sqrt{d_k}}\right) V \tag{2}$$

	Comp. complexity	# Parameters
QKV	$2nd^2$	$2d^2$
KV	nd^2	d^2
KV+pos	$nd^2 + n^2m$	$d^2 + m$

Tab. 1. Comparison of computational complexity and number of parameters of attention mechanisms. Here, d represents the embedding dimensionality, n denotes the sequence length, and m is the dimensionality of the 2D positional encoding layer. [3]

holds true. The KV self- m. This modification transforms the matrix into oattention mechanism initially creates a symmetric structure. To introduce asymmetry, Borji [3] suggests augmenting the $n \times n$ attention matrix with 2D positional encoding of dimensionne with dimensions $n \times n \times m$. A linear layer, consisting of m neurons, is then employed to project this expanded matrix back to its original $n \times n$ size (Fig. 1b). Tab. 1 illustrates the expected advantages in complexity and computational cost associated with KV attention. The KV+Pos attention results in higher parameter and FLOPS counts, which depend on the parameter m. It is important to note that m can be set to a much lower value than d. However, a significant drawback of KV+Pos attention is that its computational complexity is dependent on n^2, which can lead to high computational costs [3]. Chen et al. [5] proposes a hybrid (CNN and transformer) model. The encoder leverages a ResNet-50 architecture [6] to extract high-level features from input images. Instead of splitting the image into patches, TransUNet applies patch embedding to the feature maps generated by the CNN, creating feature patches as the transformer input. This approach allows for better preservation of spatial information and captures fine-grained details. The transformer layers then process these patches to model long-range dependencies, enhancing the network's ability to integrate global context with local features. Wu et al. [7] introduce the convolutional vision transformer (CvT), a hybrid model that enhances the ViT by integrating two key convolutional operations: token em-

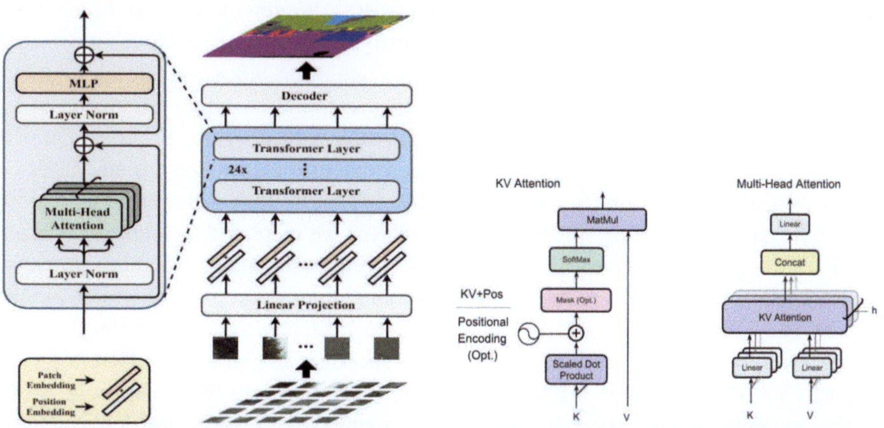

(a) The standard SETR architecture [4]. **(b)** KV version of multi-head attention [3].

Fig. 1. We implemented an SETR encoder as well as a variant with KV multi-head attention.

bedding and projection. In CvT, convolutional token embedding replaces ViT's patch splitting by applying convolutional layers. This approach allows the model to effectively leverage local information by applying multiple filters that slide over the entire image. The resulting feature maps maintain the spatial structure of the image while reducing its dimensionality. Convolutional projection applies further convolutions to the feature maps prior to passing them to the self-attention mechanism. This hybrid approach boosts accuracy, reduces parameter count, and enhances computational efficiency compared to the original ViT, particularly for image classification tasks.

2 Materials and methods

2.1 Dataset

We used the UW-Madison GI Tract Image Segmentation dataset[1] which consists of abdominal MRI slices. Annotations of the three classes (large bowel, small bowel, stomach) are provided in the form of run-length encoded organ segmentations. During preprocessing, we transformed the RLE ground truth data into 2D greyscale multi-class masks. Moreover, the dataset was split into training, validation, and test sets with a ratio of $80 : 16 : 4$ $(13238 : 2649 : 703)$.

2.2 Model architectures

To explore KV attention across different architectures, we implemented several models with KV and QKV attention variants, as detailed below. All models share a convolutional decoder adapted from SETR (Sec. 1.2). We modified the decoder to halve the feature dimensions during upsampling, reducing the overall parameter count (Fig. 2). We began by implementing the SETR encoder as outlined in [4], using a ViT-B/16 backbone with the feature dimension $D = 768$, number of heads $H = 12$, and number of layers $L = 12$ with both QKV and KV attention mechanisms. We refer to these architectures as SETR-QKV and SETR-KV, respectively. Furthermore, we explore SETR-KV-pos, where we introduce positional encoding within the KV attention block to create asymmetry, following the approach proposed in [3]. The 2D positional encoding dimension m was set to 50. Additionally, we constructed two models with a hybrid encoder. Drawing inspiration from TransUNet [5], we integrated the first four convolutional layers of the ResNet-50 architecture [6] into our encoder to capture higher-dimensional features before the patch embedding stage. In the fourth layer, we increased the number of blocks from six to nine to improve feature extraction while maintaining a feature dimension of 1024. Unlike the approach in [5], no skip connections were used. We refer to these models as SETR-QKV-CE and SETR-KV-CE, respectively. Finally, we developed an additional hybrid model using a CvT [7] as the encoder. The models SETR-CVT-QKV and SETR-CVT-KV utilize a CvT-13 encoder, with the multi-head attention (MHA) in the convolutional transformer blocks implemented with QKV and KV attention, respectively.

[1] `https://kaggle.com/competitions/uw-madison-gi-tract-image-segmentation`

2.3 Experiments

All models described in Sec. 2.2 were trained for 100 Epochs without early stopping to ensure comparable results. The input resolution was set at 224×224 and a fixed patch size of 16×16 was chosen. The AdamW optimizer with a learning rate of 10^{-4} and polynomial learning rate scheduling with factor 0.9 were used. Furthermore, a batch size of 32 was chosen for training. During training, on-the-fly data augmentation was applied, namely horizontal flipping, vertical flipping, shift scale rotate, coarse dropout, and random bright contrast, each having 50 % probability of being applied. All models were trained on the dataset described in Sec. 2.1 without using any pretrained backbones.

3 Results

The performance metrics computed for the tested architectures are the Jaccard index and the weighted Jaccard index, which are effective for evaluating segmentation overlap. Model complexity is represented by the number of learnable parameters, while computational efficiency is assessed by the number of multiply-accumulate operations (MACs) (collected through the `torchinfo` and `ptflops` python modules). Our results indicate that all KV variants perform comparably well or slightly better than their corresponding QKV implementations, while also demonstrating a reduction in both parameter count and MACs between 5% and 10% (Tab. 2).

4 Discussion

Our results indicate that KV transformers demonstrate competitive performance on segmentation tasks compared to their QKV attention counterparts. The computational cost and complexity outlined in Tab. 1 were not realized in our experiments, as the inclusion

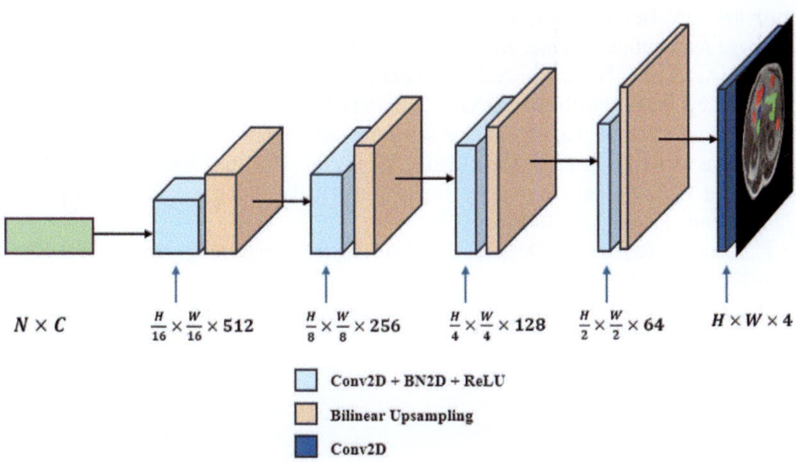

Fig. 2. We adapted the SETR-PUP decoder to also reduce feature dimensions during upsampling.

Tab. 2. The results of our experiments. We observe no performance decrease among most of the KV variants, while simultaneously seeing a reduction in parameter count and MACs. The asterisk (*) indicates that the MACs calculation requires further revision, as it does not account for the calculations related to 2D positional encoding.

	Jaccard	Weighted Jaccard	# Parameters (M)	MACs (G)
SETR-QKV	0.8718	0.8653	91.04	21.07
SETR-KV	0.8727	0.8667	83.96	19.68
SETR-KV-pos	0.8750	0.8691	83.96	19.97*
SETR-QKV-CE	0.8990	0.8946	103.14	25.02
SETR-KV-CE	0.9015	0.8960	96.05	23.68
SETR-QKV-CVT	0.8846	0.8786	22.9	9.86
SETR-KV-CVT	0.8807	0.8755	21.3	9.49

of convolutional elements in the decoders increases both of these metrics. Nonetheless, the reduction in MACs and parameters could hold practical implications in resource constrained clinical setting, such as mobile real-time disease screenings. Since the primary architectural change in KV attention takes place within the MHA block of the transformer, it could be adapted to various ViT-like architectures, presenting opportunities for additional research into the robustness of this design. In conclusion, we have examined the use of KV transformer architectures for segmentation tasks, particularly in the context of medical imaging. While our findings demonstrate that the evaluated KV variants exhibit similar performance compared to their QKV counterparts, it is important to note that these results are specific to the datasets and tasks explored in this study. Additionally, a hyperparameter search and experiments with diverse datasets are required to determine the broader applicability and generalizability of these conclusions.

References

1. Dosovitskiy A, Beyer L, Kolesnikov A et al. An image is worth 16x16 words: transformers for image recognition at scale. arXiv: 2010.11929. 2021.
2. Vaswani A, Shazeer N, Parmar N et al. Attention is all you need. Proc NIPS. 2017:6000–10.
3. Borji A. Key-value transformer. arXiv: 2305.19129. 2023.
4. Zheng S, Lu J, Zhao H et al. Rethinking semantic segmentation from a sequence-to-sequence perspective with transformers. Proc IEEE CVF CVPR. 2021:6877–86.
5. Chen J, Lu Y, Yu Q et al. TransUNet: transformers make strong encoders for medical image segmentation. arXiv: 2102.04306. 2021.
6. He K, Zhang X, Ren S et al. Deep residual learning for image recognition. Proc IEEE CVPR. 2016:770–8.
7. Wu H, Xiao B, Codella NCF et al. CvT: introducing convolutions to vision transformers. Proc IEEE CVF ICCV. 2021:22–31.

Category-fragment Segmentation Framework for Pelvic Fracture Segmentation in X-ray Images

Daiqi Liu, Fuxin Fan, Andreas Maier

Pattern Recognition Lab, Friedrich-Alexander-Universität Erlangen-Nürnberg
daiqi.deutschfau.liu@fau.de

Abstract. Pelvic fractures, often caused by high-impact trauma, frequently require surgical intervention. Imaging techniques such as CT and 2D X-ray imaging are used to transfer the surgical plan to the operating room through image registration, enabling quick intraoperative adjustments. Specifically, segmenting pelvic fractures from 2D X-ray imaging can assist in accurately positioning bone fragments and guiding the placement of screws or metal plates. In this study, we propose a novel deep learning-based category and fragment segmentation (CFS) framework for the automatic segmentation of pelvic bone fragments in 2D X-ray images. This framework consists of three consecutive steps. First, the category segmentation network extracts the left and right ilia and sacrum from X-ray images. Then, the fragment segmentation network further isolates the fragments in each masked bone region. Finally, the initially predicted bone fragments are reordered and refined through post-processing operations to form the final prediction. In the best-performing model, segmentation of pelvic fracture fragments achieves an intersection over union (IoU) of 0.91 for anatomical structures and 0.78 for fracture segmentation. Experimental results demonstrate that our CFS framework is effective in segmenting pelvic categories and fragments. For further research and development, the source code are publicly available at https://github.com/DaE-plz/CFSSegNet.

1 Introduction

Pelvic fractures, often caused by high-energy impacts like motor vehicle accidents or falls, can result in mortality rates exceeding 50% in severe cases [1, 2]. Accurate segmentation of pelvic fractures in 3D scans and X-ray images is essential, as it enables precise localization of fracture sites and guides both manual and automated reduction planning to restore pelvic anatomy [3]. While 3D CT scans provide detailed anatomical insights and are widely used for preoperative planning, 2D X-rays images are vital for intraoperative guidance and surgical plan execution. However, the projection nature of X-ray imaging complicates the automatic segmentation of pelvic bone fragments due to overlapping anatomy, fracture displacement, and complex pelvic morphology.

Most existing methods for pelvic fracture segmentation focus on CT data due to its volumetric nature and high contrast resolution [4, 5] . Deep learning approaches have been successfully applied to segment pelvic bones and detect fractures in CT scans, leveraging the rich spatial information available in 3D data [6]. In contrast, there is a lack of research on the automatic segmentation of pelvic fractures in X-ray images. Traditional image processing techniques, such as edge detection and thresholding, struggle with the

C. Palm et al. (Hrsg.), *Bildverarbeitung für die Medizin 2025*, Informatik aktuell,
https://doi.org/10.1007/978-3-658-47422-5_72

complexity and variability of pelvic anatomy in 2D projections [7, 8]. Some studies have explored convolutional neural networks (CNNs) for bone segmentation in X-ray images [9]. Additionally, recent studies have utilized deep learning for fracture detection in X-ray images, but they typically do not provide detailed segmentation of individual bone fragments [10–12].

This paper presents a deep learning-based method to automatically segment pelvic fracture categories and fragments from preoperative X-ray images. Our major contributions are as follows: (1) Our pipeline is proposed a category and fragment segmentation pipeline for pelvic fracture segmentation on X-ray images that achieves high accuracy in segmenting bone fragments. (2) During the data preparation stage, zero-padding is applied to both images and masks. (3) As a post-processing step, the predicted bone fragment masks are multiplied by the category masks to refine the final output.

2 Materials and methods

Our study aims to automatically segment the fragments in different categories of pelvic bones (the left and right ilia and the sacrum) from X-ray images. The whole CFS framework consists of three steps (Fig. 1).

The first step aims to segment each part of the pelvic bones from X-ray images. We utilize three separate category segmentation networks, each based on the Swin UNETR [13] architecture, to extract the left ilium, right ilium, and sacrum. The second step tries to isolate the bone fragments within each segmented bone region. We employ three separate fragment segmentation networks, each based on the Mask R-CNN [14] architecture, which not only performs segmentation but also integrates object detection through bounding box prediction and classification. These networks take both the X-ray images and the binary masks generated in the first step as input channels, allowing the

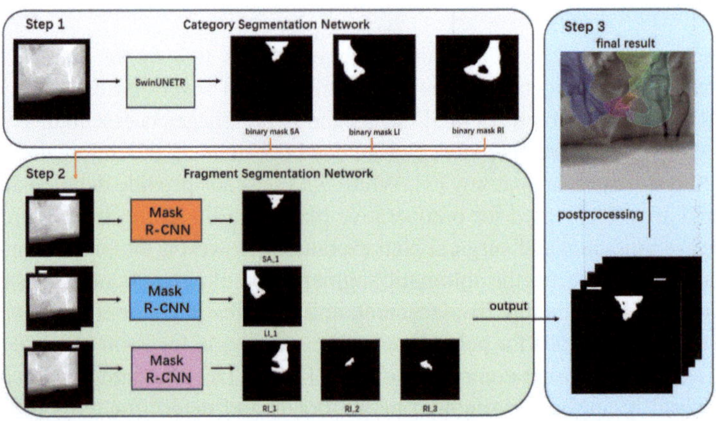

Fig. 1. Overview of the proposed pelvic fracture segmentation framework. The framework is divided into three main components: category segmentation, fragment segmentation, and post-processing.

Tab. 1. Segmentation results of different architectures used for category segmentation in the CFS framework. Swin UNETR +p represents the effect of adding zero padding operation on the experiment. The evaluation metrics are presented as mean with standard deviation (SD) for IoU, ASSD, and HD95 (on a test set of 5,000 cases). -C indicates the result of category segmentation, -F indicates the result of fragment segmentation.

Model	IOU-C	ASSD-C	HD95-C	IOU-F	ASSD-F	HD95-F
nnU-Net	0.890	4.46	15.24	0.734	11.14	43.64
	(0.07)	(0.79)	(3.02)	(0.16)	(3.08)	(4.35)
UNet++	0.896	4.45	15.23	0.736	10.55	41.49
	(0.07)	(0.72)	(2.49)	(0.15)	(2.54)	(3.98)
Attention U-Net	0.898	3.25	14.78	0.745	10.35	40.87
	(0.06)	(0.70)	(2.61)	(0.15)	(2.69)	(4.04)
VM-UNet	0.871	5.76	17.85	0.724	11.36	42.99
	(0.09)	(1.14)	(3.52)	(0.17)	(3.54)	(4.63)
Swin UNETR	0.901	3.02	14.56	0.753	9.83	40.25
	(0.07)	(0.70)	(2.26)	(0.11)	(2.35)	(3.74)
Swin UNETR +p	0.914	2.25	13.28	0.775	9.53	38.65
	(0.06)	(0.49)	(2.21)	(0.10)	(2.28)	(3.44)

model to focus on specific bone regions. During inference, the network predicts multiple bounding boxes, each associated with a confidence score. Only boxes with a confidence score above a predefined threshold, which is 0.8 in this work, are selected as potential bone fragments. In the third step, post-processing techniques are applied. The category masks from the first step are multiplied by the fragment segmentation masks from the second step. Additionally, the predicted masks are reordered according to predefined indices to ensure consistency in the output.

The dataset used in this work is sourced from the MICCAI challenge, PENGWIN[1], which provides both 2D X-ray images and 3D CT scans with annotated labels for pelvic category and fragment segmentation. The 2D X-ray images are generated from 3D CT data using DeepDRR [15], a tool that produces highly realistic images by accurately simulating physical properties and clinical detail, including anatomical features, intensity, and noise patterns. The final dataset consists of 50,000 X-ray images generated from 100 CT volumes, with each CT volume producing 500 images from different angles. The input images and masks have a resolution of 448 × 448 pixels. For each X-ray image, the dataset provides binary masks for all bone fragments within each pelvic category, with the number of fragments varying across cases.

All models were implemented using PyTorch 2.1.2. The experiments were performed on an Nvidia A100 GPU. The comprehensive code are provided at our GitHub repository[2].

[1] https://data.niaid.nih.gov/resources?id=zenodo_10913195
[2] https://github.com/DaE-plz/CFSSegNet

3 Results

Tab. 1 presents the performance comparison of various neural network architectures used for category segmentation in Step 1 of the CFS framework on a test set of 5,000 images. The architectures tested include nnU-Net [16, 17], UNet++ [18], Attention U-Net [19], VM-UNet [20] and Swin UNETR [13]. Additionally, we conducted experiments to assess the impact of using zero-padding within the CFS framework, specifically with the Swin UNETR architecture (Swin UNETR +p).

For category segmentation, the results show that nnU-Net and UNet++ achieve comparable performance, with both models exhibiting a similar intersection over union (IoU) score of approximately 0.89. Attention U-Net demonstrates a slightly better performance in category segmentation, with an IoU of 0.898 and lower ASSD and HD95 values. Swin UNETR further improves the category segmentation results, delivering an IoU of 0.901. The Swin UNETR +p model performs the best among all architectures, achieving the highest IoU (0.914) with the SD of 0.06 and the lowest ASSD and HD95 scores, making it the most effective for category segmentation.

For fragment segmentation, overall performance is generally lower compared to category segmentation, as seen in the lower IoU and higher ASSD and HD95 values. However, the models follow a similar trend as in category segmentation. Swin UNETR +p again demonstrates the best performance, achieving an IoU of 0.775 with the SD of 0.10 and providing more accurate fragment segmentation, as indicated by the lowest ASSD (9.53) and HD95 (38.65) values.

We used 250 X-ray images generated from a single CT volume. With the left hipbone as a reference, the overlap ratio (the proportion of the left hipbone area that is overlapped) was calculated for each image. The images were subsequently sorted by overlap ratio, from highest to lowest. For each sorted image, IoU scores were computed for fragment segmentation of the sacrum, right hipbone, and left hipbone. The left side of Fig. 2 presents the IoU scores for bone fragment segmentation corresponding to each X-ray image, with the X-axis representing the image index and the Y-axis representing the IoU

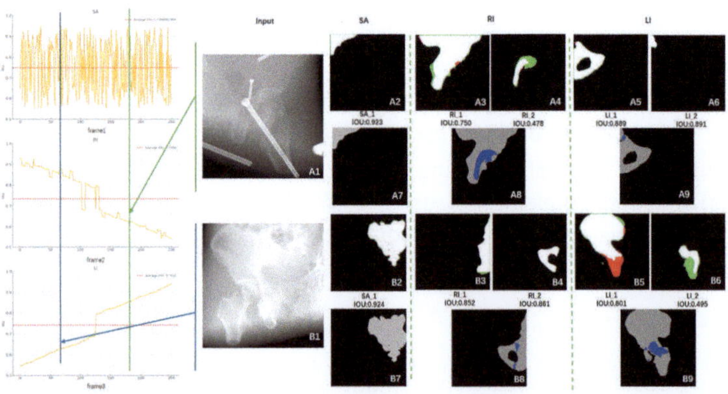

Fig. 2. Relationship between anatomical overlap and segmentation performance. blue represents the overlapping regions, red indicates false positives, and green indicates false negatives.

score for each bone fragment. On the right side of Fig. 2, two representative examples are shown, labeled A1 to A9 (top) and B1 to B9 (bottom). Each example consists of two rows: the upper row displays the predicted segmentation masks, where green areas indicate false negatives and red areas represent false positives. The lower row highlights the overlapping regions between bone fragments, shown in blue.

In the example labeled A, image A8 shows a large overlapping area at RI, with an IoU score of 0.478 for the bone fragment RI_2, while image A9 shows minimal overlap at LI, achieving an IoU score of 0.889 for the fragment LI_1. In the example labeled B, image B8 has minimal overlap in the RI region with an IoU score of 0.852 for RI_1, whereas image B9 shows large overlap in the LI region with an IoU score of 0.495 for LI_2.

4 Discussion

The results from Tab. 1 demonstrate that models incorporating more advanced architectures, such as attention mechanisms (Attention U-Net) or transformer-based structures (Swin UNETR), enhance segmentation performance, particularly in capturing boundary details. However, the complexity of a model does not necessarily correlate with improved segmentation performance. For instance, VM-UNet, despite its complexity, did not perform well for pelvic bone segmentation. When examining the effect of zero-padding on segmentation performance, we observed that using padded images and masks for training improved boundary segmentation accuracy and led to better overall performance. Additionally, using our best model for testing, the SD of IoU in fragment segmentation (0.10) was higher than that in category segmentation (0.06), indicating bigger inconsistency. This larger SD suggests that the model is less stable when segmenting bone fragments compared to category segmentation.

From Fig. 2, the results indicate that images with higher overlap ratios tend lower IoU scores for fragment segmentation. This analysis underscores the challenge that anatomical overlap poses for bone fragment segmentation, increased overlap in X-ray projections obscures the boundaries between bone fragments, making it more difficult for the network to achieve accurate segmentation. For future work, we plan to explore whether pre-segmenting overlapping regions can improve the overall performance of bone fragment segmentation.

Acknowledgement. The authors gratefully acknowledge the scientific support and HPC resources provided by the Erlangen National High Performance Computing Center (NHR@FAU) of the Friedrich-Alexander-Universität Erlangen-Nürnberg (FAU). The hardware is funded by the German Research Foundation (DFG).

References

1. Kowal J, Langlotz F, Nolte LP. Basics of computer-assisted orthopaedic surgery. Navigation and MIS in Orthopedic Surgery. Springer, 2007:2–8.

2. Sugano N. Computer-assisted orthopaedic surgery and robotic surgery in total hip arthroplasty. Clin Orthop Surg. 2013;5(1):1–9.
3. Liu J, Li H, Zeng B et al. An end-to-end geometry-based pipeline for automatic preoperative surgical planning of pelvic fracture reduction and fixation. IEEE Trans Med Imaging. 2024.
4. Wu J. Segmentation and fracture detection in CT images for traumatic pelvic injuries. Virginia Commonwealth University, Richmond, 2012.
5. Pandey P, Guy P, Hodgson AJ et al. Fast and automatic bone segmentation and registration of 3D ultrasound to CT for the full pelvic anatomy: a comparative study. Int J Comput Assist Radiol Surg. 2018;13:1515–24.
6. Liu Y, Yibulayimu S, Sang Y et al. Pelvic fracture segmentation using a multi-scale distance-weighted neural network. Proc MICCAI. 2023:312–21.
7. Fornaro J, Székely G, Harders M. Semi-automatic segmentation of fractured pelvic bones for surgical planning. Proc ISBMS. 2010:82–9.
8. Irwansyah, Lai JY, Essomba T et al. Algorithm for segmentation and reduction of fractured bones in computer-aided preoperative surgery. Proc ICBBE. 2016:12–8.
9. Cernazanu-Glavan C, Holban S. Segmentation of bone structure in X-ray images using convolutional neural network. Adv Electr Comput Eng. 2013;13(1):87–94.
10. Tomita N, Cheung YY, Hassanpour S. Deep neural networks for automatic detection of osteoporotic vertebral fractures on CT scans. Comput Biol Med. 2018;98:8–15.
11. Ukai K, Rahman R, Yagi N et al. Detecting pelvic fracture on 3D-CT using deep convolutional neural networks with multi-orientated slab images. Sci Rep. 2021;11(1):11716.
12. Yamamoto N, Rahman R, Yagi N et al. An automated fracture detection from pelvic CT images with 3-D convolutional neural networks. Proc IEEE CcS. 2020:1–6.
13. Hatamizadeh A, Nath V, Tang Y et al. Swin UNETR: swin transformers for semantic segmentation of brain tumors in MRI images. Proc MICCAI. 2021:272–84.
14. He K, Gkioxari G, Dollár P et al. Mask r-CNN. Proc IEEE ICCV. 2017:2961–9.
15. Unberath M, Zaech JN, Lee SC et al. DeepDRR – a catalyst for machine learning in fluoroscopy-guided procedures. Proc MICCAI. 2018:98–106.
16. Isensee F, Jäger PF, Kohl SA et al. Automated design of deep learning methods for biomedical image segmentation. arXiv: 1904.08128. 2019.
17. Isensee F, Jaeger PF, Kohl SA et al. nnU-Net: a self-configuring method for deep learning-based biomedical image segmentation. Nat Methods. 2021;18(2):203–11.
18. Zhou Z, Rahman Siddiquee MM, Tajbakhsh N et al. UNet++: a nested U-Net architecture for medical image segmentation. Proc DLMIA. 2018:3–11.
19. Oktay O, Schlemper J, Folgoc LL et al. Attention U-Net: learning where to look for the pancreas. arXiv: 1804.03999. 2018.
20. Ruan J, Xiang S. VM-UNet: vision mamba UNet for medical image segmentation. arXiv: 2402.02491. 2024.

DualPath-FFNet

Dynamic Fusion of Pre-trained Features with Sigmoid-gated Attention for Improved Medical Image Segmentation

Sadat H. Chowdhury[1], Mohamed Y. Jabarulla[1], Hinrich B. Winther[2], Steffen Oeltze-Jafra[1]

[1]Peter L. Reichertz Institute for Medical Informatics, Hannover Medical School, Germany
[2]Institute of Diagnostic and Interventional Radiology, Hannover Medical School, Germany
Chowdhury.sadat@mh-hannover.de

Abstract. In medical imaging, accurate image segmentation is essential for precise diagnosis and treatment planning. However, challenges such as image quality variations, complex anatomical structures, and the impracticality of traditional segmentation methods require extensive, source-specific feature extraction. In this study, we introduce DualPath-FFNet, a novel deep-learning architecture for medical image segmentation. The architecture utilizes DenseNet201 and EfficientNetV2 pre-trained networks as encoders to extract diverse feature representations from input images. Two decoders generate intermediate outputs, refined with the original input image and further enhanced by skip connections. A Sigmoid gated attention (SGA) module dynamically fuses features, prioritizing task-specific information. A third encoder aggregates information from previous stages, integrating skip connections and utilizing the SGA module. This dynamic fusion, combined with multi-view encoding and skip connections, promotes robust and informative representation learning. The performance of this model was comparatively evaluated using dice coefficient and Intersection over Union metrics over 5 different types of medical image data set against three other relavant models. DualPath-FF Net achieves an average Dice score of 0.914 across multiple datasets, demonstrating robust performance and generalizability.

1 Introduction

Medical image segmentation plays a pivotal role in computer-aided diagnosis, treatment planning, and image-guided interventions [1]. Accurate delineation of anatomical structures is crucial for clinical decision-making, and the demand for robust segmentation algorithms continues to grow with the increasing availability and complexity of medical imaging data [2]. Traditional methods often struggle with the inherent variability in medical images, including variations in image quality, noise, and anatomical diversity across different modalities [3].

Recent advancements in deep learning have spurred a significant transformation in medical image segmentation, marked by the remarkable performance of convolutional neural networks (CNNs) [4]. These CNNs have emerged as the forefront tools, achieving state-of-the-art results in segmenting medical images. Notably, pre-trained CNNs, originally trained on extensive image datasets like ImageNet, have showcased exceptional adaptability and versatility in learning hierarchical features across various image

C. Palm et al. (Hrsg.), *Bildverarbeitung für die Medizin 2025*, Informatik aktuell,
https://doi.org/10.1007/978-3-658-47422-5_73

domains [5]. Despite these achievements, the direct application of pre-trained models to specific medical imaging tasks presents substantial challenges [6].

The unique characteristics of medical images present significant challenges for integrating pre-trained models. In contrast to datasets like ImageNet [7], which contain vast quantities of labeled images across diverse categories, medical imaging datasets are often limited in number and meticulously annotated. This scarcity hinders the effective training and fine-tuning of pre-trained models, impeding their performance when applied to medical imaging tasks. Additionally, another substantial challenge arises from domain shifts within medical images. These images often exhibit distinct statistical properties and various imaging modalities, leading to a misalignment between the feature distributions learned by pre-trained models on generic image datasets and those found in medical images. As a result, directly transferring pre-trained models to medical imaging tasks can lead to suboptimal performance and reduced generalization capabilities.

To address these challenges, we propose DualPath-FFNet, a novel deep learning architecture that leverages the strengths of both pre-trained features and a dynamic attention mechanism. Our model aims to provide a generalized solution for medical image segmentation, capable of effectively handling diverse datasets and modalities. DualPath-FFNet incorporates a unique dual-path structure, enabling the model to: (1) exploit pre-trained features for efficient representation learning and (2) capture task-specific information through a dedicated path. A key innovation is the integration of a Sigmoid-gated attention mechanism, which dynamically fuses features from both paths while selectively focusing on relevant regions of interest within the medical image. We evaluate the effectiveness of the DualPath-FFNet architecture on various medical imaging datasets, comparing its performance against state-of-the-art segmentation models.

2 Methodology

As illustrated in Figure 1, the architecture employs a dual-path strategy that involves two distinct pre-trained networks: EfficientNetV2 [8] and DenseNet201 [9]. The name 'DualPath' derives from the incorporation of these two networks, while 'FF' signifies feature fusion achieved through a Sigmoid attention gate. The DualPath-FFNet is a combination of three different U-Net architectures. The first network employs EfficientNetV2 pre-trained on ImageNet as the encoder, while the second network uses DenseNet201 pre-trained on ImageNet as its encoder. Skip connections from these encoders are selected based on matching layer shapes. The proposed DualPath-FFNet architecture follows a systematic four-stage approach: (a) Feature Extraction and Preprocessing, leveraging pre-trained encoders on ImageNet to extract vital features for accurate segmentation; (b) Feature Fusion, strategically combining extracted features with a Sigmoid attention gate to enhance discriminative power; (c) Hierarchical Feature Extraction, refining segmentation through a third set of features extracted by Encoder 3, reinforced with skip connections; and (d) Incorporation of a Sigmoid attention gate, dynamically weighting contributions from various paths to sharpen focus on pertinent information. Currently, the model can only accept an input image of size $128 \times 128 \times 3$ and produces a binary output of the region of interest.

3 Experimental setup and results

3.1 Data collection and pre-processing

To evaluate the performance of DualPath-FFNet, we collected five different types of datasets. These includes skin lesion data from the International Skin Imaging Collaboration (ISIC) 2016 challenge [10], gastrointestinal polyp segmentation of Kvasir-SEG dataset [11], Brain MRI for tumor segmentation, Cardiac MRI for heart segmentation, and lung CT images for tumor segmentation were collected from the Medical Decathlon Challenge [12]. All the images were resized according to model's input requirement, and the intensity values were normalized.

3.2 Training details

The segmentation performance of DualPath-FFnet was evaluated against U-Net [13], RESL-U-Net [14] and Double U-Net [15]. These three models were selected due to their relevance to the developed DualPath-FFnet. These models were trained separately on each data set maintaining an uniform model compilation parameter for the training. The training process comprised 50 epochs, where the binary cross-entropy loss function was employed in conjunction with the Adam optimizer, utilizing a learning rate of 1×10^{-4}. To ensure a comprehensive evaluation, the dataset images and corresponding labels were partitioned into three subsets: training, validation, and testing, following a split ratio of 7:2:1. All segmentation models were trained using a High Performance Computing Cluster environment provided by Hannover Medical School (MHH).

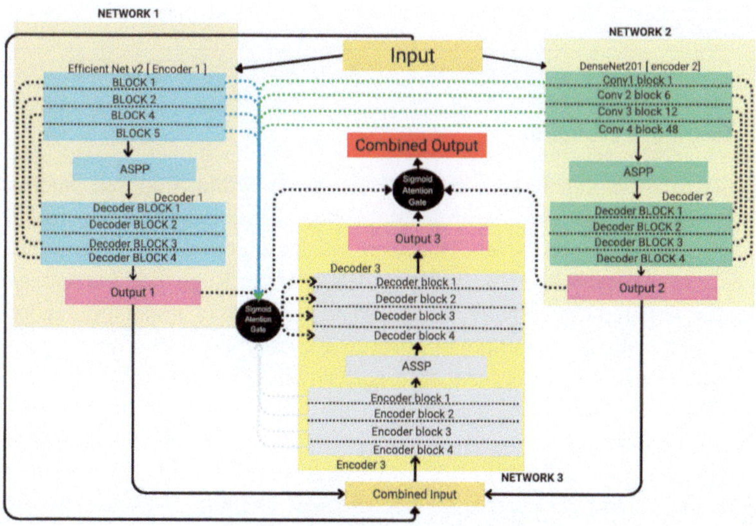

Fig. 1. DualPath-FFnet architecture.

Tab. 1. Segmentation prediction results and Dice score for different datasets and models.

	Images	Ground Truth	DualPath-FF net	Double U-Net	U-Net	RESL U-Net
Skin lesion	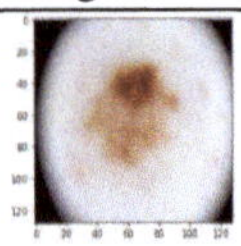	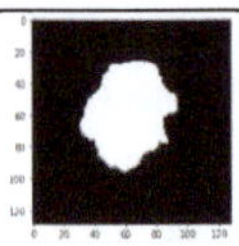	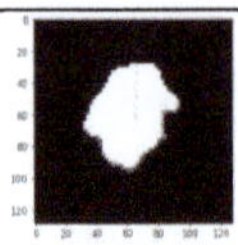	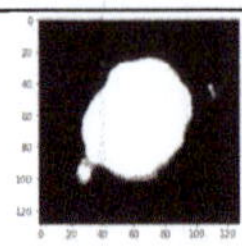	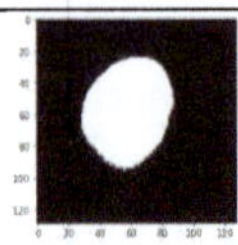	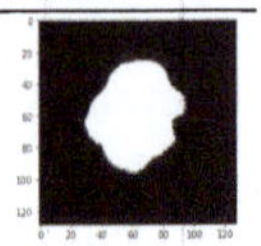
Dice			**0.96**	0.87	0.87	0.93
Polyp image	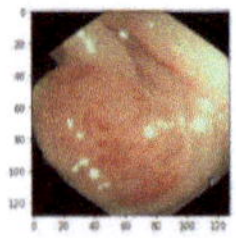	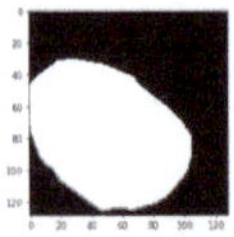	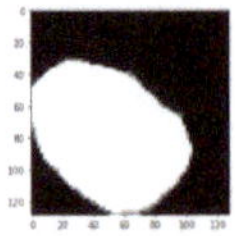	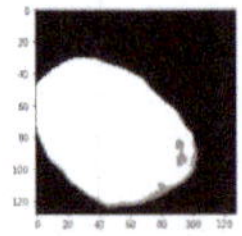	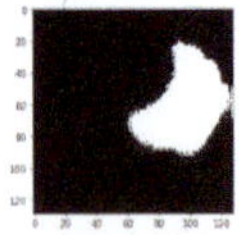	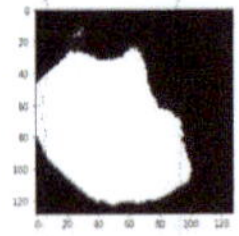
Dice			**0.96**	0.92	0.51	0.90
Lung CT	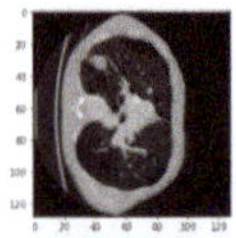	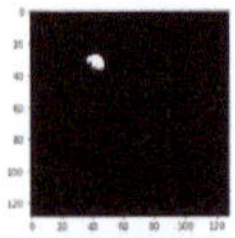	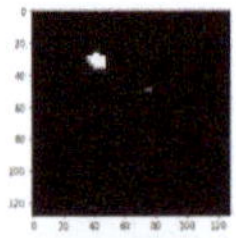	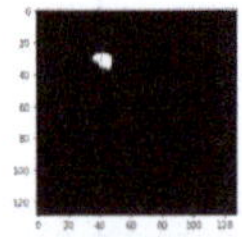	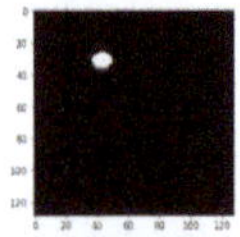	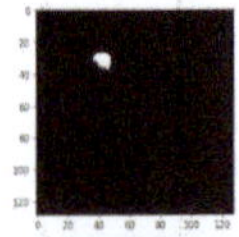
Dice			**0.84**	0.83	0.63	0.79
Brain MRI	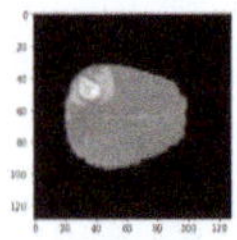	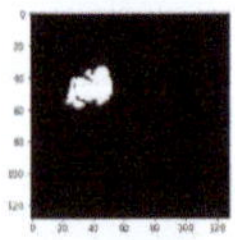	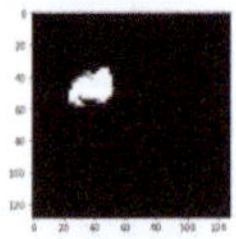	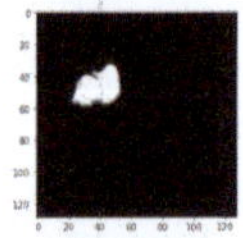	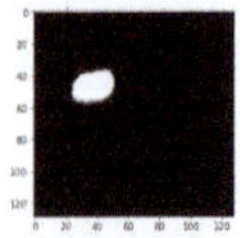	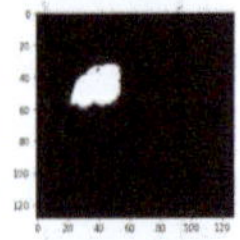
Dice			0.91	**0.94**	0.82	0.87
Heart MRI	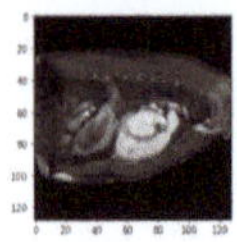	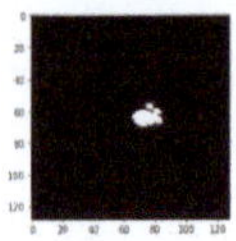	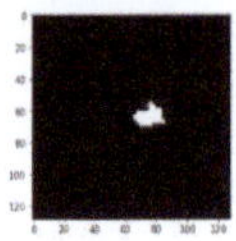	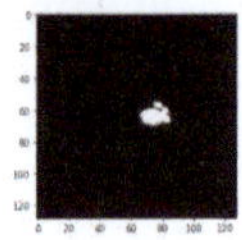	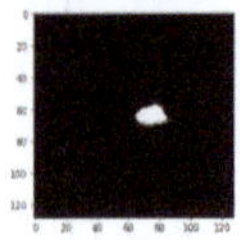	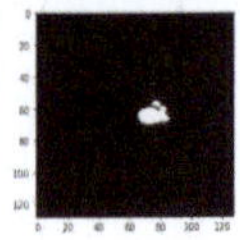
Dice			0.90	**0.96**	0.88	0.94

3.3 Performance evaluation

We conducted a comprehensive comparative analysis of our proposed medical image segmentation model against three well-established segmentation architectures: U-Net, RESL U-Net, and Double U-Net. The result of the analysis is presented in Table 1. Notably, our model exhibits enhanced delineation of the Region of Interest, providing finer details compared to alternative models. The predicted contours align more closely with the ground truth, demonstrating improved accuracy along the edges.

To quantitatively assess segmentation performance, we employed Dice coefficient (DSC) metrics. The dice score presented in the table represents the overall average, providing a consolidated measure of the performance of the models (Tab. 1). Our segmentation model, DualPath-FFNet, was systematically compared with three other state-of-the-art models across five diverse medical imaging datasets. The evaluation was based on Dice scores, offering insights into the models' proficiency in accurately delineating regions of interest.

DualPath-FFNet achieves the highest Dice scores for skin lesion (0.96), polyp (0.96), and lung CT (0.84), indicating its strong overall performance.In the case of heart and brain MRI images, Double U-Net achieved higher Dice scores compared to DualPath-FFNet. This discrepancy may stem from the increased depth and complexity of the training datasets for these modalities, which could require more careful hyperparameter tuning and a more tailored training protocol. By contrast, our approach employed a uniform training strategy across all models and datasets, including a single learning rate, which may not have been optimal for these more extensive datasets.

4 Conclusion

In this study, we integrated DenseNet201 and EfficientNetV2 as encoders, leveraging their pre-trained weights to capture diverse feature representations. Additionally, we included a custom designed encoders to extract hierarchical features. We introduced dynamic feature fusion through a Sigmoid gated attention (SGA) module to prioritize task-specific information and enhance discriminative power. The incorporation of skip connections ensures the propagation of fine-grained details across network layers. By combining these techniques, our architecture aims to overcome the limitations of existing models and provide a robust solution for medical image segmentation tasks. Through extensive experimentation and evaluation on multiple publicly available datasets, we demonstrate the effectiveness of DualPath-FFNet in achieving high segmentation accuracy. In clinical applications, the proposed DualPath-FFNet architecture holds promise for various medical imaging tasks, including tumor delineation, organ localization, and lesion detection. Its ability to capture both global context and fine-grained details makes it invaluable for assisting clinicians in making accurate diagnoses and treatment plans. Future research efforts should focus on developing strategies to mitigate these challenges, thereby enhancing the applicability and scalability of the proposed methodology for diverse clinical applications. The model was trained separately on different types of data-set. In the future, a combined dataset containing various types of medical images will be used to train the model.

Acknowledgement. This work was supported by the German Federal Ministry of Education and Research (BMBF) under the funding codes 01ZZ2315A-P as part of the Open Medical Inference (OMI) project.

References

1. Litjens G, Kooi T, Bejnordi BE et al. A survey on deep learning in medical image analysis. Med Image Anal. 2017;42:60–88.
2. Liu X, Song L, Liu S et al. A review of deep-learning-based medical image segmentation methods. Sustainability. 2021;13(3):1224.
3. Yu Y, Wang C, Fu Q et al. Techniques and challenges of image segmentation: a review. Electronics. 2023;12(5):1199.
4. Li M, Jiang Y, Zhang Y et al. Medical image analysis using deep learning algorithms. Front Public Health. 2023;11.
5. He K, Zhang X, Ren S et al. Deep residual learning for image recognition. arXiv: 1512.03385. 2015.

6. Wen Y, Chen L, Deng Y et al. Rethinking pre-training on medical imaging. J Vis Commun Image Represent. 2021;78:103145.
7. Deng J, Dong W, Socher R et al. ImageNet: a large-scale hierarchical image database. Proc IEEE CVPR. 2009:248–55.
8. Tan M, Le QV. EfficientNetV2: smaller models and faster training. arXiv: 2104.00298. 2021.
9. Huang G, Liu Z, Maaten L van der et al. Densely connected convolutional networks. arXiv: 1608.06993. 2018.
10. Gutman D, Codella NCF, Celebi E et al. Skin lesion analysis toward melanoma detection: a challenge at the international symposium on biomedical imaging (ISBI) 2016, hosted by the international skin imaging collaboration (ISIC). arXiv: 1605.01397. 2016.
11. Jha D, Smedsrud PH, Riegler MA et al. Kvasir-SEG: a segmented polyp dataset. Proc ICMM. 2020:451–62.
12. Simpson AL, Antonelli M, Bakas S et al. A large annotated medical image dataset for the development and evaluation of segmentation algorithms. arXiv: 1902.09063. 2019.
13. Ronneberger O, Fischer P, Brox T. U-Net: convolutional networks for biomedical image segmentation. arXiv: 1505.04597. 2015.
14. Khanna A, Londhe N, Gupta S et al. A deep residual U-Net convolutional neural network for automated lung segmentation in computed tomography images. Biocybern Biomed Eng. 2020;40:1314–27.
15. Jha D, Riegler MA, Johansen D et al. DoubleU-Net: a deep convolutional neural network for medical image segmentation. arXiv: 2006.04868. 2020.

Abstract: Longitudinal Segmentation of MS Lesions via Temporal Difference Weighting

Maximilian R. Rokuss[1,2], Yannick Kirchhoff[1,2,3], Saikat Roy[1,2], Balint Kovacs[1,4], Constantin Ulrich[1,4], Tassilo Wald[1,2,5], Maximilian Zenk[1,4], Stefan Denner[1,4], Fabian Isensee[1,5], Philipp Vollmuth[1,6,7], Jens Kleesiek[8,9], Klaus Maier-Hein[1,10]

[1]German Cancer Research Center (DKFZ), Heidelberg, Division of Medical Image Computing, Germany
[2]Faculty of Mathematics and Computer Science, Heidelberg University, Germany
[3]HIDSS4Health - Helmholtz Information and Data Science School for Health, Karlsruhe/Heidelberg, Germany
[4]Medical Faculty Heidelberg, Heidelberg University, Heidelberg, Germany
[5]Helmholtz Imaging, German Cancer Research Center, Heidelberg, Germany
[6]Department of Neuroradiology, Heidelberg University Hospital, Heidelberg, Germany
[7]Division for Computational Neuroimaging, Department of Neuroradiology, Heidelberg University Hospital, Heidelberg, Germany
[8]Institute for Artificial Intelligence in Medicine (IKIM), University Hospital Essen, Essen, Germany
[9]Cancer Research Center Cologne Essen (CCCE), West German Cancer Center Essen, University Hospital Essen, Essen, Germany
[10]Pattern Analysis and Learning Group, Department of Radiation Oncology, Heidelberg University Hospital

maximilian.rokuss@dkfz-heidelberg.de

Accurate segmentation of multiple sclerosis (MS) lesions in longitudinal MRI scans is crucial for monitoring disease progression and treatment efficacy. Although changes across time are taken into account when assessing images in clinical practice, most existing deep learning methods treat scans from different timepoints separately. Among studies utilizing longitudinal images, a simple channel-wise concatenation is the primary albeit suboptimal method employed to integrate timepoints. We introduce a novel approach that explicitly incorporates temporal differences between baseline and follow-up scans through a unique architectural inductive bias called difference weighting block [1]. It merges features from two timepoints, emphasizing changes between scans. We achieve superior scores in lesion segmentation (Dice score, Hausdorff distance) as well as lesion detection (lesion-level F_1 score) as compared to state-of-the-art longitudinal and single timepoint models across two datasets. Our code is made publicly available at GitHub[1].

References

1. Rokuss M, Kirchhoff Y, Roy S et al. Longitudinal segmentation of MS lesions via temporal difference weighting. Proc MICCAI. 2025;15401.

[1]www.github.com/MIC-DKFZ/Longitudinal-Difference-Weighting

C. Palm et al. (Hrsg.), *Bildverarbeitung für die Medizin 2025*, Informatik aktuell,
https://doi.org/10.1007/978-3-658-47422-5_74

Internal Organ Localization using Depth Images
A Framework for Automated MRI Patient Positioning

Eytan Kats[1], Kai Geißler[2], Jochen G. Hirsch[2], Stefan Heldman[2], Mattias P. Heinrich[1]

[1]Institute of Medical Informatics, University of Lubeck
[2]Fraunhofer Institute for Digital Medicine MEVIS, Bremen
eytan.kats@uni-luebeck.de

Abstract. Automated patient positioning is a crucial step in streamlining MRI workflows and enhancing patient throughput. RGB-D camera-based systems offer a promising approach to automate this process by leveraging depth information to estimate internal organ positions. This paper investigates the feasibility of a learning-based framework to infer approximate internal organ positions from the body surface. Our approach utilizes a large-scale dataset of MRI scans to train a deep learning model capable of accurately predicting organ positions and shapes from depth images alone. We demonstrate the effectiveness of our method in localization of multiple internal organs, including bones and soft tissues. Our findings suggest that RGB-D camera-based systems integrated into MRI workflows have the potential to streamline scanning procedures and improve patient experience by enabling accurate and automated patient positioning.

1 Introduction

The growing demand for magnetic resonance imaging (MRI) examinations underscores the need to optimize scanning procedures to reduce patient wait times and improve operational efficiency. A critical, yet time-intensive, aspect of this process is the patient preparation and planning phase, which is essential for optimizing image quality and diagnostic accuracy [1]. This phase typically involves manual positioning of the patient followed by scout imaging to facilitate detailed geometric planning for subsequent diagnostic scans [2]. Automated patient positioning systems, capable of accurately identifying and localizing the anatomical region of interest, offer the potential to streamline this process by automatically adjusting the patient table to the correct position. Such systems could substantially reduce the time spent on manual adjustments, minimize positioning errors, and enhance workflow efficiency within radiology departments.

RGB-D camera-based systems have emerged as innovative tools in radiology workflows, particularly in enhancing patient setup and positioning processes. These systems provide precise mapping of the patient's external body surface. Studies by Incetan et al. [3] and Karanam et al. [4] demonstrate the effectiveness of these systems in automated patient positioning by localizing key anatomical landmarks on the body surface, such as the head, thorax, and knee. Researchers have shown that predicting internal anatomical structures from the outer surface is also possible. Wu et al. [5] proposes a learning-based framework to generate a volumetric phantom, including the skeleton and lungs, from a detailed mesh representation of the patient's body surface. Recent line of works [6–8]

C. Palm et al. (Hrsg.), *Bildverarbeitung für die Medizin 2025*, Informatik aktuell,
https://doi.org/10.1007/978-3-658-47422-5_75

integrate shape representation of internal organs into the popular skinned multi-person linear (SMPL) model [9] that provides a flexible statistical framework to capture human pose and shape deformations. The SMPL-A method [6] estimates the deformation of organs as a patient moves, but the organs' initial shapes are obtained by a scan of the patient. OSSO [7] and BOSS [8] demonstrate the ability to infer skeletal and organ shape from the body surface. Although these methods show promising results, they rely on initial body surface mesh generation, which introduces additional processing time. Moreover, SMPL-based approaches require fitting the acquired surface mesh to obtain accurate model parameters, adding a further step to the inference process. In contrast, Teixeira et al. [10] propose a method that leverages depth camera images to directly estimate key patient scanning parameters, including lung position, isocenter, and water-equivalent diameter.

We investigate the feasibility of a learning-based framework to estimate approximate internal organ positions using simulated depth images derived from MRI scans. By leveraging depth information, the trained model infers organ locations, enabling the dynamic adjustment of patient table positioning and scan parameters, offering a potential solution to streamline radiological workflows. To ensure broad generalizability, we train our model on a large-scale dataset of approximately 10,000 full-body patient scans from the National German Cohort (NAKO) dataset [11]. Our experiments demonstrate the efficacy of the proposed solution in estimating the positions of 11 internal anatomical structures, including bones and soft tissue organs.

Our main contributions are as follows: (1) We demonstrate the efficacy of a learning-based framework in estimating internal organ locations solely from depth images. (2) We showcase the model's generalizability across diverse body types and anatomical variations through training on a large-scale dataset.

2 Materials and methods

In our study, we utilize approximately 10,000 full-body MRI scans from the NAKO dataset [11]. This extensive collection of images enables us to model anatomical information across a diverse range of anatomical variations within the population.

To simulate depth images, we normalize the MRI images to a range of 0 to 1 and apply a threshold of 0.02 to obtain a binary mask. Subsequently, we employ binary morphological opening to remove noise. Next, we extract a 2D orthographic depth image in the coronal plane by isolating the skin surface. After normalizing the depth image to a range of 0 to 1, we set to 0 all values smaller than 0.3 to eliminate table artifacts that are located far from the simulated camera position. Finally, we further denoise the resulting grayscale image using grayscale morphological opening. The resulting images are visualized in left column of Fig.1.

To ensure a representative evaluation dataset, we selected 30 cases based on criteria such as study center, patient sex, age, weight, and height. Three radiologic technologists created segmentation masks for multiple structures within these cases. To obtain the segmentation masks for training, we employed the TotalSegmentator (TS) version for MRI images [12] to process the remaining scans. We then generated binary 2D masks by projecting the volumetric segmentations of each organ onto the coronal plane. Each organ was projected separately to account for potential overlap in the 2D plane, resulting in distinct binary masks for each structure. These masks encompass 11 internal organs, including three bone structures (hips, femurs, and a vertebra), two thoracic organs (heart and lungs), and six abdominal organs (kidneys, liver, pancreas, spleen, stomach, and urinary bladder).

For training, we employ a U-Net-based architecture that takes generated depth images of the body surface as input and outputs segmentation masks of internal organs. Ground truth segmentation masks are generated using TS. We train our model in a multi-label setting using a sigmoid activation function. We utilize a weighted combination of Dice loss and binary cross-entropy loss, with equal weighting of 0.5. During training, we employ a batch size of 16 and the Adam optimizer with an initial learning rate of 0.002, which is decayed using a cosine annealing schedule.

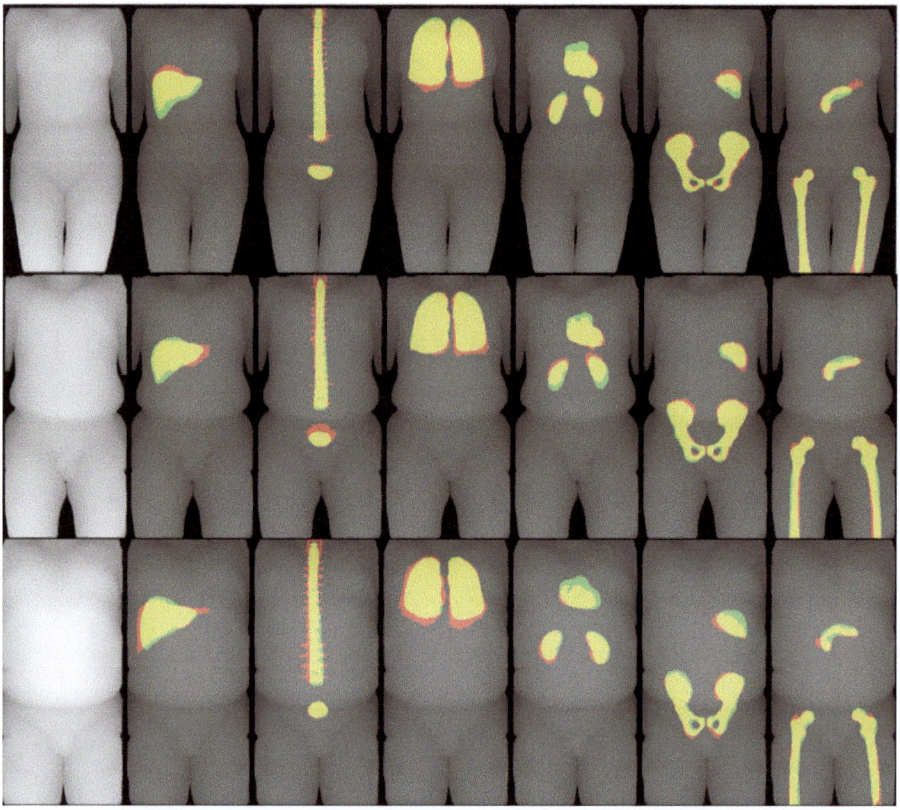

Fig. 1. Comparison of predicted and ground truth segmentations for internal organs. To enhance visualization clarity and address potential overlaps of 2D projections, organs are presented in a separate images. From left to right: depth image derived from MRI scan, liver, vertebrae and urinary bladder, lungs, heart and kidneys, spleen and hips, femurs and pancreas. Red - ground truth mask, green - model prediction, yellow - overlap between ground truth and predicted mask.

Tab. 1. The model's performance for internal organ segmentation from body surface depth images is evaluated using the mean value of the following metrics across 11 anatomical structures: Dice coefficient, ASSD, and percentile 95 of DOE. Results are reported for a manually labeled data and an automatically generated masks using TS.

Training examples	Dice Manual	Dice TS	ASSD [mm] Manual	ASSD [mm] TS	DOE [mm] Manual	DOE [mm] TS
100	72.44 ± 7.01	75.66 ± 6.4	10.11 ± 3.33	9.66 ± 3.32	48.95	40.0
1000	76.01 ± 4.42	78.82 ± 5.03	8.93 ± 1.74	8.87 ± 3.34	42.33	31.0
10000	79.44 ± 3.55	81.46 ± 4.52	7.94 ± 1.49	8.5 ± 3.43	36.0	29.0

3 Results

We evaluate the performance of the trained models on two distinct sets of ground truth segmentation masks. The first set comprises 30 images manually labeled by expert radiologic technologists, providing high-quality annotations. The second set is a hold-out collection of 696 masks generated by TS, similar to those used for the model training. Evaluation on manually labeled data assesses the model's ability to align with the 'gold standard' ground truth. Testing on additional automatically generated masks reveals its consistency with the training data and helps identify any biases introduced by the automated annotation process. The dual evaluation helps to assess the model's generalization capabilities and identify potential domain shifts between manually labeled and automatically generated data.

To evaluate the model's ability to accurately predict organ shape, we compute the average symmetric surface distance (ASSD) between predicted and actual organ boundaries. We use the Dice coefficient to assess segmentation performance. Additionally, we derive bounding boxes from the segmentation masks and calculate the detection offset error (DOE), defined as the distance between the corresponding sides of the ground truth and predicted bounding boxes. For each detected organ, we use the maximum value among the top, bottom, left, and right offsets in our calculations. This metric is particularly relevant for scanning procedures, as it quantifies the margin needed for precise patient table positioning to ensure complete coverage of the target organ during scanning. Chosen metrics provide a comprehensive evaluation of both localization accuracy and shape fidelity, enabling an assessment of the model's clinical potential.

We investigate the correlation between external body surface and internal organ location and shape. To this end, we train our model on incrementally larger datasets, tracking performance improvements for 11 anatomical structures (Tab.1). As expected, model performance improves with increasing training data, with each incremental improvement confirmed as statistically significant by a Wilcoxon signed-rank test when $p < 0.0001$. However, surprisingly, even with only 100 training examples, the model can capture variations in organ location and shape across the population.

We observed a performance gap between the model's performance on manually annotated data and automatically generated data from TS (Tab. 1). However, this gap is relatively small, suggesting that automatically generated masks can be effectively utilized to train robust models for clinical applications.

Quantitative analysis based on the DOE demonstrates the model's ability to accurately predict internal organ location (Fig.2). For most structures, the 95th percentile of the DOE is below 30mm. However, precise localization of the urinary bladder (Fig.1, middle row) and left liver lobe tip (Fig.1, bottom row) remains challenging due to variability across population.

Qualitative analysis reveals the model's ability to infer organ shapes, with particularly intriguing results for soft-tissue organs (Fig.1). Notably, the model captures natural variations in liver shape and accurately localizes the kidneys, despite their relative position variations across individuals.

These findings suggest that body surface depth information can provide valuable insights into internal organ anatomy, demonstrating the potential of integrating camera-based organ localization into radiological workflows.

4 Discussion

In this study, we present an approach to automate patient positioning using depth images. Our results demonstrate the feasibility of using depth images to estimate organ positions and shapes. The model's ability to accurately predict organ locations suggests its potential to streamline the patient setup process and reduce the time required for manual adjustments, thereby improving the overall efficiency of MRI examinations.

However, it's important to note that the depth images used in this study were derived from MRI scans, which may not perfectly represent real-world depth camera images. Real-world images can exhibit variations in lighting conditions, noise, patient movement and patient clothing, potentially impacting the model's performance. Addressing this domain gap between simulated and real-world data is a crucial area for future research.

Furthermore, exploring the potential of 3D organ shape prediction and localization can further enhance the accuracy and clinical utility of automated patient positioning

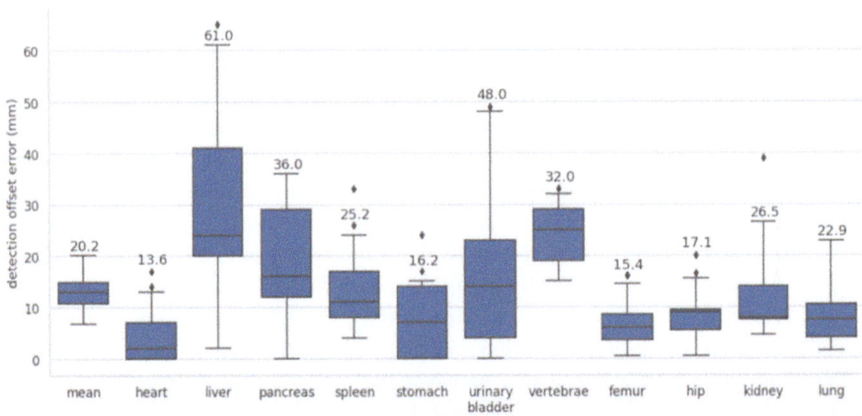

Fig. 2. Detection offset error (DOE) for anatomical structures in 30 manually segmented MRI scans. The value above each box corresponds to 95 percentile of DOE.

systems. By predicting the 3D shape and position of organs, we can gain a more comprehensive understanding of their spatial relationships and improve the precision of patient positioning.

Acknowledgement. We gratefully acknowledge the financial support by German Research Foundation (DFG), HE 7364/10-1, project number 500498869.

References

1. Van Rooyen MB, Pitcher RD. The Cinderellas of the scanner: magnetic resonance imaging pre-scan and post-scan times: their determinants and impact on patient throughput. SA J Radiol. 2020;24(1):1–6.
2. Koken P, Dries SP, Keupp J et al. Towards automatic patient positioning and scan planning using continuously moving table MR imaging. Magn Reson Med. 2009;62(4):1067–72.
3. İncetan K, Mohan R, Stoutjesdijk H et al. RGB-D camera-based clinical workflow optimization for rotational angiography. IEEE Sens J. 2020;20(15):8867–74.
4. Karanam S, Li R, Yang F et al. Towards contactless patient positioning. IEEE Trans Med Imaging. 2020;39(8):2701–10.
5. Wu Y, Singh V, Teixeira B et al. Towards generating personalized volumetric phantom from patient's surface geometry. Proc MICCAI. 2018:171–9.
6. Guo H, Planche B, Zheng M et al. SMPL-A: modeling person-specific deformable anatomy. Proc IEEE CVF CVPR. 2022:20814–23.
7. Keller M, Zuffi S, Black MJ et al. OSSO: obtaining skeletal shape from outside. Proc IEEE CVF CVPR. 2022:20492–501.
8. Shetty K, Birkhold A, Jaganathan S et al. BOSS: bones, organs and skin shape model. Comput Biol Med. 2023;165:107383.
9. Loper M, Mahmood N, Romero J et al. SMPL: a skinned multi-person linear model. ACM Trans Graph. 2015;34(6):1–16.
10. Teixeira B, Singh V, Tamersoy B et al. Automated CT lung cancer screening workflow using 3D camera. Proc MICCAI. 2023:423–31.
11. Bamberg F. Whole-body magnetic resonance imaging in the German National Cohort (NAKO): design & current status. Eur J Public Health. 2022;32(Supplement_3):ckac129–029.
12. D'Antonoli TA, Berger LK, Indrakanti AK et al. TotalSegmentator MRI: sequence-independent segmentation of 59 anatomical structures in MR images. arXiv: 2405.19492. 2024.

Leveraging Multiple Total Body Segmentators and Anatomy-informed Post-processing for Segmenting Bones in Lung CTs

Lukas Förner[1,2], Kartikay Tehlan[1,2], Constantin Bauer[1], Josua A. Decker[1], Thomas Wendler[1,2,3]

[1]Department of Diagnostic and Interventional Radiology and Neuroradiology, University Hospital Augsburg, Augsburg, Germany
[2]Computer-Aided Medical Procedures and Augmented Reality, Technical University of Munich, Garching near Munich, Germany
[3]Institute of Digital Medicine, University Hospital Augsburg, Neusaess, Germany
lukas.foerner@uk-augsburg.de

Abstract. Accurate segmentation of structures in CT is essential for clinical tasks such as tumour staging, radiotherapy planning, fracture assessment, and monitoring of disease progression. Current deep learning-based automated "segmentators" face challenges due to variability in scanner parameters, anatomical regions, and training data, which impact performance consistency across diverse datasets. We evaluated various total body segmentators on publicly available lung CT data excluded from their training sets. We found that these segmentators exhibit label mixing within individual ribs and vertebrae, often requiring anatomy-informed post-processing steps to improve accuracy. Combining multiple models and incorporating anatomical information enhances segmentation outcomes compared to using single models, highlighting the complementary strengths of different segmentation approaches and task-dependent a priori knowledge.

1 Introduction

Segmentation of anatomical structures in CT scans is vital in clinical workflows, particularly in oncology and traumatology. Accurate lung segmentation aids in quantifying lung cancer burden, and planning radiotherapy [1, 2], while thoracic bone segmentation supports fracture diagnosis, bone integrity evaluation, and provides stable references for longitudinal analyses, including tumor tracking and adaptive planning [3–5]. Automated segmentation methods for lung CTs must address challenges like variable resolution, scan ranges, scanner types, and anatomical variability [6]. However, evaluations of total-body segmentators on smaller anatomical regions like the thorax remain limited, typically focusing on single organs (e.g., vertebrae [7]) or extracted features [8].

The contribution of this work is threefold: (1) we evaluate common total-body segmentators on a dataset excluded from their training data, (2) we analyze the impact of combining these models, and (3) we incorporate a priori anatomical information to refine the automated segmentations.

C. Palm et al. (Hrsg.), *Bildverarbeitung für die Medizin 2025*, Informatik aktuell,
https://doi.org/10.1007/978-3-658-47422-5_76

2 Method and materials

2.1 Dataset

The evaluation of the segmentators was conducted using the publicly available Lung CT dataset from the Learn2Reg Challenge 2020 [9]. This dataset consists of pairs of 3D high-resolution computed tomography scans of the thorax (inspiration and expiration) for 30 subjects. Notably, the expiration scans do not provide a full view of the lungs. Two cases with breathing artifacts were excluded from the analysis. A radiologist confirmed that no significant anatomical abnormalities were present in the remaining dataset.

Although the challenge provided automatic lung segmentations for the dataset, these were not used in our experiments as the focus of this work is on segmenting bones.

2.2 Multiorgan segmentation models and label correction

A total of eight models were evaluated that were trained on four different datasets. Training a new model on these datasets lies outside the scope of this work.

TotalSegmentator [10] is a nnU-Net- based model [11] trained on the TotalSegmentator dataset[1]. This dataset consists of 1,228 CT images with 117 segmented anatomical structures. For the comparison, the total model (TS_TOTAL) was used. The same dataset was used by Lasso et al.[2] to train multiple MONAI Auto3dseg[3] models. From this range of models, four were evaluated: "Vertebrae TS2 (v2.0.0)" (TS_A3D_VERT), "Ribs TS2 (v2.0.0)" (TS_A3D_RIBS) and "Whole Body TS2 (v2.0.1)" (TS_A3D_TOTAL). Similar to TotalSegmentator, MOOSE [12] offers multiple nnU-Net models trained on over 1,700 whole-body CT images[4] with 120 segmented tissue and bone structures. For this evaluation, we used the "clin_ct_ribs" (M_RIBS) and the "clin_ct_vertebrae" (M_VERT) models. Jaus et al. presented a method for generating automated anatomy segmentation datasets and applied their method to the AutoPET dataset to generate the Dense Anatomical Prediction (DAP) Atlas dataset [13] consisting of 533 CT images with 142 segmented anatomical structures. The authors then trained two nnU-Nets on this dataset, from which we use the Atlas prediction model V2 (APM2).

For segmenting the spine we also used the winning model of the Verse2019 and the runner-up of the Verse2020 challenge [4] by Payer et al. [14] (VP). The Verse dataset [15] used for training consists of 160 CT images with segmented vertebrae.

For further assessment on how to improve the out of the box results, we split the task into segmentation and classification, evaluating each separately. In this process, all segmented ribs are merged into a single label and the segmentation is analyzed. In a second step to evaluate the classification performance, each connected component is assigned the label with the largest voxel contribution.

[1] https://zenodo.org/records/10047292

[2] https://github.com/lassoan/SlicerMONAIAuto3DSeg

[3] https://docs.monai.io/en/stable/auto3dseg.html

[4] https://github.com/enhance-pet/moose

2.3 Anatomy-informed post-processing

For post-processing, following the fact that bones are single continuous instances, first a connected component analysis is performed on the masks, and the largest label inside the connected component is assigned to the entire component. In the case of utilizing multiple models, a connected component analysis on the union of all rib labels is performed. To build a correspondence between vertebra and rib, the rib masks are skeletonized with Lee's method [16]. Then an adjacency graph of neighbouring voxels is created and for each voxel pair the shortest path is calculated. For extracting the endpoints of the rib, the longest shortest path per rib is taken and the end and start of the path are considered to be the start and end point of the rib. For each of the points, the distance to each vertebra is calculated. Following human anatomy, the two vertebrae with the lowest distance are then considered to be the vertebrae where the rib is connected to the spine. Furthermore, a threshold of 3 cm on average is used as a maximum distance to account for ribs that are cut off at the top of the image and do not have a connecting vertebra in the field of view.

2.4 Evaluation

For evaluation, the ribs were segmented by a medical student under the supervision of an expert radiologist. The segmentations of TS_TOTAL were selected as an initial segmentation and corrected. For the vertebrae, the segmentations of VP were used. Since the results of VP were visually correct, according to the expert radiologist, only the labels for mislabeled vertebrae were corrected.

The segmentation accuracy is evaluated through the standard metrics, namely, the dice score (DSC $\uparrow$), Jaccard similarity coefficient (JSC $\uparrow$), mean surface distance (MSD $\downarrow$), and Hausdorff surface distance (HSD $\downarrow$).

3 Results

For the ribs, we first calculated different segmentation metrics to assess the models' out-of-the-box capability of segmenting the ribs (Tab. 1).

Without any post-processing M_RIBS performed the best, closely followed by TS_TOTAL and TS_A3D_RIBS. For further assessment, we split the task into segmentation (Tab. 2) and classification, by evaluating them separately. The combination of different models is evaluated on the same metrics as the single models (Tab. 2). This evaluation demonstrates that as a single model APM2 outperforms all other models regarding the assessed metrics, closely followed by M_RIBS.

Label mixing within one rib is experienced by most of the models except M_RIBS. APM2 performed the worst by having up to four labels within one rib. All other models mixed two labels at most. Therefore, in a second step to evaluate the performance, we perform connected component analysis and keep the label which occurs the most within that component. For this, the accuracy of the different models was calculated. M_RIBS performed the best with an accuracy of 0.97 closely followed by TS_TOTAL (0.96) and TS_A3D_RIBS (0.95). With 0.85 APM2 performed worse, while TS_A3D_TOTAL performed the worst (0.22), having issues with mixing right and left ribs.

Tab. 1. Mean metrics for rib labels of each single model and our proposed combination with post processing . DSC: Dice score; JSC: Jaccard similarity coefficient; MSD: mean surface distance; HSD: Hausdorff surface distance in millimeters; TS_X: TotalSegmentator model X; APM2: Jaus' Atlas prediction model V2; M_X: Moose model X.

Mask Type	DSC ↑[1]	JSC ↑[1]	MSD ↓	HSD ↓
TS_A3D_RIBS	0.7417 ± 0.1767	0.6134 ± 0.1729	1.0358 ± 0.0407	20.7844 ± 12.6656
APM2	0.6677 ± 02208	0.5365 ± 0.2163	1.0156 ± 0.0187	49.6950 ± 43.0670
M_RIBS	0.7983 ± 0.1445	0.6809 ± 0.1409	1.0362 ± 0.0268	6.5105 ± 9.0790
TS_TOTAL	0.7549 ± 0.1766	0.6313 ± 0.1805	1.0396 ± 0.0388	20.0848 ± 10.3419
TS_A3D_TOTAL	0.2245 ± 0.3343	0.1813 ± 0.2841	1.0206 ± 0.0223	58.3069 ± 41.8075
APM2 + M_RIBS + TS_TOTAL	**0.8153±0.2485**	**0.7363±0.2310**	**1.0089±0.0142**	**4.7671±7.0133**

Tab. 2. Mean metrics for selected models and combinations with all ribs treated as one single label. DSC: Dice score; JSC: Jaccard similarity coefficient; MSD: mean surface distance; HSD: Hausdorff surface distance in millimeters; TS_X: TotalSegmentator model X; APM2: Jaus' Atlas prediction model V2; M_X: Moose model X.

Mask Type	DSC ↑[1]	JSC ↑[1]	MSD ↓	HSD ↓
TS_A3D_RIBS	0.8051	0.6755	1.0316	27.1512
APM2	0.8649	0.7627	1.0129	15.5540
M_RIBS	0.8314	0.7124	1.0223	17.3068
TS_TOTAL	0.8134	0.6879	1.0362	26.2734
TS_A3D_TOTAL	0.8061	0.6767	1.0300	26.9598
TS_A3D_RIBS + APM2	0.8805	0.7872	1.0126	15.8893
TS_A3D_RIBS + M_RIBS	0.8771	0.7819	1.0148	14.6982
TS_A3D_RIBS + TS_TOTAL	0.8422	0.7288	1.0243	26.1962
TS_A3D_RIBS + TS_A3D_TOTAL	0.8189	0.6947	1.0276	26.8034
APM2 + M_RIBS	0.8843	0.7933	1.0080	11.3962
APM2 + TS_TOTAL	0.8892	0.8012	1.0109	14.5024
M_RIBS + TS_TOTAL	0.8804	0.7873	1.0178	12.3176
M_RIBS + TS_A3D_TOTAL	0.8775	0.7825	1.0141	16.1563
TS_A3D_RIBS + APM2 + M_RIBS	0.8894	0.8015	1.0076	13.8194
TS_A3D_RIBS + APM2 + TS_TOTAL	0.8923	0.8062	1.0103	16.0523
TS_A3D_RIBS + M_RIBS + TS_TOTAL	0.8923	0.8064	1.0130	14.6188
APM2 + M_RIBS + TS_TOTAL	0.8946	0.8100	1.0071	**10.9343**
TS_A3D_RIBS + APM2 + M_RIBS + TS_TOTAL + TS_A3D_TOTAL	**0.8965**	**0.8132**	**1.0065**	16.6755

Regarding spine segmentation, our manual segmentation revealed that in 49 instances the labels of VP were shifted by one. With our method of matching the rib to corresponding vertebrae, we reduce the instances of mislabeled vertebrae by 48, leaving only one mislabeled case. For our proposed post-processing, we use APM2 + M_RIBS + TS_TOTAL as it keeps a good balance between segmentation performance and the number of models. For the spine, we use VP (Fig. 1).

Fig. 1. Segmentation results of various models showing label mixing and shifting as well as missing segmentation of last part of rib connecting to the spine in some models.

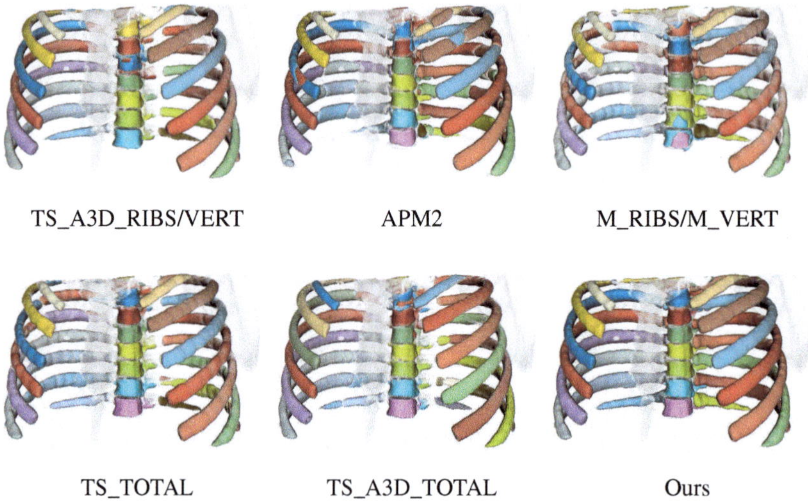

4 Discussion

This study evaluated various total body segmentators on lung CT data with normal rib anatomy to highlight their potential and limitations in delineating thoracic bones. Limitations in training data influenced performance, with APM2 and M_RIBS outperforming others due to including the rib neck, emphasizing the need for representative training data. The analysis revealed label mixing in individual rib segmentations across most models, requiring anatomy-informed post-processing, such as the method proposed here, to improve accuracy. Additionally, combining models proved more effective than individual ones by leveraging their strengths in specific regions. Understanding these automated methods' capabilities will enhance their application in medical imaging tasks such as feature extraction, volume estimation, and longitudinal tracking.

Acknowledgement. This research was partially funded by the Bavarian Ministry of Economic Affairs, Regional Development and Energy (StMWi) under grant number DIK-2310-0004// DIK0556/02.

References

1. Mansoor A, Bagci U, Foster B et al. Segmentation and image analysis of abnormal lungs at CT: current approaches, challenges, and future trends. Radiographics. 2015;35(4):1056–76.
2. Primakov SP, Ibrahim A, Timmeren JE van et al. Automated detection and segmentation of non-small cell lung cancer computed tomography images. Nat Commun. 2022;13(1):3423.

3. Jin L, Yang J, Kuang K et al. Deep-learning-assisted detection and segmentation of rib fractures from CT scans: development and validation of FracNet. EBioMedicine. 2020;62.
4. Sekuboyina A, Husseini ME, Bayat A et al. VerSe: a vertebrae labelling and segmentation benchmark for multi-detector CT images. Med Image Anal. 2021;73:102166.
5. Kim ST, Goli L, Paschali M et al. Longitudinal quantitative assessment of covid-19 infection progression from chest cts. Proc MICCAI. 2021:273–82.
6. Liebl H, Schinz D, Sekuboyina A et al. A computed tomography vertebral segmentation dataset with anatomical variations and multi-vendor scanner data. Sci Data. 2021;8(1):284.
7. Altini N, De Giosa G, Fragasso N et al. Segmentation and identification of vertebrae in CT scans using CNN, k-means clustering and k-NN. Informatics. 2021;8(2):40.
8. Julie A, Sundar LKS, Seban RD et al. MOOSE vs TotalSegmentator: comparison of feature values of segmented anatomical regions in [18F] FDG PET/CT images. Soc Nuclear Med. 2024.
9. Hering A, Murphy K, Ginneken B van. Learn2Reg challenge: CT lung registration training data. 2020.
10. Wasserthal J, Breit HC, Meyer MT et al. TotalSegmentator: robust segmentation of 104 anatomic structures in CT images. Radiol: Artif Intell. 2023;5(5):e230024.
11. Isensee F, Jaeger PF, Kohl SAA et al. nnU-Net: a self-configuring method for deep learning-based biomedical image segmentation. Nat Methods. 2021;18(2):203–11.
12. Sundar LKS, Yu J, Muzik O et al. Fully automated, semantic segmentation of whole-body ^{18} F-FDG PET/CT images based on data-centric artificial intelligence. Eur J Nucl Med. 2022;63(12):1941–8.
13. Jaus A, Seibold C, Hermann K et al. Towards unifying anatomy segmentation: automated generation of a full-body CT dataset via knowledge aggregation and anatomical guidelines. arXiv: 2307.13375. 2023.
14. Payer C, Stern D, Bischof H et al. Coarse to fine vertebrae localization and segmentation with SpatialConfiguration-Net and U-Net. Proc VISIGRAPP VISAPP. 2020:124–33.
15. Löffler MT, Sekuboyina A, Jacob A et al. A vertebral segmentation dataset with fracture grading. Radiol: Artif Intell. 2020;2(4):e190138.
16. Lee TC, Kashyap RL, Chu CN. Building skeleton models via 3-D medial surface axis thinning algorithms. CVGIP: Graphical Models and Image Processing. 1994;56(6):462–78.

Evaluation of TransUNet for the Segmentation of Retinal Structures in OCT-A

Leonie Schüßler[1,2], Anna-Sophia Hertlein[1,2], Alexander K. Schuster[3], Stefan Wesarg[1]

[1]Fraunhofer Institute for Computer Graphics Research IGD
[2]Technical University of Darmstadt
[3]Dept. of Ophthalmology, University Medical Center, Johannes Gutenberg-University, Mainz
leonie.schuessler@igd.fraunhofer.de

Abstract. Optical coherence tomography angiography (OCT-A) is a novel, non-invasive technology for visualizing retinal structures. Segmentation of these structures can indicate ophthalmic diseases such as diabetic retinopathy or glaucoma to aid diagnosis. However, limited data availability and artifacts make this task challenging. Adapted from other domains, transformer-based models yield promising results in medical image segmentation, challenging U-Net as the de facto standard method. This work evaluates TransUNet, a hybrid transformer and convolution-based architecture against U-Net in the task of segmenting retinal structures in OCT-A in a multifaceted comparison. Robustness under a reduced training volume and the effect of varying degrees of data augmentation, including noise simulations specific to OCT-A, are included as further aspects of comparison. Although no significant advantage in overall segmentation performance was found, TransUNet outperformed U-Net in the data-reduced setting and showed a better aptitude to capitalize on augmented data.

1 Introduction

Ophthalmic diseases are widespread among the population and can result in vision loss if not treated early. For diagnosis, retinal imaging techniques are a crucial component to visualize disease-related structural changes of the retina. Optical coherence tomography angiography (OCT-A) has become a popular tool for non-invasive and rapid retinal imaging and has proven useful in the diagnosis of glaucoma, diabetic retinopathy and age-related macular degeneration [1, 2]. As a functional extension of OCT, OCT-A measures the reflection of laser light of red blood cells, enabling visualization of the blood vessel movement in the eye [2]. For the extraction of disease-indicating parameters, an accurate segmentation of retinal structures is indispensable. Since the advance of deep learning, Convolutional Neural Networks, especially U-Nets, have become the primarily adopted approach to solve the issue of medical image segmentation as they have proven immensely successful in a wide range of applications [3]. Yet, in recent years, the advance of vision transformers in other domains has launched research to exploit the their benefits for the medical field, as well [4]. These attention-based models have the ability to capture long-range dependencies and global context in the image [5]. However, vision transformers have to learn image characteristics from scratch and thus require an extensive training volume to avoid overfitting [5]. Since data scarcity is a prevalent problem in the medical domain, hybrid models offer a combination of

C. Palm et al. (Hrsg.), *Bildverarbeitung für die Medizin 2025*, Informatik aktuell,
https://doi.org/10.1007/978-3-658-47422-5_77

transformer modules and convolutional layers as mitigation [4]. TransUNet is one of the first works integrating a transformer module into a U-shaped architecture as a hybrid model [6]. Although the performance of vision transformers is often tied to the training target structure and image modality, TransUNet excels as a structure-independent model with strong results in various segmentation tasks, making it a promising model choice for the task of retinal segmentation [4]. Its architectural similarities with U-Net enable a systematic comparison [6]. The contribution of this work comprises a performance evaluation of TransUNet for segmenting retinal structures in OCT-A images under multiple conditions. Specifically, we investigate whether the vision transformer-based encoder in TransUNet improves segmentation performance in this context over the purely convolutional encoder design of U-Net. To further assess whether the pretrained transformer encoder of TransUNet enables more efficient and robust feature learning, additional trials are conducted on smaller subsets of the training data. This work explores the models' ability to leverage data-augmentation, includeing specific artifacts in OCT-A acquisition to investigate potential improvements in robustness against such noise.

2 Materials and methods

All models were trained on the publicly available OCTA-500 dataset [7] with a split of 80% training, 10% validation, and 10% testing. OCTA-500 consists of 500 2D en-face OCT-A images of sizes 304 × 304 and 400 × 400 pixels with manually labeled segmentation masks of capillaries, large vessels, arteries, veins and foveal avascular zone (FAZ) (Fig. 2 (D)(i)). Additionally, we performed inference on a second dataset from the Gutenberg Premature Eye Study, granted by the Department of Ophthalmology of the University Medical Center Mainz, referred to as OCTA-Mainz in the following. This dataset contains 442 en-face OCT-A images of size 512 × 512 pixels with a field

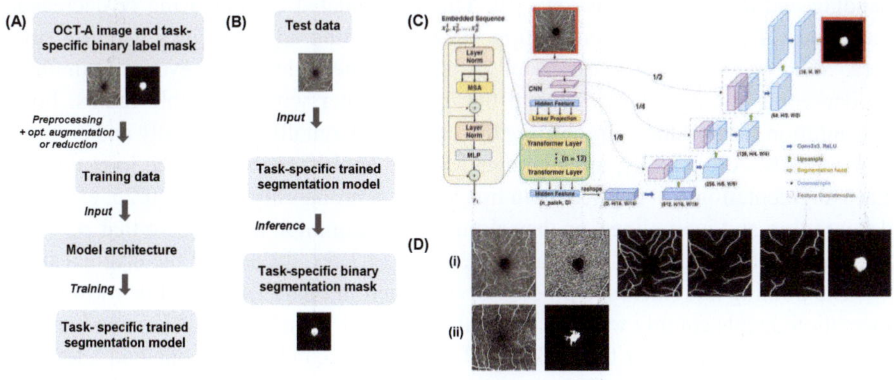

Fig. 1. (A) Training procedure with an exemplary mask. (B) Inference procedure. (C) TransUNet architecture. Source: Adapted from [6]. The red frames denote the changed elements. (D) (i) OCT-A image and corresponding ground-truth masks from OCTA-500 (from left to right: capillaries, large vessel, vein, artery, FAZ) (ii) OCT-A image and FAZ ground-truth from OCTA-Mainz.

of view of $10^\circ \times 10^\circ$ and manually-labelled FAZ masks only (Fig. 1 (D)(ii)), resized during preprocessing to 400×400 pixels.

U-Net and TransUNet are trained to segment a retinal structure as a binary mask. We use the U-Net architecture as described by [8] and TransUNet as implemented by [6]. Its architecture draws similarities to the U-Net model by combining a contracting and an expansive path (Fig. 1 (C)). Additionally, it contains a pre-trained transformer module, consisting of several layers of multi-headed self-attention and multi-layer perceptron blocks in the encoder. In the expansive path, a cascaded upsampler decodes the feature representation into a dense output prediction, supplemented by skip-connections to propagate low-level spatial information into the upsampling process [6].

Three experimental conditions are deployed. First, in the *regular* condition, the performance in the segmentation of all retinal structures in OCTA-500 is compared with the above mentioned data split. Secondly, we evaluate the performance of FAZ segmentation under a reduced training volume (50% and 25%). Finally, in the third experimental condition, different data augmentation strategies are trialed to evaluate the abilities to harness augmented data. Here, simple photo- and geometric transformations (random rotation, centered cropping, intensity-and contrast change), referred to as type *simple*, are used in comparison to specific augmentations simulating artifacts occurring during OCT-A acquisition, referred to as *noise* (Fig. 2). This includes artifacts caused

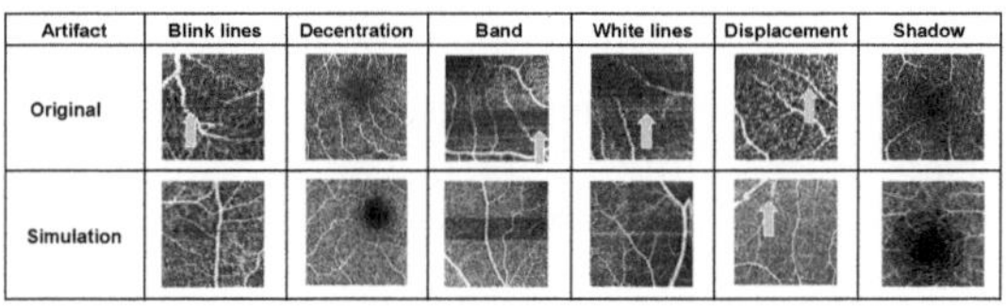

Fig. 2. Artifacts in OCT-A images. Top row: original (taken from OCTA-Mainz). Bottom row: simulation (on OCTA-500).

by eye movement such as black blink lines, white lines from rapid eye movement, banding and displacement of rows [9]. This is simulated by increasing or decreasing the values of pixels in one or multiple rows or shifting adjacent lines within a small area. Shadow artifacts, caused by obstruction of the light in the eye, are simulated by darkening a circular area around the image center with a variable radius. Fovea decentration is reproduced by shifting the image horizontally or vertically and cropping it afterwards. Additionally, all augmentations are applied together in the joint type *all*. Each augmentation a is applied to an image with a probability of $p_a = 0.25$, except for decentration and white lines, as they simulate less common artifacts, so that $p_a = 0.1$ was chosen here. This results in dataset volumes of 1.5×, 2× and 4× the original size.

The training and inference process is visualized in Fig. 1 (A-B). While most implementation details comply with the original U-Net and TransUNet [6, 8], some hyperparameters were adapted for this task. For TransUNet, a batch size of one and a learning rate of $1e-2$ was used. The U-Net was trained with batch size eight and a learning rate of $1e-4$. For both, training was conducted for 100 epochs with a hybrid Dice and binary Cross-Entropy loss in tasks capillary and FAZ and Dice loss for the remaining tasks. The TransUNet architecture comprised 105 million trainable parameters, whereas U-Net had 17 million parameters. For quantitative assessment of segmentation performance,

Dice similarity coefficient (DSC) is deployed. Since DSC is less effective for small targets with fine boundary delineation, such as intricate retinal structures in OCT-A, the spatial-distance based average Hausdorff distance (AHD) is used supplementary. AHD calculates the maximum distance between corresponding prediction pixel coordinates and ground-truth pixel coordinates, averaged over all distances between point pairs.

3 Results

In the regular trials, TransUNet performed with a mean DSC of 0.87 ± 0.03 and a mean AHD of 1.6 ± 1.21, while U-Net achieved a mean DSC of 0.87 ± 0.04 and a mean AHD of 1.78 ± 1.17 (Tab. 1). A Wilcoxon signed rank test ($\alpha = 0.05$) did not find sufficient evidence for a significant difference in performance between the models for either metric. FAZ segmentation reveals the highest performance in DSC, while the best AHD performance was found for capillary segmentation. The largest disparity between the models can be observed in FAZ segmentation, where TransUNet achieves an AHD score 0.5x smaller than U-Net. Fig. 3 shows an exemplary FAZ segmentation result.

	DSC		AHD	
	TransUNet	U-Net	TransUNet	U-Net
Capillary	0.86 ± 0.05	0.87 ± 0.04	0.42 ± 0.52	0.35 ± 0.37
FAZ	0.92 ± 0.1	0.91 ± 0.19	1.02 ± 2.49	2.05 ± 8.32
Large Vessel	0.88 ± 0.03	0.88 ± 0.03	0.77 ± 0.42	0.78 ± 0.47
Artery	0.85 ± 0.04	0.84 ± 0.05	2.68 ± 2.94	2.62 ± 2.08
Vein	0.83 ± 0.06	0.83 ± 0.07	3.1 ± 3.44	3.08 ± 3.79
Mean	0.87 ± 0.03	0.87 ± 0.04	1.60 ± 1.21	1.78 ± 1.17

Tab. 1. TransUNet and U-Net in the regular trials on the OCTA-500 test set.

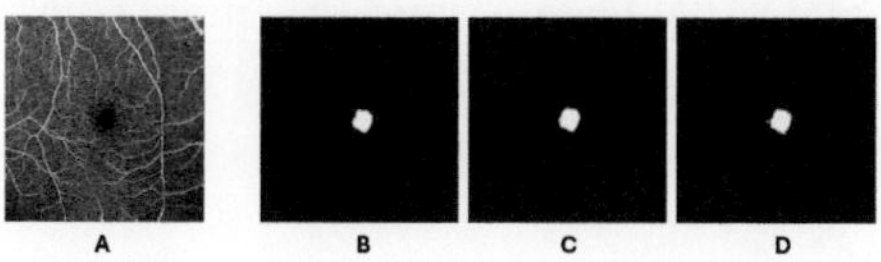

Fig. 3. OCT-A image (A), FAZ ground truth (B), Predicted FAZ segmentation mask of TransUNet (C) and U-Net (D).

With a 50% reduction of the training volume, both TransUNet and U-Net exhibit a similar decline, as can be seen in Fig. 4 (A). However, with 25% of the data, TransUNet performs higher than U-Net. In some cases, U-Net was not able to predict the target structure at all, classifying the entire image as background. These failed predictions were especially prominent in the 25% reduction on OCTA-Mainz, where 236 failures were recorded, constituting more than half of the available images.

Regarding the effect of data augmentation, a significant difference between TransUNet and U-Net is present in DSC and AHD on OCTA-500. Here, TransUNet improves performance, while U-Net deteriorates with increased augmentation. On OCTA-Mainz both models show increased performance. On average, TransUNet failed in four predictions and U-Net failed in 29 predictions on OCTA-Mainz. Simple augmentations yielded the best scores for both models over both datasets and metrics (Fig. 4 (B)). On OCTA-500, TransUNet peaked in the 2x condition, while U-Net peaked in the 1.5x condition. For OCTA-Mainz, the 4x condition worked best for TransUNet; the best augmentation condition varies between AHD and DSC for the U-Net.

4 Discussion

Although there was no significant performance gap between TransUNet and U-Net in the regular trials, their performances exhibited variability across tasks. The trials of data reduction entailed a decline in segmentation performance for both models. TransUNet demonstrated a considerable degree of stability in its performance across the reduction trials, while U-Net exhibited a pronounced decline in prediction performance and an accelerated increase in the number of failed predictions. The discrepancy between the two models is especially evident on OCTA-Mainz dataset, where U-Net becomes essentially unusable at the 25% reduction, unable to make any prediction in over half of the cases. Here, the reduced dataset size did not result in TransUNet exhibiting overfitting, but rather demonstrating a robust and precise prediction ability. This could indicate that the transformer-based encoder enables TransUNet to learn features more efficiently and robustly even in low-data settings.

Regarding data augmentation, TransUNet was able to benefit on OCTA-500, while U-Net degraded, resulting in a significant performance difference between the two models. However, even though TransUNet outperformed U-Net, both models benefited from the augmentation on OCTA-Mainz, proving the general effectiveness of the strategies. Considering all trialed augmentation strategies, TransUNet has an increased susceptibility for augmented training, as it is consistently improving across all conditions. This is especially useful in the data-starved medical domain. In general, all augmentation strategies increased performance, though more pronounced on OCTA-Mainz, which could be due to the fact that its images contain more noise and initial performance was lower, leaving more room for substantial improvement. OCTA-Mainz comprises retinal scans of adults having been born prematurely, thus potentially exhibiting structural variations

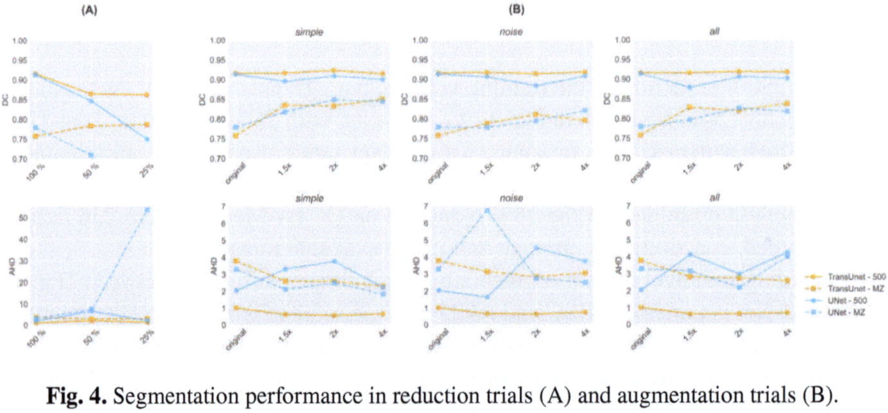

Fig. 4. Segmentation performance in reduction trials (A) and augmentation trials (B).

compared to non-premature born adult OCT-A images, which might cause a distribution shift and therefore varying performance between the datasets. While no universally optimal quantity of augmentation was found, TransUNet performance peaked more often with the highest quantity of augmentation than U-Net. This indicates that more augmented data helps TransUNet to grasp more information, which makes sense regarding that the superiority of the transformer architecture is usually enabled by an increased number of data points. Simple augmentation leads to the best results, surpassing the combination of simple and noise augmentation. This demonstrates that the interactions between the augmentation techniques are complex and hard to predict. Our artificial noise augmentations did also prove effective in increasing performance. Further analysis is needed to identify which noise-simulation techniques are most beneficial, or which need to be revised. TransUNet is computationally more expensive to train and deploy than U-Net, which should be considered for on-device inference and industrial applications. On par performance with U-Net was found for regular training, TransUNet proved successful in upholding performance on reduced training volumes and an increased capability to harness data augmentation. This shows the impact of the transformer-based encoder and renders TransUNet a valid choice for the segmentation of retinal structures in OCT-A, highlighting its ability to yield commendable results without task-specific modifications. This also suggest that transformer-based models hold potential for further improvements in the medical field, warranting additional research.

Acknowledgement. We would like to thank Prof. Dr. Achim Fieß and his team for acquiring and providing the image data from the Gutenberg Prematurity Eye Study.

References

1. Tan X, Chen X, Meng Q et al. OCT2Former: A retinal OCT-angiography vessel segmentation transformer. Comput Methods Programs Biomed. 2023:107454.
2. Rao HL, Pradhan ZS, Suh MH et al. Optical coherence tomography angiography in glaucoma. J Glaucoma. 2020:312–231.
3. Li J, Chen J, Tang Y et al. Transforming medical imaging with transformers? a comparative review of key properties, current progresses, and future perspectives. arXiv: 2206.01136. 2022.
4. Xiao H, Li L, Liu Q et al. Transformers in medical image segmentation: A review. Biomed Signal Process Control. 2023:104791.
5. Dosovitskiy A, Beyer L, Kolesnikov A et al. An image is worth 16x16 words: transformers for image recognition at scale. arXiv: 2010.11929. 2021.
6. Chen J, Lu Y, Yu Q et al. TransUNet: transformers make strong encoders for medical image segmentation. arXiv: 2102.04306. 2021.
7. Li M, Huang K, Xu Q et al. OCTA-500: A retinal dataset for optical coherence tomography angiography study. Med Image Anal. 2024;93:103092.
8. Ronneberger O, Fischer P, Brox T. U-Net: Convolutional networks for biomedical image segmentation. Proc MICCAI. 2015:234–41.
9. Anvari P, Ashrafkhorasani M, Habibi A et al. Artifacts in optical coherence tomography angiography. J Ophthalmic Vis Res. 2021:271–86.

Camera-based Guide Wire Tracking for a Hybrid Neurovascular Intervention Training System

Sonja Wichelmann[1], Roman Leonov[2], Claudia Rittmüller[2], Torben Pätz[1]

[1]Fraunhofer Institute for Digital Medicine MEVIS, Lübeck / Bremen
[2]Fraunhofer Research Institution for Individualized and Cell-Based Medical Engineering IMTE, Lübeck
sonja.wichelmann@mevis.fraunhofer.de

Abstract. Currently, there are completely virtual training simulators as well as 3D printed vessel phantoms available to train neuroradiology interventions. With this work, we aim to combine both approaches by a camera-based guide wire tracking for the first time. To achieve this, the camera has to be calibrated to the mask of the 3D printed vessel phantom. Then, the guide wire is segmented in the camera image, its 3D position is estimated, and then it is projected into a virtual projection of a whole-body CT scan. A resulting example of our approach is shown, and further necessary future work is discussed.

1 Introduction

Training simulators are currently available on the market that provide a fully virtual simulation of neurovascular interventions, e.g., Mentice [1]. Usually, these systems include a projection image of a simulated patient, the feedback of the inserted instruments, and contrast agent administration is simulated. However, a box instead of a realistic patient phantom with vessels inside lies in front of the surgeon, which might not be a completely realistic setting.

For this purpose, phantom-based training systems are available that allow a more realistic training and education for endovascular procedures [2, 3]. Here, the vascular anatomy is three-dimensionally (3D) printed and a pump system simulates the blood flow in a real patient. However, an angiosuite or an imaging system is needed to train a neuroradiology intervention on such a phantom system. In addition, further equipment, for example, for radiation protection is necessary.

In our project, our aim is to overcome this disadvantage and offer a hybrid training system by combining a realistic phantom model with a virtual C-arm and a pump system for realistic fluid flow. The position of the inserted instruments in the phantom will be tracked with cameras and transferred to the virtual C-Arm. In this work, the first implementation of a camera-based guide wire tracking is presented. This includes the camera-to-vessel model calibration, the guide wire segmentation in the camera image, and the 3D position estimation. Also, the results of our first setup are presented, and the current limitation as well as necessary future steps are discussed.

C. Palm et al. (Hrsg.), *Bildverarbeitung für die Medizin 2025*, Informatik aktuell,
https://doi.org/10.1007/978-3-658-47422-5_78

2 Material and methods

2.1 Materials

For the physical setup, we built a light table that serves as a homogeneous bright background. In this design, a number of LED stripes have been arranged underneath a tarnished plate to diffuse light from below. In addition, item profiles were used as an outer frame of the table and a fixture was used to mount a standard consumer webcam (Logitech(TM) C925E). A medical data set of computer tomography (CT) scans with contrast agent (CTA) was used as a basis for the phantom design of the vessels (ethic reference number: 20-121A, 03.04.2020, Universtiy Hospital Schleswig-Holstein). The iliac arteries and the aorta were segmented, and fluidic connections were added by using computer-aided design (CAD) software (Solidworks 2023). The vessels were then 3D printed with clear resin (Formlabs 3B printer). The wall thickness was chosen to be 2 mm. A thinner wall might lead to less distortions caused by refractions at the wall sides, but at the same time the walls would become too fragile and might break during handling.

2.2 Methods

Two calibration steps must be performed for the camera-based guide wire tracking: The camera itself is calibrated, and afterwards the resulting camera model is 2D3D registered to the vessel model. The camera-based tracking itself consists of the following steps: A segmentation in the 2D image is performed and a 3D position is estimated with

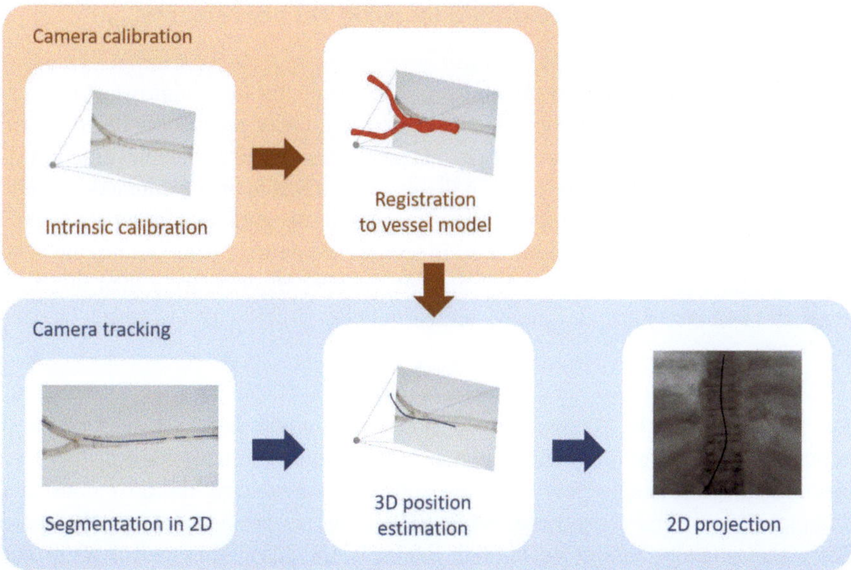

Fig. 1. Overview over all guide wire tracking steps.

a backprojection. Finally, the instrument shape is projected into and visualized in a projection image from a human CT image. Each step is visualized in Fig. 1, and described in more detail in the following subsections. All software components were developed as modules in MeVisLab[1] in Python and C++ to achieve an efficient, real-time-capable computation.

2.2.1 Camera to vessel calibration. A camera calibration using the OpenCV library [4] is performed, and the obtained focal length f_x, f_y and the optical center c_x, c_y of the camera are used to generate the world matrix W of the camera image dependent on the z−dimension

$$W = \begin{pmatrix} \frac{z}{f_x} & 0 & 0 & -\frac{c_x}{f_x}z \\ 0 & \frac{z}{f_y} & 0 & -\frac{c_y}{f_y}z \\ 0 & 0 & 1 & z \\ 0 & 0 & 0 & 1 \end{pmatrix} \tag{1}$$

Based on the focal point $f = (0, 0, 0)$ and the world matrix of the camera above, a 2D3D registration between the camera and the vessel phantom can be conducted by transforming the camera image and the focal point such that the projected 3D vessel mask fits to the vessel phantom part shown in the image. This 2D3D registration step yields the rigid transformation T_C^M and is currently done manually by visually comparing the real camera image with the overlayed projected vessel mask.

2.2.2 2D guide wire segmentation in the camera image. The camera image is masked by the 3D vessel mask projected into the camera image. Then, an intensity threshold is used to extract pixels belonging to the guide wire. Finally, the image mask is converted to a point list by determining the guide wire pixel positions.

2.2.3 3D guide wire position estimation. The 3D center line point list of the vessel mask is projected into the camera image and the translation of each center line point from the projected camera image position to its 3D position are used as depth estimation. The 3D position of each guide wire point in the camera image is then estimated by finding the nearest center line point in the camera image and using its translations into the 3D vessel mask. The center line is also used to sort the guide wire points along the vessel. Afterwards, false positive guide wire points are detected by comparing their distance to other points and are removed. Finally, an interpolation is performed to have a full guide wire shape.

2.2.4 Visualization in 2D projection. Based on a whole body CT scan of the visible human project[2] and projection geometry assumptions suitable for a C-Arm, a 2D projection image is created by using the approach for creating digital reconstructed radiographs [5–7]. The vessel mask is manually transformed so that it is in the approximately anatomically correct position in the body CT scan. This causes no problem

[1] `https://www.mevislab.de/`

[2] `https://www.nlm.nih.gov/research/visible/visible_human.html`

for the projection creation, since the CT image contains no contrasted blood vessel. Afterwards, the 3D positions of the tracked guide wire can be projected into the virtual projection image and visualized as a black line.

2.3 Evaluation setup

Before the evaluation setup, the camera is calibrated with a checkerboard as described in the OpenCV library, and the resulting matrix W is determined and saved later.

The open ends of the 3D printed vessel phantom are closed, water is added, and a small hole in the iliac artery is used as entrance for the guide wire similar to neuroradiological interventions. Our pumping system as in [8] is not used in this setup, as this experiment serves as an initial evaluation of the camera-based tracking. The camera and the 3D printed vessel model are arranged and fixated such that the iliac artery and aorta are clearly visible in the camera image. Then, the vessel mask is calibrated to the camera image and the resulting transformation T_C^M is saved for later.

Afterwards, a thin, flexible, black guide wire with a J-shaped tip is inserted through the hole of the filled vessel phantom at the right iliac artery. A camera image is captured by using OpenCV and saved. Then, the guide wire is tracked as described with the camera-based approach and the computation time of each step was measured.

3 Results

The evaluation setup of the table, the camera and the phantom is shown in Fig. 2a. We place the camera and the vessel phantom such that the iliac arteries as well as the first parts of the abdominal aorta are visible. Fig. 2b shows that the iliac arteries and the bifurcation match to a high degree, whereas differences of the abdominal aorta parts are visible.

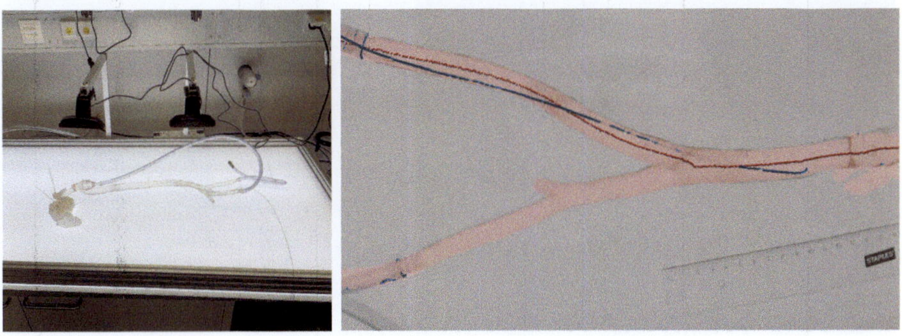

(a) (b)

Fig. 2. The evaluation setup (a) and the camera image (b) with the projected vessel mask (light red) after registration, the projected vessel center line (red) and the guide wire after segmentation (blue) .

The threshold-based segmentation segmented the guide wire and also some false positive pixels, because some parts of the vessel walls also have an intensity below the threshold. With the 3D position estimation, all those points are removed and the 3D point list contains only points of the guide wire.

The camera model manually registered to the vessel mask is illustrated in Fig. 3a, and in Fig. 3b a virtual anterior-posterior (AP) projection through the abdominal part of the whole body CT scan as well as the projection of the estimated 3D positions of the tracked guide wire is shown. Our impression is that the resulting virtual projection looks comparable to real projections.

We also measured the computation times and obtained 3.43 ms for the 2D segmentation, 4.39 ms for the 3D point estimation and 12.31 ms for the projection visualization of the visible guide wire. In total, the overall tracking pipeline took 20.13 ms, which shows the real-time capability of this first setup.

4 Discussion

With this work, we provide a first proof-of-concept of combining a 3D printed vessel phantom with a virtual C-arm by tracking a guide wire inside the phantom. The very first results show that a guide wire tracking is possible and can be realistically visualized in the virtual projection. However, the current setup also has limitations: For the treshold-based segmentation, it was difficult to choose a suitable threshold and the chosen threshold of 90 resulted in several false-positive pixels. The current tracking pipeline works only with rigid 3D printed vessels, because the 2D3D registration is done only once before tracking and no intraoperative correction is done. Furthermore, it allows only the tracking of one

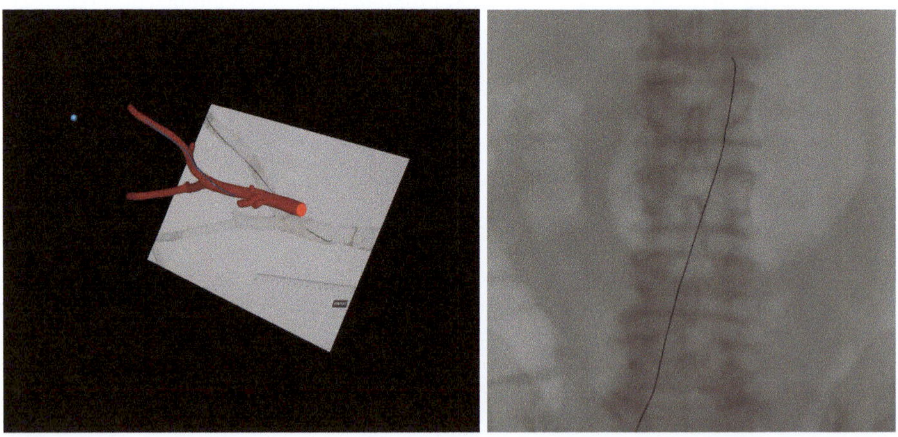

(a) (b)

Fig. 3. The 3D scene (a) with the focal point (blue), the camera image, the registered vessel mask (red) and the estimated 3D positions of the guide wire (blue) and the resulting virtual AP projection of the human body CT with the projected shape of the tracked guide wire (b).

instrument in the aorta and further developments are planned to reach a full hybrid training system:

First, multiple cameras have to be arranged along the full length of the aorta, the carotides, and at the cerebral arteries to enable tracking in the whole vessel phantom. In addition, the tracking algorithms need to be adapted so that they can segment and estimate the 3D position of different inserted instruments. Also, visualizations of other instruments, e.g. catheters, sheats, need to be created as they are in real fluoroscopy images. In addition, the whole tracking of the inserted instruments still has to work in real-time, and the calibration steps of the camera to the vessel should be more automatic.

Also, the phantom setup needs to be improved to enable a more stable tracking: Air bubbles (as visible in the camera image in Fig. 2) have to be avoided in the phantom models because they cause a different light refraction and disturb the tracked instrument. Additionally, the smoothness of phantom vessel walls needs to be increased to avoid regions where the inserted guide wire is invisible. Using more than one camera can also reduce the error of the 3D position estimation error caused by the backprojection.

In addition, a broader validation of the tracking accuracy has to be performed in order to proof how realistic the resulting C-Arm projections are and to evaluate how suitable the system for neurovascular trainings is.

Acknowledgement. This work was supported by the Fraunhofer Internal Programs under Grant No. SME 40-08039.

References

1. Schneider MS, Sandve KO, Kurz KD et al. Metric based virtual simulation training for endovascular thrombectomy improves interventional neuroradiologists' simulator performance. Interv Neuroradiol. 2023;29(5):577–82.
2. Spallek J, Kuhl J, Wortmann N et al. Design for mass adaptation of the neurointerventional training model HANNES with patient-specific aneurysm models. Proc ICED. 2019;1(1):897–906.
3. Schwenke H, Kemmling A, Schramm P. High-precision, patient-specific 3D models of brain aneurysms for therapy planning and training in interventional neuroradiology. Transactions on Additive Manufacturing Meets Medicine. 2019;1(1).
4. Bradski G. The OpenCV library. Dr. Dobb's J Softw Tools. 2000.
5. Goitein M, Abrams M, Rowell D et al. Multi-dimensional treatment planning: II. beam's eye-view, back projection, and projection through CT sections. Int J Radiat Oncol Biol Phys. 1983;9(6):789–97.
6. Russakoff D, Rohlfing T, Mori K et al. Fast generation of digitally reconstructed radiographs using attenuation fields with application to 2D-3D image registration. IEEE Trans Med Imaging. 2005;24(11):1441–54.
7. Lange A, Heldmann S. Intensity-based 2D-3D registration using normalized gradient fields. Proc BVM. 2020:163–8.
8. Paulsen BA, Schwenke H, Schramm P et al. Towards dual-use training simulator in interventional neuroradiology. Proc CDBME. 2023;9(1):447–50.

Abstract: Learned Image Compression for HE-stained Histopathological Images via Stain Deconvolution

Maximilian Fischer[1,2,3], Peter Neher[1,2,4], Tassilo Wald[1,5], Constantin Ulrich[1,3], Peter Schüffler[6,7], Shuhan Xiao[1,5], Silvia Dias Almeida[1,3], Alexander Muckenhuber[6], Rickmer Braren[8], Michael Götz[1,9], Jens Kleesiek[10,11], Marco Nolden[1,4], Klaus Maier-Hein[1,3,4,5,12]

[1]German Cancer Research Center (DKFZ) Heidelberg, Division of Medical Image Computing, Germany
[2]German Cancer Consortium (DKTK), partner site Heidelberg
[3]Medical Faculty, Heidelberg University, Heidelberg, Germany
[4]Pattern Analysis and Learning Group, Department of Radiation Oncology, Heidelberg University Hospital, Heidelberg, Germany
[5]Faculty of Mathematics and Computer Science, Heidelberg University, Heidelberg, Germany
[6]TUM School of Medicine and Health, Institute of Pathology, Technical University of Munich, Munich, Germany
[7]TUM School of Computation, Information and Technology, Technical University of Munich, Munich, Germany
[8]Department of Diagnostic and Interventional Radiology, Faculty of Medicine, Technical University of Munich, Munich, Germany
[9]Clinic of Diagnostics and Interventional Radiology, Section Experimental Radiology, Ulm University Medical Centre, Ulm, Germany
[10]Institute for AI in Medicine (IKIM), University Medicine Essen, Essen, Germany
[11]German Cancer Consortium (DKTK), partner site Essen
[12]National Center for Tumor Diseases (NCT), NCT Heidelberg, a partnership between DKFZ and University Medical Center Heidelberg

maximilian.fischer@dkfz-heidelberg.de

Processing histopathological whole slide images (WSI) leads to massive storage requirements for clinics worldwide. Even after lossy image compression during image acquisition, additional lossy compression is frequently possible without substantially affecting the performance of deep learning-based (DL) downstream tasks. In this paper, we show that the commonly used JPEG algorithm is not best suited for further compression and we propose stain quantized latent compression (*SQLC*), a novel DL based histopathology data compression approach. *SQLC* compresses staining and RGB channels before passing it through a compression autoencoder (*CAE*) in order to obtain quantized latent representations for maximizing the compression. We show that our approach yields superior performance in a classification downstream task, compared to traditional approaches like JPEG, while image quality metrics like the multi-scale structural similarity index (MS-SSIM) is largely preserved. Our method is online available[1] [1].

[1]https://anonymous.4open.science/r/SQLC-2E8C/

C. Palm et al. (Hrsg.), *Bildverarbeitung für die Medizin 2025*, Informatik aktuell,
https://doi.org/10.1007/978-3-658-47422-5_79

References

1. Fischer M, Neher P, Wald T et al. Learned image compression for HE-stained histopathological images via stain deconvolution. Proc MICCAI. 2024.

Erratum zu: Bildverarbeitung für die Medizin 2025

Christoph Palm, Katharina Breininger, Thomas M. Deserno, Heinz Handels, Andreas Maier, Klaus Maier-Hein, Thomas Tolxdorff

Erratum zu:
C. Palm et al. (Hrsg.), *Bildverarbeitung für die Medizin 2025*, Informatik aktuell, https://doi.org/10.1007/978-3-658-47422-5

Dieses Werk wurde durch die Universität Augsburg und das Bayerische Staatsministerium für Wirtschaft, Landesentwicklung und Energie (Förderkennzeichen: DIK-2310-0004// DIK0556/02) finanziell gefördert. Ursprünglich war diese Information leider nicht verfügbar, sie wurde nun auf der Copyright-Seite aufgenommen.

Die aktualisierte Version des Buches finden Sie unter
https://doi.org/10.1007/978-3-658-47422-5

C. Palm et al. (Hrsg.), *Bildverarbeitung für die Medizin 2025*, Informatik aktuell,
https://doi.org/10.1007/978-3-658-47422-5_80

Autorenverzeichnis

C. Palm et al. (Hrsg.), *Bildverarbeitung für die Medizin 2025*, Informatik aktuell,
https://doi.org/10.1007/978-3-658-47422-5

MIX
Papier aus verantwortungsvollen Quellen
Paper from responsible sources
FSC® C105338

If you have any concerns about our products,
you can contact us on
ProductSafety@springernature.com

In case Publisher is established outside the EU,
the EU authorized representative is:
Springer Nature Customer Service Center GmbH
Europaplatz 3, 69115 Heidelberg, Germany

Printed by Libri Plureos GmbH
in Hamburg, Germany